Board Review Series

PSYCHIATRY

Roderick Shaner, M.D.

Associate Professor of Clinical Psychiatry
Director, Medical Student Education in Psychiatry
University of Southern California School of Medicine
Los Angeles, CA

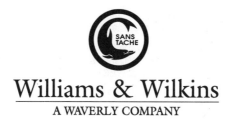

Williams & Wilkins
A WAVERLY COMPANY

BALTIMORE • PHILADELPHIA • LONDON • PARIS • BANGKOK
BUENOS AIRES • HONG KONG • MUNICH • SYDNEY • TOKYO • WROCLAW

Editor: Elizabeth A. Nieginski
Managing Editor: Amy G. Dinkel
Development Editor: Beth Goldner
Production Coordinator: Felecia R. Weber
Cover Designer: Cathy Cotter
Typesetter: Maryland Composition
Printer: Port City Press
Binder: Port City Press

351 West Camden Street
Baltimore, Maryland 21201-2436 USA

Rose Tree Corporate Center
1400 North Providence Road
Building II, Suite 5025
Media, Pennsylvania 19063-2043 USA

Accurate indications, adverse reactions and dosage schedules for drugs are provided in this book, but it is possible that they may change. The reader is urged to review the package information data of the manufacturers of the medications mentioned.

Printed in the United States of America

Diagnostic and Statistical Manual of Mental Disorders, 4th ed. (DSM-IV) diagnostic descriptions and criteria are referred to in, or have been adapted for, this book with permission of the American Psychiatric Association.

Library of Congress Cataloging-in-Publication Data

Shaner, Roderick.
    Psychiatry / Roderick Shaner.—1st ed.
        p.   cm.—(Board review series)
    Includes index.
    ISBN 0-683-07674-4
    1.   Psychiatry—Examinations, questions, etc.   2. Psychiatry—
Handbooks, manuals, etc.   I. Title.   II. Series.
    [DNLM: 1. Mental Disorders—diagnosis—examination questions   WM
18.2 S528p 1996]
RC457.S53   1996
616.89′0076—dc20
DNLM/DLC
for Library of Congress   96-20247
                                                                            CIP

The publishers have made every effort to trace the copyright holders for borrowed material. If they have inadvertently overlooked any, they will be pleased to make the necessary arrangements at the first opportunity.

To purchase additional copies of this book, call our customer service department at **(800) 638-0672** or fax orders to **(800) 447-8438.** For other book services, including chapter reprints and large quantity sales, ask for the Special Sales department.

Canadian customers should call **(800) 268-4178,** or fax **(905) 470-6780.** For all other calls originating outside of the United States, please call **(410) 528-4223** or fax us at **(410) 528-8550.**

Visit Williams & Wilkins on the Internet: http://www.wwilkins.com or contact our customer service department at **custserv@wwilkins.com.** Williams & Wilkins customer service representatives are available from 8:30 am to 6:00 pm, EST, Monday through Friday, for telephone access.

                                                                97 98 99
                                                3 4 5 6 7 8 9 10

Contents

Part Two: Psychiatric Disorders 33

Part Three: Clinical Psychopharmacology 239

Preface

This book is a concise summary of psychiatric diagnoses, guidelines for psychiatric treatment, and important psychiatric facts. It is not a comprehensive reference work.

Psychiatric diagnoses help us acquire and organize clinical information and rationally plan treatment. These diagnoses also tell us about the probable clinical course of individuals with psychiatric disorders.

Treatment guidelines organize our clinical knowledge for the purpose of healing patients. Treatment guidelines facilitate medical education and provide yardsticks by which we can measure quality and appropriateness of care. Treatment guidelines also facilitate comparison of alternative therapeutic regimens.

Psychiatric facts are useful for diagnosis, treatment planning and assessment, and patient education. Facts about epidemiology, etiology, and clinical course are useful to researchers as a rationale for the development of diagnostic criteria and treatment guidelines. Because the clinician-scientist is part of the core identity that health care professionals have assumed, a broad mastery of medical data is important in these professions. A mastery of medical facts also suggests competence in clinical skills. Therefore, this knowledge is tested on licensing examinations.

This book is useful if you want a quick and basic review of the information a clinician must know about psychiatric diagnosis and treatment to be an effective general physician or other mental health care professional. It is also useful if you want to know the facts that are most often asked on exams to measure mastery of psychiatric knowledge.

This book is divided into five sections:

- **The process of diagnosis.** The psychiatric diagnostic interview and the assessment of child development are described.
- **Psychiatric disorders.** Major classes of mental disorders are described, including epidemiology, etiology, diagnostic criteria, associated features, differential diagnoses, and treatment guidelines.
- **Clinical psychopharmacology.** The clinical use of major classes of psychiatric medications is described, including antipsychotics, anxiolytics, antidepressants, and mood stabilizers.
- **Psychotherapies.** Basic theories, techniques, and clinical indications are described for major types of psychotherapies, including psychodynamic, behavioral, cognitive, and humanistic therapies.
- **Special issues.** Psychiatric emergencies, psychiatric aspects of general medical conditions, forensic and ethical issues, and geriatric issues are outlined.

Included in each chapter are case-based examination questions with explanations. A case-based comprehensive examination with explanations for each answer is also provided.

Use of DSM-IV material

The diagnostic features described for specific mental disorders in this book are based on DSM-IV criteria sets, but are simplified in many cases. Threshold and boundary criteria (i.e., technical descriptions of symptom severity and detailed distinctions among disorders with similar symptoms), unless unusual, are not specifically described for many disorders discussed in this book. Specifiers (i.e., additional criteria used to more specifically delineate some DSM-IV diagnoses) are simplified and often informally described as types or subtypes of mental disorders. Mental disorder not otherwise specified (NOS), and other residual categories in DSM-IV, are not specifically described in this book.

Acknowledgments

The author wishes to thank his students, his colleagues, and the staff of Williams & Wilkins for their valuable comments, suggestions, and help.

Part One

The Process of Diagnosis

1

Overview of the DSM-IV and Psychiatric Diagnosis

I. Overview

A. **The Diagnostic and Statistical Manual of Mental Disorders, 4th edition (DSM-IV),** is the **official diagnostic nomenclature of the American Psychiatric Association.**

B. **The structure and conventions** of the DSM-IV have a profound effect on the way clinicians diagnose and discuss mental disorders and **are closely followed in the diagnostic descriptions in this book.**

II. The Significance of the DSM-IV

A. DSM-IV criteria

1. The DSM-IV contains **sets of criteria for determining the presence of various mental disorders** in individuals with disturbances of thought, emotion, or behavior.
2. The **diagnostic criteria are largely based on the presence, duration, and course of various physical and psychological signs and symptoms.** Specific etiologies or test results also are part of the diagnostic criteria for some mental disorders.
3. It is important to remember that DSM-IV criteria are useful for classifying various mental disorders, but are not meant to classify the human beings who suffer from them.

B. Selection of treatment. DSM-IV classification is a **useful tool for rational selection of treatment.** Diagnoses made by these criteria often have predictive value about how individuals will respond to specific treatments and about the probable course of illness.

C. DSM-IV disorders are defined on the basis of available clinical knowledge. As more information is learned about mental disorders, criteria will be updated in subsequent editions.

D. Debate continues about the most useful and accurate ways to diagnose mental disorders; the DSM-IV serves as a common language in which to debate such topics.

III. Contents of the DSM-IV

A. The DSM-IV contains an **introduction, sets of instructions for use of the manual, diagnostic descriptions for mental disorders,** and **appendices.**

    1. The **diagnostic descriptions for mental disorders are divided into 17 categories** based on shared features (e.g., mood disorders, anxiety disorders, personality disorders).

    2. The appendices include a glossary of psychiatric terms, a description of culture-bound syndromes, and a set of diagnostic trees.

B. **Multi-axial assessment.** A complete DSM-IV **diagnostic formulation contains assessment based on five axes,** each of which refers to a different domain of information. Axes provide a comprehensive clinical picture and facilitate treatment planning.

    1. **Axis I** is the site for **recording most clinical diagnoses.**

    2. **Axis II** is the site for **recording personality disorders and mental retardation.**

    3. **Axis III** is the site for **recording general medical conditions** that have relevance to the diagnosis or treatment of disorders on Axes I or II.

    4. **Axis IV** is a list of **relevant psychosocial and environmental problems.**

    5. **Axis V** is a scale [Global Assessment of Function (GAF)] for **rating the overall functional level.**

C. **Criteria sets.** Each disorder in DSM-IV is associated with a discrete set of criteria that is necessary for making a diagnosis.

    1. The criteria may include **clinical course, duration, current and past symptoms,** and **etiology.**

    2. The criteria set for a specific mental disorder has two purposes:

        a. To define the major clinical features of the disorder

        b. To define those clinical features that help distinguish it from other disorders

    3. Some criteria have special purposes:

        a. **Threshold criteria** determine whether symptoms are significant enough to warrant diagnosis.

        b. **Exclusionary (boundary) criteria** determine which of several disorders with overlapping symptoms should be diagnosed.

D. **Specifiers** are short descriptions added to DSM-IV diagnoses to more **sharply define subtype, severity, or course.**

E. **Description of mental disorders.** The DSM-IV uses a standardized, self-explanatory outline to describe mental disorders:

    1. **Diagnostic features,** which describe the defining features of the mental disorder

    2. **Specifiers** (see III D)

    3. **Criteria** (see III C)

    4. **Coding and recording procedures,** which, based on the International Classification of Diseases (ICD-9-CM), describe the specific numeric code for the disorder that is used in statistical reporting

    5. **Associated features and diagnoses include:**

        a. Associated descriptive features and mental disorders, which include associated clinical findings that are not part of the criteria set

        b. Associated laboratory findings

        c. Associated physical examination findings and general medical conditions

    6. **Specific culture, age, and gender features** associated with the disorder

    7. **Prevalence** of the disorder in general or specific populations

    8. **Course** of the disorder

    9. **Familial pattern** of the disorder

   10. **Differential diagnosis,** which describes other diagnoses that may account for the clinical findings

IV. Diagnostic Uncertainty and the DSM-IV

A. General information

    1. **In some cases, there is not enough information available** to determine whether all necessary diagnostic criteria for a disorder are present (e.g., during an emergency assessment or when there is no information about history).

    2. **In cases of diagnostic uncertainty,** the clinician uses diagnoses with a lower level of **"diagnostic specificity,"** and may mention more specific diagnoses as **"rule-outs."**

B. The DSM-IV conventions for conveying diagnostic uncertainty in order of increasing specificity are:

    1. **Diagnosis deferred.** Information is inadequate to make a diagnostic judgment.

    2. **Unspecified mental disorder (nonpsychotic).** Information is sufficient to rule out psychosis, but not adequate for further specification.

    3. **Psychotic disorder not otherwise specified (NOS).** Information is sufficient to determine presence of psychosis, but not adequate for further specification.

    4. **Category of disorder NOS.** Information is sufficient to determine category of disorder present, but not adequate for further specification.

    5. **Specific diagnosis (provisional).** Information is sufficient to form a **"working diagnosis,"** but diagnostic uncertainty remains.

Review Test

Directions: The numbered item or incomplete statement in this section is followed by answers or by completions of the statement. Select the ONE lettered answer or completion that is BEST for this case.

1. An 18-year-old man suffering from hallucinations and delusions is brought to the emergency room. The patient is unable to give any meaningful history regarding the onset, duration, and course of his symptoms, and no other sources of information are available. Which of the following is the most appropriate level of diagnostic specificity?

(A) Brief psychotic disorder
(B) Diagnosis deferred
(C) Psychotic disorder not otherwise specified (NOS)
(D) Schizophrenia, paranoid type (provisional)
(E) Unspecified mental disorder

Directions: Each set of matching questions in this section consists of a list of four to twenty-six lettered options (some of which may be in figures) followed by several numbered items. For each numbered item, select the ONE lettered option that is most closely associated with it. To avoid spending too much time on matching sets with large numbers of options, it is generally advisable to begin each set by reading the list of options. Then, for each item in the set, try to generate the correct answer and locate it in the option list, rather than evaluating each option individually. Each lettered option may be selected once, more than once, or not at all.

Questions 2–3

Match each patient described with the most appropriate DSM-IV axis for recording the supplied clinical information.

(A) Axis I
(B) Axis II
(C) Axis III
(D) Axis IV
(E) Axis V

2. A 30-year-old man with an onset of visual deficits and right lower extremity weakness

3. A 45-year-old man, recently widowed, and facing severe economic hardship

Questions 4–5

Match each of the criterion types with the appropriate diagnostic criterion.

(A) During a 2-year period, the patient has not been without symptoms for more than 2 months at a time.
(B) The disturbance causes clinically significant impairment in social, occupational, or other important area of functioning.
(C) The disturbance is not better accounted for by another mental disorder.
(D) The patient avoids occupational activities that involve significant interpersonal contact.
(E) There is evidence from the history, physical examination, or laboratory data that the findings are due to a general medical condition.

4. Exclusionary (boundary) criterion

5. Threshold criterion

Answers and Explanations

1–C. Psychotic disorder not otherwise specified (NOS) indicates that there is adequate clinical information to determine the presence of psychosis, but that there is insufficient information to make a more specific diagnosis, as in this case. Diagnosis deferred indicates that there is adequate information to determine the presence of a mental disorder, but the presence or absence of psychosis cannot be determined. Unspecified mental disorder indicates that there is adequate clinical information to determine that psychosis is absent, but there is insufficient information to make a more specific diagnosis. Schizophrenia, paranoid type (provisional), indicates that there is adequate clinical information to determine that the diagnosis is most likely schizophrenia. Brief psychotic disorder indicates that there is enough clinical information to determine that all criteria for this disorder are met.

2–3. The answers are: 2-C, 3-D. Axis III is the site for recording general medical conditions, such as sensory and motor deficits, which have relevance to the diagnosis or treatment of disorders on axis I or II. Axis IV is a list of relevant psychosocial and environmental problems, such as death of a spouse or economic problems. Axis I is the site for recording most clinical diagnoses. Axis II is the site for recording personality disorders and mental retardation. Axis V is a scale [Global Assessment of Function (GAF)] for rating the overall functional level.

4–5. The answers are: 4-C, 5-B. Exclusionary (boundary) criteria determine which of several disorders with overlapping symptoms should be diagnosed. Threshold criteria determine whether symptoms are significant enough to warrant diagnosis. The other criteria do not relate to threshold or exclusions.

2

The Diagnostic Interview

I. Overview

A. Goals of the psychiatric interview may be to **clarify diagnosis, assess behavior, encourage emotional release, facilitate behavioral change, impart information, and foster self-understanding.**

B. Psychiatric interviews vary widely in both style and content because clinicians use different kinds of information, emphasize different interview goals, and use differing interview techniques to accomplish these goals.

C. Goals of the diagnostic interview

    1. Obtain useful information. The clinician must ask the questions and make the observations necessary for diagnosis and a psychosocial formulation, often using DSM-IV criteria.

    2. Be therapeutic. The clinician must help the patient feel comfortable and hopeful.

        a. Demonstrate concern and empathy

        b. Demonstrate interest

        c. Appear competent

        d. Supply useful information

    3. Demonstrate social regard. The patient is entitled to respect.

    4. Be ethical. The clinician must **avoid unethical ways of obtaining information,** or otherwise compromising the patient's best interests.

    5. Be efficient. The clinician must **phrase questions well and make observations parsimoniously,** usually within approximately 45 minutes.

II. Obtaining Clinical Information

A. Types of information available to the interviewing clinician include:

    1. History obtained from the patient, the patient's family, and knowledgeable others

    2. Findings from examination

        a. Physical examination

        b. Mental status examination

        c. Patient–clinician interaction

B. **Inductive and deductive data gathering**

   1. **Deductive data gathering is dependent on knowledge of psychiatric diagnoses.** The clinician deduces the correct diagnosis based on knowledge of what information is necessary to obtain.
   2. **Inductive data gathering** is dependent on the information that key questions and observations yield. Key questions and observations should always be explored because they often yield important information.
   3. Often, the results of inductive questions will lead to deductive questioning.

C. **The manner in which information is gathered may affect the information obtained.** An unstructured interview may yield different information from that gathered from a formally structured interview.

III. Components of the Diagnostic Interview. There are **three principal components of a diagnostic interview.**

A. **History from patient, family, and others**

   1. Information must be gathered both inductively and deductively.
   2. Gathering history requires both open-ended and closed-ended questions.

B. **Mental status examination**

   1. The mental status examination starts immediately during a diagnostic interview, well before history taking.
   2. The mental status examination consists of **keen observation of the patient's manner and behavior** in relating history and interacting with the clinician.
   3. **Specific mental status questions and tests may be used to obtain more precise information** or to quantify findings.
   4. **Mental status examination tests must be performed correctly** if their results are to have any meaning for those who interpret them.

C. **"Process" observations.** The manner in which a patient relates to the clinician and the **themes of his conversation (often referred to as the "process" of the interview)** may have important diagnostic significance.

IV. High-Yield Inductive History Questions

A. **Presenting problems**

   1. What brings you to the hospital?
   2. How long has this been a problem?
   3. Did it happen suddenly, or has it been gradually getting worse?

B. **Treatment History**

   1. Have you ever seen a psychiatrist or counselor before?
   2. Have you ever had a psychiatric hospitalization?
   3. What kind of previous diagnoses and treatments have you received?
   4. Have you had any serious medical problems?
   5. What kinds of recreational drugs, over-the-counter drugs, and prescribed medications have you taken?
   6. Have you had any problems with alcohol or drugs?

C. **Family history.** Is there any history of psychiatric hospitalization, alcoholism, suicide, or legal problems in your family?

D. Social history

1. How was your childhood?
2. Did you have any school problems?
3. How have you gotten along with others?
4. Have you had any long term relationships?
5. What kind of work have you done?

E. Current social situation

1. What is your current living arrangement?
2. How are you supported?
3. What kind of stress have you recently experienced?

V. The Mental Status Examination

A. Overview

1. The mental status examination has diagnostic significance because **different mental disorders affect consciousness in characteristic ways.**
2. For the purposes of psychiatric diagnosis, **the clinician is interested in those parts of consciousness that can demonstrate psychopathology.**

   a. **Arousal.** Is the patient able to focus, maintain, and shift attention?

   b. **Psychomotor activity.** Are the patient's movements (including speech) normal, purposeful, and coordinated?

   c. **Mood.** What is the emotional state of the patient?

   d. **Memory and other cognitive functions.** Is the patient able to encode and recall information, use language, recognize surroundings, complete complex motor behaviors, and plan and execute tasks?

   e. **Thought processing.** Is the patient able to abstract and correctly interpret the environment?

   f. **Thought content.** What is the patient thinking about?

3. **Overview of observations and tests.** The results of sophisticated observations and specific tests in the mental status examination allow the clinician to make inferences about the clinically important areas of consciousness.

   a. **Observations.** Knowing what to observe comes from an understanding of psychiatric diagnostic criteria.

   b. **Tests.** Tests are used to elicit further psychopathology that was not fully evaluated by observation alone, or to quantify observed findings. Standard tests such as **Digit Span, Three Objects at Five Minutes,** and **Proverb Interpretation** must be performed correctly if their results are to be correctly interpreted by others.

B. Observations and tests during mental status examination

1. **Physical appearance**

   a. Does the patient have any physical signs of illness?

   b. Is the patient dressed appropriately?

   c. Is the patient neatly groomed?

2. Arousal and attention

    a. Is the patient hyperalert, alert, lethargic, stuporous, or in a coma?

    b. Can the patient focus and sustain attention on questions and tasks?

    c. Serial Sevens Test. Ask the patient to perform sequential subtractions. ("I'd like to test a little more closely your ability to concentrate. Would you please start at 100 and count backward by seven?")

3. Psychomotor activity

    a. Quantity. Does the patient exhibit increased, normal, or decreased psychomotor activity?

    b. Quality

        (1) Is the patient's psychomotor activity appropriate or inappropriate?

        (2) Motor pathology. Is there evidence of focal deficits, incoordination, or abnormal movements?

        (3) Speech (see V B 4)

    c. Handshake test. By greeting the patient with a standing handshake, the clinician can observe problems with coordination, motor strength in upper and lower extremities, and abnormal movements.

4. Speech

    a. Coordination. Is the patient's speech clear or slurred?

    b. Quantity of psychomotor activity. Is the patient's speech pressured (i.e., speeded up), of normal rate and rhythm, dysarthric, or sparse?

    c. Thought processing. Is the patient coherent or incoherent?

    d. Intelligence. Is the patient's vocabulary in native language superior, normal, or impoverished?

5. Mood

    a. Mood is inferred by **level of psychomotor activity, self-report,** and **facial expressions.**

    b. Moods have diagnostic significance. Is the patient's mood euphoric (i.e., elevated), expansive, irritable, dysphoric, depressed, anxious, or neutral?

6. Affect

    a. Definition. Affect is the **moment-to-moment modulation of psychomotor activity,** as revealed by facial expressions, voice intonation, and fine motor activity.

    b. Quality. Is the patient's affect appropriate or inappropriate?

    c. Range. Is the patient's affect flat (i.e., no modulation), blunted (i.e., slight modulation), normal, or labile (i.e., overly modulated)?

    d. Intensity. Is the patient's affect bland (i.e., overly unconcerned), normal, or constricted (i.e., overly intense)?

7. Memory and other cognitive functions

    a. The patient's ability to relate her history is the best indicator of an intact memory.

    b. Memory function is usually clinically described as **immediate memory, recent memory,** or **long-term memory. Other cognitive func-**

tions include the ability to understand language and communicate, recognize persons and objects, perform complex motor behaviors, and plan and execute tasks.

c. **Tests**

   (1) Immediate memory. Digit Span is the standard test for immediate memory.

      (a) The patient is presented with seven random digits and asked to immediately repeat them.

      (b) Phone numbers are useful for this test.

   (2) Recent memory

      (a) Orientation test. The degree of orientation to correct time, date, and place is the standard test for a patient's recent memory function.

      (b) Three Objects at Five Minutes. Asking the patient to remember three discrete random objects is the standard test for ability to encode and recall information.

   (3) Long-term memory

      (a) Demographic information is often the only verifiable data that the clinician can use to test long-term memory. The clinician can ask for information such as the patient's name, date of birth, names of parents, name of spouse, names of children, date of marriage, and current address. Information that the patient has acquired at earlier ages is most resistant to loss.

      (b) Language. The clinician can detect aphasia by asking the patient to identify common objects or by assessing the patient's comprehension of spoken or written instructions.

      (c) Recognition. The clinician can detect agnosia by asking the patient if he recognizes familiar people or objects (e.g., keys, wristwatch).

      (d) Complex motor behavior. The clinician can detect apraxia by asking the patient to demonstrate tying shoelaces or preparing food.

      (e) Ability to plan and execute tasks. The clinican can ask the patient to describe the steps involved in planning a shopping trip or mailing a package.

8. **Thought processes**

  a. **Hallucinations.** The clinician must assess presence, type, and quality of the patient's hallucinations.

   (1) Definition. Hallucinations are sensory impressions in the absence of stimuli.

   (2) Observations. Does the patient appear to be responding to hallucinations ("internal stimuli")?

   (3) High-yield question. Do you hear voices in your head or see things that aren't really present?

  b. **Delusions.** The clinician must assess presence, type, and quality of the patient's delusions.

(1) **Definition.** Delusions are patently false beliefs firmly held in spite of overwhelming evidence to the contrary.

(2) **Observations.** Does the patient appear overly suspicious, grandiose, guilty, or bizarre?

(3) **High-yield questions**

    (a) **Persecutory delusions** (i.e., delusions of being victimized). Do you believe anyone is after you or out to kill you? If so, who?

    (b) **Delusions of reference** (i.e., delusional attribution of personal significance to unrelated events). Do you believe that the radio or television is talking about you?

    (c) **Grandiose delusions** (i.e., delusions of power or self-importance). Do you believe you have any special powers?

c. **Thought associations.** Many types of thought association pathology exist: **loose** (i.e., illogical progressions of ideas), **circumstantial** (i.e., thought that is only vaguely related to a point), **tangential** (i.e., a train of thought that gradually departs from a point), **flight of ideas** (i.e., rapid jumping of thoughts through a secession of tenuously related ideas), **rambling, overinclusive** (i.e., a train of thought that becomes bogged down in the recitation of minutiae), and **concrete** (i.e., failure to grasp abstraction).

(1) **Observations.** Does the patient present history in a coherent manner?

(2) **Tests**

    (a) **Proverb interpretation.** A patient is asked to interpret one or more proverbs, and problems with thought association and abstraction are noted.

    (b) **Similarities and differences.** A patient is asked to list similarities and differences between two objects (e.g., an apple and an orange), and problems with thought association and abstraction are noted.

9. **Thought content**

a. What has the patient talked about during the interview?

b. Are specific themes or characteristics present (e.g., obsessions, fears, depressive thoughts, guilt, somatic concerns, or sexual ideation)?

c. **High-yield questions for specific thought content**

(1) **Suicidal thoughts.** Do you wish to commit suicide? Would you? How?

(2) **Homicidal thoughts.** Do you wish to kill someone? Would you? Who?

(3) **Judgment.** How much does the patient agree with the clinician about specific issues or actions?

VI. The Clinician–Patient Relationship

A. **The manner in which the patient relates to the clinician is an important source of information** about how the patient functions in an interpersonal environment.

B. **The clinician observes aspects of interpersonal relating during the diagnostic interview:**
   1. Is the patient cooperative or uncooperative with the interview?
   2. Does the patient assume an active or passive role?
   3. Is the patient open or guarded?
   4. Is the patient friendly, hostile, or neutral?
   5. Does the patient relate to the interviewer in a role of submissiveness or assertiveness?

C. **Generalizations about interpersonal style** that are based on the diagnostic interview must be made with caution because characteristics of the clinician or the interview situation may strongly influence the findings.

D. **A good clinician must be aware of his own interpersonal characteristics** and how they affect patients.

Review Test

Directions: The numbered item or incomplete statement in this section is followed by answers or by completions of the statement. Select the ONE lettered answer or completion that is BEST for this case.

1. Which of the following statements about inductive data gathering is most accurate?

(A) An unstructured interview format is essential to gather data inductively
(B) Effective inductive data gathering is dependent on a clinician having formed a clearly defined differential diagnosis for a patient's presenting complaint
(C) Inductive data gathering refers chiefly to the observations made that are based on clinician–patient interaction
(D) Inductive data gathering is dependent on the knowledge that certain key questions and observations should always be explored, because they often yield important information
(E) Inductive questions must be open ended

2. During a psychiatric diagnostic interview, which of the following is the best time to initiate the mental status examination?

(A) After clinical rapport is established
(B) After the clinician introduces himself to the patient
(C) After the clinical history is obtained
(D) Before the patient develops a transference reaction to the clinician
(E) Before the clinician begins speaking to the patient

3. Which of the following is the most accurate definition of "process" observations?

(A) Information obtained by the clinician through specific mental status examination questions
(B) Observations regarding the etiology of psychopathology that may be uncovered during the diagnostic interview
(C) Observations about the way a patient organizes sensory information to create abstract concepts
(D) Observations regarding the manner in which a patient relates to the clinician and the themes of his conversation
(E) Observations regarding the way a clinician conducts a diagnostic interview, including mental status examination

Directions: The set of matching questions in this section consists of a list of four to twenty-six lettered options (some of which may be in figures) followed by several numbered items. For each numbered item, select the ONE lettered option that is most closely associated with it. To avoid spending too much time on matching sets with large numbers of options, it is generally advisable to begin each set by reading the list of options. Then, for each item in the set, try to generate the correct answer and locate it in the option list, rather than evaluating each option individually. Each lettered option may be selected once, more than once, or not at all.

Questions 4–5

Match each of the following tests with the aspect of consciousness it assesses.

(A) Judgment
(B) Level of arousal
(C) Recent memory
(D) Attention
(E) Abstract reasoning

4. Orientation to time and place

5. Proverb interpretation

Answers and Explanations

1–D. In a diagnostic psychiatric interview, inductive data refer to that information which is gathered because it may yield important clinical material. In deductive data gathering, on the other hand, data are obtained specifically to rule in or rule out specific diagnoses. Inductive data can be gathered during a highly structured interview. Inductive questions may be open or closed ended.

2–E. The mental status examination is initiated at the beginning of the interview, starting with observations about the patient's level of arousal and manner of dress as well as physical findings. Next, observations about psychomotor activity, speech, mood, and thought processes are made. Specific mental status tests (e.g., orientation to time and place, memory of objects at 5 minutes, proverb interpretation) are usually performed later in the interview, after sufficient clinical history has been obtained and rapport is established. The patient may develop a transference reaction at the start of an interview.

3–D. "Process" refers to the underlying psychodynamics of a patient during an interview and to the interpersonal dynamics between the clinician and patient. Interpersonal dynamics may be revealed in themes of conversation as well as transference phenomena.

4–5. The answers are: 4-C, 5-E. Adequate recent memory function is essential for remaining oriented to time and place, and it is the component of consciousness assessed through questions about time and place. The ability to reason is assessed by tests such as proverb interpretation and object similarities and differences. Judgment is determined by the clinician's assessment of the patient's understanding of specific issues or actions. Level of arousal is assessed through observation of the patient's response to various verbal and physical stimuli. The ability to focus attention is assessed by tests such as serial sevens.

3

Developmental Assessment and Theory

I. **Normal Development.** The changes embodied in human development contain the meaning of our lives. These changes have captured the imaginations of both scientists and philosophers and are the genesis of many powerful theories about the human experience.

    A. **Human development** results from a lifelong interaction between biological development and environmental influence.

        1. **Endogenous biological development** is largely genetically determined.

        2. **Environmental influences** include family interactions and events (e.g., attachment, separation, loss), sociocultural influences, and psychological and social stressors.

    B. **Different aspects of development** can be arbitrarily divided:

        1. Gross motor development
        2. Fine motor development
        3. Perceptual development
        4. Speech development
        5. Cognitive development
        6. Social development
        7. Emotional development

    C. **Differences in normal development.** Different aspects of psychosocial development occur at different rates, even in the same individual. For example, speech may develop more rapidly than other skills in one child. In another child at the same overall developmental level, speech may develop more slowly.

II. **Early Developmental Milestones.** Development usually is incremental and continuous but is often described by observable milestones.

    A. **Birth to 6 months—innate behavior**

        1. **Motor.** Infant displays innate motor reflexes.

        2. **Perceptual–cognitive.** Infant attends to stimuli and moves in relation to them.

3. **Communicative.** Infant cries and coos.
4. **Emotional.** Innate emotional behavior includes negative and neutral affects.
5. **Social.** Innate social behavior includes an attraction to faces.

B. **Age 6 months—stable platform**

1. **Gross motor.** Infant sits up well and can roll over.
2. **Fine motor.** Infant can transfer objects from one hand to the other.
3. **Perceptual–cognitive.** Infant visually tracks, inspects, and discriminates among people and objects.
4. **Communicative.** Infant cries, laughs, and babbles using consonants.
5. **Emotional.** Infant derives obvious enjoyment from interacting playfully with others.
6. **Social.** Infant displays stranger anxiety.

C. **Age 1 year—movement through environment**

1. **Gross motor.** Infant walks.
2. **Fine motor.** Infant manipulates objects.
3. **Perceptual–cognitive.** Infant notes discrepancies between expected and actual events.
4. **Communicative.** First words are spoken.
5. **Emotional.** Infant is able to display pride, anger, and shame.
6. **Social.** Infant displays separation anxiety.

D. **Age 18 months—purposeful interaction with environment**

1. **Gross motor.** Infant climbs.
2. **Fine motor.** Infant uses simple objects, such as spoons and sticks.
3. **Perceptual–cognitive.** Infant identifies common objects, such as a ball or a shoe.
4. **Communicative.** Infant has a 20–100 word vocabulary.
5. **Emotional.** Infant displays complex emotion.
6. **Social.** Infant displays assertiveness and social communication.

E. **Age 2 years—shaping environment**

1. **Gross motor.** Child runs.
2. **Fine motor.** Child is able to copy a circle, and later a square and triangle.
3. **Perceptual–cognitive.** Infant is able to think abstractly and classify information.
4. **Communicative.** Child has a 200–300 word vocabulary.
5. **Emotional.** Child displays increasingly more complex emotion.
6. **Social.** Child displays complex social interaction.

F. **Age 3 years—planning environment**

1. **Gross motor.** Child jumps and is able to stand on one foot.
2. **Fine motor.** Child is able to copy a cross.
3. **Perceptual–cognitive.** Child is capable of internal reasoning.
4. **Communication.** Child has a vocabulary of 1500 words, including pronouns.
5. **Emotional.** Child displays a full range of complex emotion.
6. **Social.** Child displays complex social interactions and goal setting.

III. Developmental Assessments. In addition to clinical observation, several **assessment instruments commonly are used to quantify aspects of child development.**

    A. Developmental milestones are often assessed by the **Denver Developmental Screening Test** or the **Gesell Infant Scale.**

    B. Cognitive development is often assessed by the **Wechsler Intelligence Scale for Children-Revised (WISC-R).**

    C. Social development is often assessed by the **Vineland Adaptive Behavior Scales.**

IV. Overview of Metapsychological Developmental Theories

    A. Definition. Metapsychological developmental theories **describe the development of personality and consciousness.** These theories attempt to explain how inborn traits and subsequent experiences shape individual consciousness.

    B. Although these theories have differing assumptions, scopes, and purposes, they share some common themes.

        1. Innate mental structures and characteristics are the substrate for subsequent development.

        2. There are **specific and sequential maturational stages.**

        3. Environmental interactions and social experiences affect subsequent personality.

            a. A normal environment, especially one that provides normal social experiences, leads to a psychologically normal person.

            b. An abnormal environment, especially one that provides abnormal social experiences, often leads to psychopathology.

        4. The beginnings of consciousness arise in an understanding of the distinctions between self and nonself.

V. Psychoanalytic Theory (Freud). Freud proposed **three models of the mind,** each with a developmental perspective.

    A. Topographical model. The mind has three regions, each with a different operating system: the **unconscious, preconscious,** and **conscious.**

        1. Unconscious system. The unconscious system develops earliest and is **characterized by an irrational wish-driven type of thinking (primary process).**

        2. Preconscious system. The preconscious system **serves as a conduit of unconscious mental activity into consciousness** and is accessible to consciousness through directed attention or daydreams.

        3. Conscious system. As an infant grows, he must learn to control his activities based on subjective experience and objective reality. To accomplish this, the conscious system develops and is **characterized by rational thinking (secondary process).**

    B. Structural model. The mind is divided into three components: the **id, ego,** and **superego.** Adult personality is the result of interactions among the id, ego, and superego.

1. The **id is innate,** but the development of the ego and superego is closely linked to developmental processes and events.

   a. The id contains **mental representatives of the instinctual drives.**

   b. The id is **governed by the "pleasure principle,"** in which reality is ignored and only wishes are represented.

2. The **ego develops from the id** as a result of maturation and experience and is **governed by the "reality principle."**

   a. The ego **modulates anxiety** by using repression and defense mechanisms.

   b. The ego **regulates instinctual drives** to permit adaptation to the external world.

3. The **superego,** or conscience, **develops as a result of the child's identification with parental authority.**

C. **Genetic model.** During childhood, the **primary source of interest and pleasure (erotogenic zone) shifts from oral to anal to phallic.** Experiences during each phase of psychosocial development are important determinants of future personality.

   1. The **oral phase** (birth to age 1 year) is characterized by the development of dependency and aggression.

   2. The **anal phase** (age 1 to 3 years) is characterized by the development of possessiveness and organization.

   3. The **phallic phase** (age 3 to 5 years) is characterized by the development of conscience and identification with the same-sex parent via the **oedipal conflict.**

   4. The **latency period** (age 5 to 12 years) is characterized by the development of adaptation skills

   5. **Adolescence** (age 12 to 18 years) is characterized by the reemergence of sexual interest and identification with peers and adult roles.

VI. Post-Freudian Psychoanalytic Theories

A. **Differentiation (Mahler).** The most important process of human development is the **gradual individuation and separation of the infant from the mother** through a series of phases. This process **culminates in "psychological birth" or "hatching."**

   1. **Autistic phase** (birth). The child does not differentiate self from nonself.

   2. **Symbiotic phase** (age 2 to 6 months). The child differentiates self from the rest of the environment but does not understand the nature of the difference.

   3. **Separation and individuation** (age 6 months to 3 years). The child gradually becomes enamored of the world and recognizes the mother as a separate human being (**object constancy**).

B. **Epigenetic cycle (Erik Erikson).** The life cycle is characterized by stages of personality development, each concerning the resolution of a different emotional conflict.

1. Trust versus mistrust (birth)
2. Autonomy versus shame and doubt (age 1 year)
3. Initiative versus guilt (age 3 years)
4. Industry versus inferiority (age 5 years)
5. Identity versus identity diffusion (age 12 years)
6. Intimacy versus self-absorption or isolation (age 18 years)
7. Generativity versus stagnation (age 30 years)
8. Integrity versus despair and isolation (age 55 years)

VII. Temperament Theory (Chess and Thomas)

A. **Overview.** Human **infants have different innate characteristics** (e.g., activity level, adaptability, quality of mood, and response to novelty).
B. **These characteristics generate a basic temperament** that profoundly affects subsequent development of personality.
   1. **Easy babies** (75%) are happy, adaptable, and have regular rhythms of activity.
   2. **Slow to warm up babies** (15%) are inactive and withdrawn in new situations but adapt well after repeated or prolonged exposure.
   3. **Difficult babies** (10%) are fussy, intense, avoid novel situations, and have irregular rhythms of activity.

VIII. Genetic Epistemology (Piaget)

A. **Overview.** Piaget's theory of cognitive development centers around the question of **how one's knowledge of the world develops.** The process of interaction with the world is described by **assimilation of an experience, accommodation to the experience,** and, ultimately, **adaptation to the experience.** Out of this process, mental schemata develop and are constantly changed.
B. **Developmental stages**
   1. **Sensori-motor** (birth to age 2 years). Objects are not perceived as separate from action, and gradually the concept of cause and effect develops.
   2. **Preoperational** (age 2 to 7 years). Mental representations of objects develop, and objects are manipulated.
   3. **Concrete operational** (age 7 to 14 years). Rules and classifications are realized.
   4. **Formal operational** (age 14 years and older). Reasoning and abstraction develop.

IX. Attachment Theory (Bowlby)

A. **Overview. Infants have innate behaviors that produce an attachment to maternal figures.** These behaviors include clinging, crying, and smiling.
   1. **Infants show pleasure when close to the maternal figure,** but during separation they emit a series of responses, including protest, despair, grief, and denial.
   2. These behaviors "bond" the maternal figure to the infant.

B. **Quality of attachment.** The temperament of the infant, the personality of the mother, and the types of separations that they experience determine the quality of attachment.

1. The quality of early attachment determines the way an infant will attach and relate to other people throughout life.
2. Some forms of psychopathology, especially depression, are caused by insecure early attachment.

Review Test

Directions: The numbered item or incomplete statement in this section is followed by answers or by completions of the statement. Select the ONE lettered answer or completion that is BEST in this case.

1. An infant believes that his sensation of hunger causes the mother to appear with milk. According to psychoanalytic theory, this form of thought is characteristic of which of the following periods of psychological development?

(A) Autistic phase
(B) Symbiotic phase
(C) Oedipal phase
(D) Anal phase
(E) Phallic phase

Directions: Each set of matching questions in this section consists of a list of four to twenty-six lettered options (some of which may be in figures) followed by several numbered items. For each numbered item, select the ONE lettered option that is most closely associated with it. To avoid spending too much time on matching sets with large numbers of options, it is generally advisable to begin each set by reading the list of options. Then, for each item in the set, try to generate the correct answer and locate it in the option list, rather than evaluating each option individually. Each lettered option may be selected once, more than once, or not at all.

Questions 2–3

Match each of the following milestones with the usual age at which it is accomplished.

(A) Birth
(B) Age 6 months
(C) Age 1 year
(D) Age 18 months
(E) Age 2 years

2. Walking

3. Vocabulary of 200–300 words

Questions 4–5

Match each developmental theory with the associated theorist(s).

(A) Bowlby
(B) Chess and Thomas
(C) Erikson
(D) Freud
(E) Piaget

4. Knowledge of the world develops through a process of assimilation, accommodation, and adaptation to experience

5. Innate behavioral characteristics generate a basic temperament that forms the substrate for the development of personality

Answers and Explanations

1–B. During the symbiotic phase of development, which is most extensively described by **Mahler**, the infant differentiates himself from the rest of the environment but does not yet understand the nature of the disconnection. This phase is normal from approximately 3 to 6 months of age. The symbiotic phase follows the autistic phase, during which no differentiation between self and environment occurs. Anal, phallic, and oedipal phases are later periods described in psychoanalytic theory and are all characterized by the ability to distinguish self from environment.

2–3. The answers are: 2-C, 3-E. Walking first occurs at approximately 1 year of age, followed by climbing at 18 months of age, running at 2 years of age, and jumping and hopping at 2 years of age and older. A vocabulary of 200–300 words usually is mastered at approximately 2 years of age, along with simple 2- or 3-word sentences.

4–5. The answers are: 4-E, 5-A. Piaget developed the theory of genetic epistemology, which is a theory of cognitive development that centers around the question of how one's knowledge of the world develops. The process of interaction with the world is described by assimilation of an experience, accommodation to the experience, and ultimately by adaptation to the experience. Chess and Thomas developed temperament theory, which is a theory of personality development that postulates that infants have different innate characteristics (e.g., activity level, adaptability, quality of mood, and response to novelty) that generate a basic temperament that profoundly affects subsequent development of personality. Bowlby elaborated attachment theory, which describes the effect of early bonding experiences on later personality. Erikson is associated with an epigenetic cycle theory of personality development that is composed of discrete stages characterized by the resolution of different emotional conflicts. Freud developed three psychoanalytic theories of personality development that emphasize the effect of early emotional experiences on later personality.

4
Overview of Childhood Psychiatric Diagnosis

I. Special Childhood Diagnostic Problems

A. Child development

1. **Assessing normality or diagnosing pathology** of childhood behavior requires a detailed knowledge of psychosocial development.
2. In adults, pathologic behavior may endure over long periods of time, but **in children, behavior is constantly evolving.**
3. **A psychiatric illness may have different signs and symptoms** during different stages of child development.
   a. It may be difficult to distinguish the clinical course of an illness from changes resulting from ongoing psychosocial development.
   b. Intercurrent psychiatric illness may have downstream effects on psychosocial development. Developmental lag that resulted from a time-limited episode of pathology may be apparent later in childhood.
   c. It may be difficult to distinguish the effects of a therapeutic intervention from the effects of further development.

B. Sensitivity to environment

1. In adults, enduring patterns of behavior make it easier to distinguish inherent behavior from immediate environmental influence.
2. **Children are much more sensitive to environmental influence.** They have less trait stability across different settings.
3. **Two environments are especially pervasive in childhood: family and school.**
   a. **The family environment.** The family is the most universal childhood environment.
      (1) It may be impossible to distinguish the pathology of a family from the pathology of an identified child patient.
      (2) **Family pathology may create psychiatric problems in a child.** Likewise, psychiatric problems in a child may create family problems.

       (3) **"Goodness of fit"** is a concept that attempts to explain how the interaction between temperament (inherent childhood traits) and environment produces psychological health or psychopathology.

    b. **The school environment**

       (1) It is often difficult to distinguish the problems in a school or classroom from problems in a child.

       (2) **The peak age of incidence for many childhood disorders is 5 years of age** (school enrollment). Many **disorders resolve at approximately 16–18 years of age** (school completion).

  4. The way childhood complaints present to clinical attention is usually different from that of adults. Children rarely make appointments with psychiatrists; people in the child's environment (e.g., parents, teachers) perceive a problem and bring it to clinical attention.

C. Ethical concerns. Psychiatric or other medical treatment in childhood involves special ethical concerns.

  1. Often, **the child's target symptoms are more disturbing to others** than to the patient.

  2. Obtaining consent to treatment is more complicated in childhood. Because children may not be considered completely competent to give consent, guardians may be involved in the process.

  3. Consent for participation in research protocols is even more problematic, making the study of child psychiatric diagnosis and treatment more difficult.

II. Diagnostic Systems in Child Psychiatry

A. Past diagnostic systems in child psychiatry have often been unsatisfactory for clinical practice because they were based more heavily on metapsychological developmental theory than on clinical usefulness.

B. The **DSM-IV diagnostic framework** reflects the rapid and ongoing changes in the understanding and treatment of childhood mental disorders.

III. Overview of DSM-IV Childhood Diagnosis

A. Many psychiatric disorders that occur in adults also occur in children; however, these disorders may cause different symptoms during childhood. For example:

  1. **Major depressive disorder.** The child's mood may be irritable instead of depressed.

  2. **Posttraumatic stress disorder.** The child's response to a traumatic event may be disorganization and agitation instead of fear, helplessness, or horror.

B. Descriptive classification of childhood psychopathology. Disorders that usually first appear in childhood are grouped together in the DSM-IV.

  1. **Mental retardation** is a general delay in the acquisition of cognitive skills and resultant problems with adaptation.

  2. **Learning, motor skills, and communication disorders** are delays in the development of specific cognitive, motor, and language skills.

3. **Pervasive developmental disorders** are qualitative distortion of normal development, including **autistic disorder, Rett disorder, childhood disintegrative disorder,** and **Asperger disorder.**

4. **Attention deficit and disruptive behavior disorders** are characterized by behavior that is socially disruptive. These disorders include **attention deficit hyperactivity disorder (ADHD), conduct disorder,** and **oppositional defiant disorder.**

5. **Feeding and eating disorders of childhood** are persistent feeding and eating disturbances, including **pica, rumination disorder,** and **feeding disorder of infancy or early childhood.**

6. **Tic disorders** are characterized by sudden involuntary movements and vocalizations, including **Tourette disorder,** and **chronic and transient tic disorders.**

7. **Elimination disorders** include inappropriate defecation (**encopresis**) and inappropriate urination (**enuresis**).

8. **Other disorders** include **separation anxiety disorder** and other emotional conditions.

Review Test

Directions: Each of the numbered items or incomplete statements in this section is followed by answers or by completion of the statement. Select the ONE lettered answer or completion that is BEST in each case.

1. Which of the following factors is the most responsible for difficulties with identifying psychiatric disorders in children?

(A) Childhood behavior is more sensitive to environmental influences than is the behavior of adults
(B) Children are less likely than adults to be seen by skilled clinicians
(C) Children have less prominent psychopathology than adults
(D) The effects of medication are more unpredictable in children than in adults
(E) There is less interest in research of childhood mental disorders

2. Which of the following statements most accurately characterizes mental retardation?

(A) Mental retardation is a delay in acquisition of cognitive skills that results exclusively from chromosomal or genetic abnormalities or from prenatal or perinatal insults to the central nervous system (CNS)
(B) Mental retardation is a lifelong condition
(C) Mental retardation is characterized by disproportionate delays in specific cognitive skills, relative to other developmental skills
(D) Mental retardation is characterized by a general delay in the acquisition of cognitive skills and resultant problems in adaptation
(E) The formal diagnosis of mental retardation depends exclusively on the presence of an IQ of less than 70

3. A 3-year-old girl is referred for evaluation of her apparent disinterest in others (including her parents), failure to develop speech, peculiar mannerisms, and occasional head-banging. She reportedly seemed "strange" since her earliest months. She has episodes where she runs around the house hitting the walls and uttering loud cries, and she sometimes huddles anxiously in corners. Which of the following is the most likely diagnosis?

(A) Attention deficit hyperactivity disorder (ADHD)
(B) Autistic disorder
(C) Learning disorder
(D) Rumination disorder
(E) Separation anxiety disorder

Directions: The set of matching questions in this section consists of a list of four to twenty-six lettered options (some of which may be in figures) followed by several numbered items. For each numbered item, select the ONE lettered option that is most closely associated with it. To avoid spending too much time on matching sets with large numbers of options, it is generally advisable to begin each set by reading the list of options. Then, for each item in the set, try to generate the correct answer and locate it in the option list, rather than evaluating each option individually. Each lettered option may be selected once, more than once, or not at all.

Questions 4–5

Match each description with the most appropriate diagnostic category.

(A) Disruptive behavior disorders
(B) Elimination disorders
(C) Feeding and eating disorders
(D) Pervasive developmental disorders

4. A 10-year-old boy repeatedly steals, lies, sets fires, and threatens younger children

5. A 6-year-old girl repeatedly defecates in her bed during the night and asks her mother to be diapered like her newborn sibling

Answers and Explanations

1–A. Because children are more sensitive to environmental influences, it is more difficult to identify behaviors that represent childhood psychopathology rather than responses to environmental problems. To make reliable diagnoses of mental disorders in children, it may be necessary to demonstrate that pathologic behavior is present in multiple settings. There are no data to suggest that children are less likely than adults to be seen by skilled clinicians, and childhood symptomatology is no less prominent than that of adults. The effects of medication are equally difficult to predict in all ages. There is currently a significant amount of interest in the research of childhood mental disorders.

2–D. The diagnosis of mental retardation depends on the demonstration of both a general delay in acquisition of cognitive skills (as measured by IQ) and resultant problems in adapting to the environment. There are other causes of mental retardation in addition to chromosomal or genetic abnormalities or prenatal or perinatal insults to the central nervous system (CNS) [e.g., environmental deprivation and CNS injuries during childhood]. Mental retardation may remit when the child's environment changes (e.g., when an individual leaves the school environment). Delays in only a few cognitive skills, such as reading or communication, may be mistaken for the more general delays of mental retardation.

3–B. This case is most suggestive of autistic disorder, a pervasive developmental disorder. Pervasive developmental disorders are characterized by qualitative impairments in social and communication skills, interests, and activities. Attention deficit hyperactivity disorder (ADHD) is characterized by inattention, impulsivity, and hyperactivity. Learning disorders are characterized by deficits in specific academic skills relative to the individual's overall achievement and abilities. Rumination disorders are characterized by persistent eating disturbances and include pica and feeding disorder of infancy or early childhood. Separation anxiety disorder is characterized by excessive anxiety about being separated from caregivers.

4–5. The answers are: 4-A, 5-B. Conduct disorder, a persistent pattern of violation of the basic rights of others and of age-appropriate societal norms, is a disruptive behavior disorder. Oppositional defiant disorder, a pattern of anger and defiant behavior toward authority, is another example of a disruptive behavior disorder. Encopresis, repeated defecation in inappropriate places such as clothing or floors after 4 years of age, is an elimination disorder. Autistic disorder is a pervasive developmental disorder, a category characterized by qualitative disturbances of development.

Part Two

Psychiatric Disorders

5

Developmental Disorders

I. Overview of Developmental Pathology

A. Developmental delays

1. Developmental delays may result from several kinds of psychopathology, and the delays themselves can lead to additional psychopathology.
2. Development may be generally delayed or be delayed only in specific areas.

B. Significance of developmental problems. A knowledge of developmental disorders and their consequences has diagnostic and therapeutic importance.

1. **General development**

   a. General developmental delays can indicate mental retardation, an adverse environment (e.g., impoverished, abusive), sensory impairment, or the presence of other mental disorders.
   b. General developmental delays can lead to problems with age-appropriate impulse control, self-esteem, and socialization.

2. **Motor development**

   a. Motor development is an easily observed, constant phenomenon that may suggest the presence of pathology in other areas.
   b. Motor development problems may generate further problems in speech and social skills.

3. **Cognitive development.** The ability to perceive, think, and adapt to the environment is uniquely developed in humans.

   a. Perceptual–cognitive problems seriously impair the ability to adapt to the environment and can generate severe psychopathology.
   b. Aberrant perceptual–cognitive development may indicate the need for intervention to correct or ameliorate underlying pathology, such as sensory deficits, learning and communication disorders, and environmental and social problems.

4. **Communication development**

   a. Communication is essential to both social behavior and cognitive ability in humans.

    b. Disorders of speech may reflect motor, sensory, perceptual, or cognitive problems.

  5. Social development. Social interaction is essential for learning and for the development of human consciousness.

  6. Emotional development

    a. A lack of emotional responsiveness may be an early sign of cognitive or environmental problems.

    b. Problems with emotional responsiveness in a child may lead to parenting failures if parents are not encouraged by signs of pleasure or love resulting from their efforts.

    c. Early intervention may be important to avert later pathology.

II. Overview of Developmental Disorders. The **predominant disturbance in developmental disorders involves the acquisition of cognitive, language, motor** or **social skills.** The disturbance may involve a general delay (e.g., mental retardation), a delay in a specific area (e.g., learning, motor skills, and communication disorders), or qualitative distortions of normal development (e.g., pervasive developmental disorders).

  A. Mental retardation is characterized by **subnormal intelligence and impaired adaptation to environment.**

  B. Learning disorders are characterized by **academic achievement levels substantially below those expected for age, intelligence, and environment.**

  C. Motor skills disorder is characterized by a **significant impairment in age-appropriate motor coordination** greater than expected for any associated general medical condition or mental retardation.

  D. Communication disorders are characterized by a **significant impairment in age-appropriate language function.**

  E. Pervasive developmental disorders are **severe, qualitative disturbances in multiple areas of development.**

III. Diagnostic Clues

  A. Presenting complaint. The child fails to master age-appropriate skills in one or more areas.

  B. History. The child's history may include **delayed developmental milestones, peculiar social behavior, failure to develop social bonds, inability to keep up with peers,** and **poor self-esteem.**

  C. Mental status examination shows delayed or aberrant age-appropriate cognitive, language, motor, or social skills and behaviors.

  D. Physical examination shows evidence of general medical conditions associated with developmental disorders (e.g., starvation, hydrocephalus).

  E. Laboratory studies show evidence of genetic or chromosomal abnormalities, metabolic errors, or toxins associated with developmental disorders.

IV. Mental Retardation

  A. Overview

    1. Mental retardation is characterized by more criteria than simply subaverage intellectual function. Another **significant feature is the impairment in adaptive function that results from decreased intelligence.**

2. **Diagnosis of mental retardation** may depend on the environmental demands placed on the individual; therefore, the diagnosis of mental retardation may be appropriate during the school years, but no longer be useful once the individual enters a less demanding intellectual environment.

3. **Mental retardation is not synonymous with dementia,** and although both conditions present with subaverage intellectual function, in general, they are usually easily distinguished clinically.

4. Because the **onset of mental retardation occurs before 18 years of age,** subsequent social development is affected, creating a **characteristic childlike clinical presentation.**

5. **Mild mental retardation** (Table 5–1)

   a. There are marked differences in the clinical presentation of mildly retarded individuals as compared with the more severely retarded individuals.

   b. The majority of retarded patients (85%) have mild retardation.

   c. Mild mental retardation is often not associated with any other general medical condition.

6. **More severe retardation** is often associated with general medical conditions such as **genetic and chromosomal abnormalities, metabolic or endocrine conditions,** or **other physical and neurologic problems** caused by intrauterine insult or postnatal trauma.

B. **Epidemiology**

1. **Occurrence.** Mental retardation is present in 1% of the population. It occurs at a **1.5:1 male to female ratio.**

2. **Cultural factors**

   a. IQ testing is notoriously sensitive to cultural factors and should be administered with great care.

   b. Some known risks factors for mental retardation are more common in lower socioeconomic environments. These risks include **intrauterine exposure to toxins and infection, poor prenatal care,** and **postnatal exposure to heavy metals and physical trauma.**

3. **Familial pattern**

   a. In mild retardation, there is no distinct familial pattern, although it may be more common in some families.

   b. In mental retardation caused by genetic and chromosomal abnormalities, there are characteristic inheritance patterns for various lesions (e.g., trisomy 21, metabolic diseases).

Table 5–1. Subtypes of Mental Retardation

Subtype	IQ	Percentage of cases
Mild	50–70	85%
Moderate	35–50	10%
Severe	20–35	4%
Profound	less than 20	1%

C. **Etiology**

1. Most cases of mild retardation are **idiopathic** in origin.
2. **Genetic and chromosomal abnormalities.** Inborn errors of metabolism (e.g., lipidoses, aminoacidurias, glycogen storage diseases) and chromosomal abnormalities (e.g., cri du chat syndrome, Down syndrome, fragile X syndrome) are causes of more severe mental retardation.
3. **Pregnancy and perinatal problems.** Exposure to toxins (e.g., alcohol), fetal hypoxia, fetal malnutrition, and fetal infections (rubella, cytomegalovirus, other viruses) can cause mental retardation.
4. **Acquired general medical conditions.** Central nervous system (CNS) infection (e.g., herpesvirus), trauma, anoxia, and exposure to toxins (e.g., lead) can cause mental retardation.
5. **Environmental factors** such as social deprivation can cause mental retardation.

D. **Diagnosis**

1. **Diagnostic features** include:

   a. Significantly subaverage intellectual function (**IQ less than 70**), as measured by a variety of IQ tests
   b. Concurrent **impairment in adapting to demands in school, work, social, and other environments**
   c. Onset before 18 years of age

2. **Subtypes** (see Table 5–1)
3. **Associated features and diagnoses**

   a. **Mild retardation**

      (1) The individual can attain academic skills to approximately the sixth grade level.
      (2) The individual can often live independently in the community or with minimal supervision and is often self-supporting.
      (3) The individual may have problems with impulse control and self-esteem.
      (4) Conduct disorders, substance-related disorders, and attention deficit hyperactivity disorder (ADHD) are more common in individials with mild retardation than in the general population.

   b. **Moderate retardation**

      (1) The individual may be able to attain academic skills to a second grade level.
      (2) The individual may be able to manage activities of daily living, work in sheltered workshops, and live in residential community settings.
      (3) The individual may have significant problems conforming to social norms.
      (4) Individuals with Down syndrome are at high risk for early development of Alzheimer disease.

   c. **Severe and profound retardation**

      (1) Little or no speech is present in cases of severe and profound retardation.

      (2) Some individuals may have limited abilities to manage self-care.

      (3) Most individuals require highly supervised care settings.

   d. Differential diagnoses include learning and communication disorders, sensory impairment, pervasive developmental disorders, borderline intellectual functioning (IQ 70–100), and environmental deprivation.

E. Clinical course

1. Overview. The course of any given case of mental retardation is dependent on the degree of retardation, the cause of retardation (e.g., if it is a static or progressive condition), the associated general medical conditions, and the environment.

2. Onset

   a. The onset of mental retardation may occur in infancy if the factors responsible are congenital and the degree of retardation is severe.

   b. In mild mental retardation, the onset is often at the beginning of schooling.

3. Developmental course

   a. Developmental milestones are almost always delayed.

   b. In mental retardation with a postnatal onset, such as occurs in association with head trauma or anoxia, the subsequent developmental course is slowed.

   c. Intercurrent problems with impulse control and self-esteem are common, and there is risk for development of other emotional and behavioral problems.

   d. In mild mental retardation, problems may attenuate after school years, and the patient may lead a relatively normal life.

F. Treatment

1. Prevention

   a. Genetic counseling, good prenatal care, and safe environments are important in primary prevention.

   b. Paracentesis may reveal chromosomal abnormalities associated with mental retardation in high-risk pregnancies (mother > 35 years of age).

   c. The effects of some inborn errors of metabolism can be avoided or attenuated with special diets or supplements [e.g., phenylalanine-free diet for phenylketonuria (PKU)].

2. Optimum treatment of associated general medical conditions may improve the individual's overall level of cognitive and adaptive function.

3. Special education services, a set of techniques for academic training, may improve the individual's ultimate level of function.

4. Behavioral guidance and attention to promoting self-esteem may improve long-term emotional adjustment.

5. A supportive environment, especially during times of stress, may prevent increased psychopathology and preserve function.

V. Learning Disorders

A. Overview

1. A significant number of school-age children have learning problems in one or more areas that are greater than expected based on their overall intellectual abilities.
2. Accurate diagnosis of learning disorders is important, as the disorder may be mistaken for mental retardation, and can lead to further learning problems, school failure, and decreased self-esteem.
3. Special education techniques usually can ensure normal learning in individuals with learning disorders.

B. Epidemiology

1. **Occurrence.** Learning disorders are present in **5% of school-age children.**
2. **Cultural factors.** The results of the academic testing necessary to diagnose learning disorders may be influenced by educational, social, and recreational experiences.
3. **Familial pattern.** There is a higher prevalence of learning disorders among relatives of individuals with learning disorders.

C. Etiology

1. Presumptively, some cases of learning disorders are due to the effects of coexisting general medical conditions on CNS function. For example, cerebral palsy may impair discrete areas of the brain that underlie associated mechanisms necessary for reading or calculation.
2. Many cases of learning disorders have no obvious etiology.

D. Diagnosis

1. **Diagnostic features**
   a. When a learning disorder is present, an individual's learning achievement in specific areas is substantially below expectations, given the patient's age, intelligence, and educational experience.
   b. If a sensory deficit is present, the learning disorder is in excess of what is typically expected. For example, a child with visual impairment may be expected to have some delay in development of reading skills, but a developmental reading disorder is not diagnosed unless the degree of the delay is in excess of what is accounted for by the visual impairment.
2. **Types of learning disorders** include **reading disorder** (which is the most common and is usually diagnosed in males), **mathematics disorder,** and **disorder of written expression.** Each type of learning disorder is often associated with other types.
3. **Associated features and diagnoses**
   a. Some general medical conditions and substance-induced conditions are associated with learning disorders, including lead poisoning and fetal alcohol syndrome.
   b. Conduct disorder, oppositional defiant disorder, and ADHD may be present.
   c. Perceptual–motor problems and other cognitive problems may be present.

      d. Poor self-esteem and social immaturity may be present.

      e. Differential diagnoses include environmental deprivation, hearing or vision impairment, mental retardation, and pervasive developmental disorders.

E. Clinical course

    1. Onset. The age of onset is usually during elementary school.

    2. School failure and behavioral disturbances may occur.

    3. The subsequent development of other conduct disturbances is related to the degree of educational help available and the presence of a normal IQ.

    4. Deficits may persist into adulthood and interfere with occupational function.

F. Treatment

    1. Special education is essential to ensure general learning and maximize skills in the deficient areas.

    2. Counseling of patients and families may be necessary to improve self-esteem, social behavior, and family functioning.

    3. Concurrent psychiatric conditions should be treated.

VI. Motor Skills Disorder: Developmental Coordination Disorder

A. Overview. Developmental coordination disorder is characterized by a **significant impairment in the development of motor coordination** that is not due to a general medical condition and not part of autistic disorder.

B. Features. Clumsiness, poor athletic skills, and **difficulty with other activities requiring fine motor coordination** are common.

    1. Learning and communication disorders are often present with a motor skills disorder.

    2. Occurrence. Motor skills disorder is present in **5% of school-age children.**

C. Clinical course. The course is variable, and deficits may become less marked in adulthood.

VII. Communication Disorders

A. Overview

    1. A variety of communication problems may become evident in childhood, including **problems with understanding speech, problems with expressive language, problems with articulation,** and **stuttering.**

    2. In some cases, communication problems may represent distinct disorders (see VII D 2) and cause significant academic and social problems.

    3. Although some deficits may remit during subsequent development, others may persist into adulthood.

B. Epidemiology

    1. Occurrence. Communication disorders are present in **approximately 5% of school-age children.**

2. **Cultural factors.** The results of diagnostic assessments of communication function may be influenced by educational and social experiences.
3. **Familial pattern.** There is a higher prevalence of learning disorders and communication disorders among relatives of individuals with communication disorders.

C. **Etiology**

1. Presumptively, **abnormal CNS function** caused by a variety of genetic or environmental insults are responsible for some cases of communication disorders.
2. **Emotional stress** may play a causative role in the development of stuttering.

D. **Diagnosis**

1. **Diagnostic features** include difficulties with age-appropriate communication skills that are in excess of those that may be explained by co-existing mental retardation, sensory or motor problems, or environmental deprivation.
2. **Types**
   a. **Expressive language disorder** is characterized by difficulty using age-appropriate vocabulary, errors in tense, and a limited ability to construct sentences.
   b. **Mixed receptive–expressive language disorder** is characterized by difficulties using age-appropriate expressive language and difficulty understanding language.
   c. **Phonological disorder** is characterized by difficulties making age-appropriate speech sounds.
   d. **Stuttering** is a characteristic disturbance in the fluency and timing of speech.
3. **Associated features and diagnoses**
   a. Multiple communication disorders may be present simultaneously, and sometimes learning disorders are present.
   b. Other behavioral problems, including conduct disturbances and social withdrawal, may be present.
   c. Evidence of broader CNS dysfunction may be present, including incoordination, other perceptual–motor problems, abnormal electroencephalographic findings, and seizure disorders.
   d. Other developmental delays may be present.
   e. **Differential diagnoses** include autistic disorder, mental retardation, hearing impairment, motor deficits that affect speech, environmental deprivation, and selective mutism.

E. **Clinical course**

1. Communication disorders may first be evident at approximately 3 years of age, depending on the severity.
2. Episodes of emotional stress may precipitate or exacerbate communication disorders, especially stuttering.
3. The course of most communication disorders is variable, with complete recovery occurring in approximately 50% of all affected individuals and varying degrees of persistent impairment for others.

4. The course may be complicated by resultant social and behavioral problems.

F. Treatment includes:

1. Speech therapies
2. Stress reduction and counseling
3. Special education techniques

VIII. Pervasive Developmental Disorders

A. Overview

1. Pervasive developmental disorders are **characterized by qualitative disturbances in development.**
2. These rare and often devastating conditions were **once referred to as "childhood psychosis."**
3. Pervasive developmental disorders are distinct from early-onset schizophrenia.

B. Autistic disorder

1. Overview

a. The essential features of autistic disorder are qualitative impairments in social interaction, communication, imaginative activities, and interests.

b. These symptoms appear differently at successive phases of development.

c. **Theories**

   (1) Autistic disorder was first described in psychodynamic terms as a syndrome that stemmed from parenting failure. This theory has been disproved.

   (2) In the 1950s, epidemiologic studies by Chess and Thomas demonstrated a relationship between intrauterine rubella and autistic disorder.

   (3) Most researchers now believe that autistic disorder is a sequelae of a wide variety of early insults to the developing CNS.

d. Associated features of autistic disorder include mental retardation, peculiar motor behavior, odd responses to sensory stimuli, peculiar emotional development, and self-injurious behavior.

e. The clinical course of autistic disorder is characterized by very early onset, which is usually first recognized by parents when the child is 2 or 3 years of age.

f. A few autistic children, especially those with normal intelligence and coherent speech by 5 years of age, may become partially functional as adults.

g. **Idiot savants,** seemingly retarded individuals with one or two outstanding talents (e.g., as portrayed in the movie *Rain Man*), usually suffer from autistic disorder or one of its variants.

h. Many children with autistic disorder ultimately become indistinguishable from adults with moderate to severe mental retardation.

i. The treatment of autistic disorder has been relatively unsuccessful, and family counseling is usually necessary.

2. Epidemiology

   a. Occurrence. Autistic disorder is present in 0.04% of the general population. It occurs at a 5:1 male to female ratio.

   b. Familial pattern. There is an increased incidence of autistic disorder among relatives of individuals with the disorder.

3. Etiology

   a. Presumptively, autistic disorder results from CNS damage due to known or unknown factors. The sites of CNS damage associated with autistic disorder are unknown.

   b. General medical conditions associated with autistic disorder include encephalitis, maternal rubella, PKU, tuberous sclerosis, fragile X syndrome, and perinatal anoxia.

   c. In many cases, there is no obvious etiology.

4. Diagnosis

   a. Diagnostic features

   (1) Qualitative impairments in social interaction include a lack of peer relationships and a failure to use nonverbal social cues.

   (2) Qualitative impairments in communication include absent or bizarre use of speech.

   (3) Restricted, repetitive, and stereotyped behavioral patterns include odd preoccupations with repetitive activities, bizarre mannerisms, and rigid adherence to purposeless rituals.

   (4) The onset of deficits occurs before 3 years of age.

   (5) Autistic disorder is diagnosed if the impairment is not better explained by other pervasive developmental disorders.

   b. Associated features and diagnoses of autistic disorder include mental retardation, peculiar motor behavior, odd responses to sensory stimuli, peculiar emotional development, and self-injurious behavior.

   (1) Mental retardation is present in 75% of patients with autistic disorder.

   (2) Self injuries may be caused by head-banging or biting.

   (3) General medical conditions associated with autistic disorder may be present (see VIII B 3 b).

   (4) Hyperserotonemia and other neurotransmitter abnormalities are sometimes reported.

   (5) There is a higher incidence of abnormal EEGs, seizures, and abnormal brain morphology among individuals with autistic disorder.

   (6) Differential diagnoses include other pervasive developmental disorders, mental retardation, hearing impairment (in infancy), environmental deprivation, and selective mutism.

5. Clinical course

   a. Onset. By definition, onset occurs before 3 years of age; however, early manifestations may be subtle.

    b. During infancy, **a lack of responsiveness** may be the most obvious feature.

    c. Failure of age-appropriate social and language development becomes more evident as the individual gets older.

    d. The course is affected by the presence of mental retardation and other disabilities associated with general medical conditions.

    e. Approximately 30% of individuals with autistic disorder become semi-independent in adulthood; however, almost all patients have severe residual disabilities.

    f. The predictors of a poor outcome are associated mental retardation and failure to develop useful speech by 5 years of age.

    g. Seizures develop by adulthood in 25% of autistic individuals.

6. Treatment includes:

    a. Family counseling and education

    b. Special education

    c. Antipsychotic medications to control some episodes of severe agitation or self-destructive behavior

C. Other pervasive developmental disorders

1. Overview. Other severe disorders of development differ from autistic disorder based on their pattern of developmental deficits, additional symptoms, or clinical course.

2. Rett disorder

    a. Rett disorder, unlike autistic disorder, is always **characterized by an initial period of normal development** and has only been described in females.

    b. After normal initial development, there is a **deceleration of head growth, loss of hand coordination and onset of peculiar hand movements, loss of social engagement, incoordination,** and **severe retardation.** These deficits remain constant.

    c. Rett disorder has a presumptive genetic etiology, and the disorder is extremely rare.

3. Childhood disintegrative disorder

    a. Childhood disintegrative disorder always has a period of normal development lasting at least 2 years.

    b. Following this period, there is a loss of previously acquired skills and the onset of autistic symptoms.

    c. This disorder is very rare and slightly more common in males.

    d. Childhood disintegrative disorder may be associated with general medical conditions that damage the CNS, but it is usually of an unknown etiology.

4. Asperger disorder

    a. Asperger disorder differs from autistic disorder in that it is always characterized by normal language and cognitive development.

    b. The relationship of this presumptively rare disorder to autistic disorder is unclear, and some clinicians believe that these disorders overlap and have similar etiologies.

Review Test

Directions: Each of the numbered items or incomplete statements in this section is followed by answers or by completions of the statement. Select the ONE lettered answer or completion that is BEST in each case.

1. A 6-year-old girl is referred by her school for evaluation of her limited speech. She reportedly has "difficulty with language" and avoids talking. Which of the following findings is most suggestive of a diagnosis of expressive language disorder?

(A) Difficulties making age-appropriate speech sounds
(B) Difficulties using age-appropriate expressive language and difficulty understanding language
(C) Difficulties with age-appropriate vocabulary, tenses, and sentence construction
(D) Disturbances in the fluency and timing of speech
(E) Persistent failure to speak in social situations

2. Which of the following statements about learning disorders is the most accurate?

(A) Learning disorders cannot be diagnosed in individuals who are mentally retarded
(B) Learning disorders occur in 10% of school-age children
(C) Multiple learning disorders rarely occur in the same individual
(D) Special education is ineffective in the treatment of learning disorders
(E) There is a higher prevalence of learning disorders among relatives of individuals with learning disorders

3. Which of the following statements about mild mental retardation is most accurate?

(A) Eighty-five percent of individuals with mental retardation have mild retardation
(B) Individuals with mild retardation usually achieve academic skills no higher than the third grade level
(C) Most cases of mild retardation are caused by perinatal insults
(D) Most individuals with mild retardation live in sheltered, group residential settings in the community
(E) Substance abuse is less common among the mild mentally retarded

Directions: Each set of matching questions in this section consists of a list of four to twenty-six lettered options (some of which may be in figures) followed by several numbered items. For each numbered item, select the ONE lettered option that is most closely associated with it. To avoid spending too much time on matching sets with large numbers of options, it is generally advisable to begin each set by reading the list of options. Then, for each item in the set, try to generate the correct answer and locate it in the option list, rather than evaluating each option individually. Each lettered option may be selected once, more than once, or not at all.

Questions 4–5

Match each of the descriptions with the most closely corresponding pervasive developmental disorder.

(A) Asperger disorder
(B) Autistic disorder
(C) Childhood disintegrative disorder
(D) Rett disorder

4. A 2 ½-year-old boy who has reached all developmental milestones on or ahead of schedule develops a gradual loss of previously acquired skills and the onset of autistic symptoms

5. A 5-year-old girl has marked qualitative impairments in social interaction and a restricted range of interests and activities, but no delay in development of cognitive or general language function

Answers and Explanations

1–C. Expressive language disorder is characterized by problems with vocabulary, tenses, and sentence construction. Phonological disorder is characterized by problems making speech sounds. Mixed receptive–expressive language disorder is characterized by problems with both expressive language and language comprehension. Stuttering is characterized by disturbances in the fluency and timing of speech. Selective mutism is characterized by the failure to speak in specific social situations.

2–E. Learning disorders appear to be more frequent among relatives of individuals with learning disorders. Learning disorders are diagnosed in individuals who are mentally retarded if the deficits are greater than can be accounted for by the general degree of retardation. Learning disorders occur in 5% of school-age children. Multiple learning disorders are often present in the same individual. Special education designed to maximize the use of learning abilities has be demonstrated to improve the outcome of learning disorders.

3–A. The majority of individuals with mental retardation have mild retardation. It may be difficult to determine the cause of a given case of mild retardation. Both environmental and polygenetic influences have been implicated. Most individuals with mild retardation live independently in the community and may attain academic skill at the sixth grade level. Substance abuse and other behavioral problems are more common in individuals with mild retardation.

4–5. The answers are: 4-C, 5-A. Childhood disintegrative disorder differs from autistic disorder in that there is a distinct history of normal development that precedes the onset of autistic symptoms. Asperger disorder differs from autistic disorder in that cognitive and language skills are unaffected. Autistic disorder is characterized by qualitative impairments in social interaction, communication, and imagination that have an onset before 3 years of age. Rett disorder is characterized by the development of autistic symptoms, deceleration of head growth, and characteristic motor symptoms; it has been described only in females.

6
Attention Deficit Hyperactivity Disorder

I. History

A. **Attention deficit hyperactivity disorder (ADHD)** has been a **controversial diagnosis** in child psychiatry because it involves social issues and chronic drug treatment.

B. **ADHD has been given a number of names** in the past, including hyperkinetic syndrome, hyperactive syndrome, minimal brain dysfunction, and attention deficit disorder.

C. **Clinical descriptions of ADHD exist from the last century,** but treatment with amphetamines was first attempted by Bradley in the 1930s for **"organic drivenness"** in postencephalitic children.

D. **Over the last 3 decades,** the occasional presence with ADHD of perceptual motor deficits ("soft neurologic signs"), histories of perinatal problems, and an association with other central nervous system (CNS) syndromes has suggested to researchers that physiologic lesions may be etiologic.

E. Because **environmental stressors can also be associated with many symptoms of ADHD,** the etiology and treatment of this disorder have remained a subject of sometimes impassioned debate.

II. Epidemiology

A. **Occurrence.** ADHD occurs at a **9:1 male to female ratio.** ADHD is present in **5% of school-age children.**

B. **Familial pattern.** ADHD is associated with an increased prevalence of the disorder, as well as mood and anxiety disorders, substance-related disorders, and antisocial personality disorder in relatives of an individual with ADHD.

III. Etiology

A. **CNS pathology** is implicated in some cases because of an association with other CNS pathology.

B. **Environmental problems,** including chaotic family and school situations, have also been implicated.

IV. Diagnosis

A. Diagnostic clues

1. **Presenting complaints** may include:
   a. The child cannot sit still (**"motor always running"**)
   b. The child cannot pay attention
   c. The child is disruptive in class
   d. The child cannot restrain impulses
2. **Clinical history** may include such problems as short attention span, constant fidgeting, inability to sit through cartoons or meals, inability to wait in lines, failure to stay quiet or sit still in class, shunning by peers, fighting, poor academic performance, carelessness, and poor relationships with siblings.
3. **Mental status examination** results are usually unremarkable.
4. **Physical examination.** Perceptual–motor problems and incoordination are occasionally present.
5. **Laboratory studies** are not diagnostic.

B. Diagnostic features

1. There is a triad of inattention, hyperactivity, and impulsivity.
2. The symptoms last for at least 6 months.
3. The onset occurs before 7 years of age.
4. Symptoms are present in multiple settings.
5. ADHD does not occur exclusively during autistic disorder or psychoses and is not better explained by another mental disorder.

C. Subtypes are based on the predominance of symptoms of inattention or of hyperactivity and impulsivity.

D. Associated features and diagnoses

1. **Symptoms may vary in type and severity,** depending on the age and different environments of the child.
2. **Minor physical abnormalities** may be more common.
3. **Common associated conditions** include low self-esteem, mood lability, conduct disorder, learning disorders, motor skills disorder, communication disorders, drug abuse, school failure, and physical trauma as a result of impulsivity.
4. **Differential diagnoses** include age-appropriate behavior, response to environmental problems, mental retardation, autistic disorder, and mood disorders.

V. Clinical course

A. The **onset is often early;** however, ADHD is usually first recognized when a child enters school.
B. **Symptoms** usually persist throughout childhood; however, gross motor symptoms attenuate.
C. **Some features of ADHD persist** into adulthood in approximately 30% of affected individuals.
D. **Conduct disorders,** oppositional defiant disorder, and antisocial personality disorder may develop later.

E. Poor prognostic signs include a low IQ, presence of conduct disorder, and behavioral problems in parents.

IV. Treatment

A. Overview

1. The **mainstays of treatment** are accurate diagnosis, pharmacotherapy, and child and family counseling.

   a. **Stimulant medications,** especially methylphenidate (Ritalin) and other amphetamines, are the medications of choice. They are usually effective in decreasing hyperactivity, inattention, and impulsivity.

   b. It is essential to **identify specific target behaviors before initiating pharmacotherapy.** Target behaviors may vary depending on the setting.

2. Because it is **important to obtain accurate behavioral information** from a variety of settings, **structured questionnaires are often given to parents and teachers** to assess both baseline behaviors and response to treatment.

B. Goals of treatment are to:

1. Improve classroom performance
2. Improve self-esteem
3. Prevent behavioral complications

C. Use of medication

1. **Methylphenidate** (Ritalin) is the most common pharmacotherapy. Other medications such as **pemoline** and **dextroamphetamine** also are effective.

2. The **mode of action is unknown,** but therapeutic effects such as increased attention span and decreased motor activity are also observed in children without ADHD who are given the medication experimentally.

3. **Complications of treatment** with amphetamines include insomnia, anorexia, liver enzyme elevation, temporary growth retardation, and exacerbation of tics.

4. **Pharmacotherapy guidelines.** The clinician must confirm diagnosis and define target symptoms before initiating treatment.

   a. **Obtain baseline laboratory information,** including liver function tests and height and weight data.

   b. **Educate** both family and patient about treatment goals and plans.

   c. **Begin medication at a low dose** and increase the dose over a few weeks. Dosage level and schedule may need to be fine-tuned to obtain the optimal response and minimize adverse effects.

   d. If possible, administer medication only on school days, and do not automatically restart medication following the patient's summer vacation.

   e. Ensure that psychological, social, and educational measures are taken to add structure and stability to the patient's home and school environments.

D. Treatment response

1. There is almost always an immediate response to treatment.
2. The medication dosage necessary for optimal response for treatment of inattention may be lower than that for hyperactivity.
3. **Improvement in impulse control** is associated with improved social behavior.
4. Pharmacotherapy for children with ADHD does not seem to predispose them to drug abuse in adulthood.

Review Test

Directions: Each of the numberred items or incomplete statements in this section is followed by answers or by completions of the statement. Select the ONE lettered answer or completion that is BEST in each case.

Questions 1–3

A 13-year-old boy is referred by his junior high school principal for evaluation of his short attention span and inability to sit quietly in class or on the school bus. He has a quick temper at school and at home, and he is teased about his temper by his peers.

1. Which of the following is most likely to be an associated finding in this case?

(A) Affectual blunting
(B) Autistic mannerisms
(C) Conduct disturbances
(D) Grandiosity and inflated self-esteem
(E) Mental retardation

2. Which of the following is most likely to characterize his clinical course?

(A) His behavior deficits will become increasingly severe in adolescence
(B) He has a 20% likelihood of developing schizophrenia by late adolescence
(C) His symptoms of inattention will likely decrease, and his symptoms of hyperactivity will likely increase
(D) If behavioral problems are also present in his parents, there may be an environmental etiology for his symptoms and, thus, there will be a more benign clinical course
(E) There is a 70% likelihood that his symptoms will remit by adulthood

3. Which of the following is the most appropriate initial pharmacologic treatment for this case?

(A) Carbamazepine
(B) Chlorpromazine
(C) Desipramine
(D) Lorazepam
(E) Pemoline

4. Which of the following most accurately reflects the prevalence of attention deficit hyperactivity disorder (ADHD) in school-age children?

(A) 0.1%
(B) 0.5%
(C) 1%
(D) 5%
(E) 10%

5. Which of the following statements regarding the diagnosis of ADHD is most accurate?

(A) Symptoms must be present for at least 2 years
(B) Symptoms must be present in multiple settings
(C) Symptoms must include poor school achievement
(D) Symptoms must include perceptual–motor problems
(E) The onset of symptoms must occur before 10 years of age

Answers and Explanations

1–C. The symptoms in this case are suggestive of attention deficit hyperactivity disorder (ADHD). Conduct disturbances are a common associated finding in individuals with ADHD; drug abuse is also more common. Affect tends to be more labile, and low self-esteem is common. Although mental retardation is seen more often in children with ADHD than in the general population, it is not a common associated finding, and this boy is at the expected grade level for his age. Autism is rarely diagnosed in individuals with ADHD.

2–E. Symptoms remit by adulthood in the majority of individuals with ADHD, although ADHD in adulthood is diagnosed at an increasing rate. Generally, symptoms of hyperactivity persist but decrease over time. Schizophrenia is not a common sequela of ADHD. The presence of behavioral problems and substance abuse in parents of individuals with ADHD is a poor prognostic finding.

3–E. Most children with ADHD are initially treated with amphetamines or related compounds, most often methylephenidate. Pemoline is an amphetamine-like medication that is useful in the treatment of ADHD. It has a longer half-life than methylphenidate, and it can be administered as a single morning dose. Although desipramine has been use to treat ADHD, most studies have not demonstrated efficacy comparable to that of stimulant medications. Carbamazepine, chlorpromazine, and lorazepam have little efficacy in the treatment of ADHD.

4–D. The prevalence of ADHD is 5% in school-age children. There is a 9:1 male to female ratio for this disorder. The prevalence of ADHD in adulthood is much lower.

5–B. A diagnosis of ADHD requires that symptoms are present in multiple settings. The presence of ADHD in multiple settings ensures that the symptoms are not merely a response to environmental problems in a specific situation. Perceptual–motor problems and poor school achievement are usually seen in individuals with ADHD, but are not necessary for diagnosis. Symptoms must be present for at least 6 months and must occur before 7 years of age. As with many disorders of childhood, the onset is usually in the initial years of schooling.

7

Disruptive Behavior Disorders

I. **Overview.** **Disruptive behavior disorders,** including **conduct disorder** and **oppositional defiant disorder,** have been controversial diagnoses in child psychiatry, as they involve social issues, legal issues, and involuntary treatment.

   A. **Conduct disorder** is characterized by **violations of basic rights** of others or of societal norms in **four areas: aggression, property destruction, deceitfulness or theft,** and **rule violations.**

      1. **Children with conduct disorder have been described as juvenile delinquents,** incorrigible, "bad seeds," psychopaths, or simply youngsters trying to survive in difficult circumstances.

      2. **Interventions** used have included incarceration, psychotherapy, structured living situations, and medications.

   B. **Oppositional defiant disorder** can superficially resemble conduct disorder, especially to the authority figure making the diagnosis. With oppositional defiant disorder, the **behavioral problems usually focus on relationships to authority.**

II. **Diagnostic Clues**

   A. **Presenting complaints** may include disruptiveness, problems with discipline, persistent lying or stealing, abusive behavior toward others, fighting, and fire setting.

   B. **History.** The individual's history may include fighting, poor school performance, incarceration or other legal problems, abusiveness and manipulation of others, property destruction, lying, and inappropriate sexual behavior.

   C. **Mental status examination** results are usually unremarkable.

   D. **Physical examination** occasionally reveals evidence of injuries from fights.

   E. **Laboratory studies** are not diagnostic.

III. Conduct Disorder

A. Epidemiology

1. **Occurrence.** Conduct disorder occurs at a **9:1 male to female ratio.** Conduct disorder is present in **10% of school-age children.**
2. **Cultural factors.** Multiple cultural factors influence the expression of aggression and patterns of acceptable behavior.
3. **Familial pattern.** There is an increased prevalence of antisocial personality disorder, conduct disorder, attention deficit hyperactivity disorder (ADHD), mood disorders, and substance-related disorders in relatives of individuals with conduct disorder.

B. Etiology

1. **Genetic influences** may play a role by affecting temperament.
2. **Chaotic family and school environments** and other social stressors have also been implicated.

C. Diagnosis

1. **Diagnostic features** include a persistent pattern of behavior that violates the basic rights of others or age-appropriate social norms in the following areas:

   a. **Aggression toward people and animals** includes bullying, fighting, cruelty to people or animals, robbery, and rape.
   b. **Destruction of property** includes vandalism and fire setting.
   c. **Deceitfulness or theft** includes lying for gain.
   d. **Serious violations of rules** include running away and school truancy.

2. **Subtypes** of conduct disorder include **childhood onset** (before 10 years of age) and **adolescent onset.**
3. **Associated features and diagnoses** include:

   a. Family pathology
   b. More aggressive symptoms in males
   c. Learning disorders and ADHD
   d. Physical injuries caused by fights and risk-taking behaviors
   e. Substance-related disorders
   f. School and occupational failures

4. **Differential diagnoses** include oppositional defiant disorder, ADHD, adjustment disorders, and response to environmental chaos.

D. Clinical course

1. **Onset** occurs most often during late childhood or early adolescence.
2. Children with a younger onset have a more severe course.
3. In most patients, the symptoms gradually remit.
4. In a significant number of patients, antisocial personality disorder, somatoform disorders, depressive disorders, and substance-related disorders are present in adulthood.

E. Treatment

1. **Prevention. Moral instruction** may have a role in primary prevention of conduct disorder.

2. **Structured living settings** can be effective, especially those settings that place value on group identification and cooperation.
3. **Punishment and incarceration** have not proved to be efficacious.

IV. Oppositional Defiant Disorder

A. Epidemiology

1. **Occurrence.** Oppositional defiant disorder occurs at a **1:1 male to female ratio.** Oppositional defiant disorder is present in **10% of school-age children.**
2. **Familial pattern** is the same as that for conduct disorder (see III A 3).

B. Etiology

1. **Innate features of temperament,** including high reactivity and increased motor behavior, may predispose a child to development of oppositional defiant disorder.
2. **Specific family problems,** including inconsistent or poor parenting, have also been implicated.

C. Diagnosis

1. **Diagnostic features.** A persistent pattern of negativistic, hostile, and defiant behaviors toward adults, including arguments, temper outbursts, vindictiveness, and deliberate annoyance, is a characteristic feature of oppositional defiant disorder.
2. **Associated features and diagnoses** include:
   a. Family conflict and school failure
   b. Low self-esteem and mood lability
   c. Early onset of substance abuse
   d. ADHD and learning disorders
3. **Differential diagnoses** include conduct disorder, age-appropriate behavior, responses to social chaos, mental retardation, communication disorders, and mood disorders.

D. Clinical course

1. **Onset** usually occurs in latency or early adolescence and may start gradually. Onset occurs later in females.
2. Family conflict often escalates after the onset of symptoms.
3. Conduct disorder often supervenes.

E. Treatment

1. **Parent education** may play a useful role by lessening family dysfunction and promoting parenting skills, which decrease the frequency and intensity of problematic behaviors.
2. Some evidence suggests that individual **psychotherapy** can be effective.
3. Finding an **alternate caregiver** for the child may be indicated in some cases.

Review Test

DIRECTIONS: Each of the numbered items or incomplete statements in this section is followed by answers or by completions of the statement. Select the ONE lettered answer or completion that is BEST in each case.

1. A 13-year-old boy has a history of argumentativeness and vindictiveness toward his parents and teachers, but no history of physical agressiveness, theft, or destruction of property. Which of the following is the most likely diagnosis?

(A) Attention deficit hyperactivity disorder (ADHD)
(B) Conduct disorder
(C) Learning disorder
(D) Mental retardation
(E) Oppositional defiant disorder

2. A 15-year-old girl has a history of fighting, truancy, alcohol and marijuana abuse, bullying, lying, and promiscuity. She comes from a single-parent family with many siblings, and her father has a history of alcohol abuse. She is described as having been difficult to manage "since she was born." Which of the following is the least characteristic aspect of this case?

(A) A family history of alcohol abuse
(B) Her history of polysubstance abuse
(C) Her difficulty getting along with peers
(D) The patient is a girl
(E) Her early history of interpersonal difficulties

3. A mother seeks advice for managing her 11-year-old son who is increasingly difficult to discipline and has been suspended numerous times from attending his sixth-grade class. Which of the following is the most appropriate first step in management of this case?

(A) Educate the mother in effective parenting techniques
(B) Initiate a trial of methylphenidate
(C) Initiate a trial of antidepressant medication
(D) Remove the child from the home
(E) Suggest that the child attend a more discipline-oriented school

4. The parents of a 12-year-old boy demand laboratory tests to determine if there is "something wrong" with their son. The boy has a 3-year history of increasing discipline problems at school, defying of his parents, associating with gang members, and stealing household possessions. He has no known medical conditions. Which of the following results would most likely be revealed by a battery of tests that included an electrolyte panel; complete blood count; thyroid, liver, and renal function tests; electroencephalogram; and magnetic resonance imaging?

(A) Decreased cerebral asymmetry
(B) Hypoglycemia
(C) No abnormal findings
(D) Temporal lobe seizure focus
(E) Ventricular enlargement

5. A 5-year-old boy is repeatedly sent home from kindergarden because of bullying and fighting with peers, deliberately breaking objects in the classroom, and killing frogs in the classroom terrarium by dropping rocks on them. Which of the following statements about the clinical course in this case is most accurate?

(A) The child is likely to have shown severe symptoms earlier than 5 years of age
(B) The clinical course is likely to be more severe due to the violent features of the child's symptoms
(C) The clinical course cannot be predicted by the age of onset of symptoms
(D) The clinical course is likely to be more severe than if the symptoms had a later onset
(E) The clinical course is likely to be less severe than if the symptoms had a later onset

Answers and Explanations

1–E. Oppositional defiant disorder is characterized by a pattern of defiance of authority in the absence of conduct disorder. Conduct disorder is characterized by a pattern of violation of major age-appropriate social norms, including aggressiveness, destruction of property, theft, and çärule breaking. Disruptive behavior disorders are more common in individuals with attention deficit hyperactivity disorder (ADHD), communication disorders, or mental retardation, but there is no evidence of these diagnoses in this boy.

2–D. This case is most suggestive of conduct disorder. The male to female ratio of conduct disorder is 9:1, making the individual's gender the most uncharacteristic aspect of the case. (In oppositional defiant disorder, the male to female ratio is 1:1.) A family history of substance abuse and antisocial behavior is common in individuals with conduct disorder. Substance abuse and difficulties with peers are also common in affected individuals. Some inborn personality traits may predispose an individual to the development of conduct disorder, and an early history of interpersonal difficulties is common.

3–A. This case suggests the presence of oppositional defiant traits. Teaching effective parenting skills has been efficacious in decreasing oppositional defiant behavior. Increased discipline is often ineffective in the treatment of oppositional defiant disorder. Although removal of a child from the home is sometimes indicated, it is usually reserved as a last resort effort. Without the presence of other pathology, medications have not been consistently effective treatments for oppositioinal defiant disorder or conduct disorder.

4–C. This case is suggestive of a conduct disorder. Laboratory studies are usually unremarkable in these cases. Toxicology studies may reveal recreactional drug use, which is common in individuals with conduct disorder. The physician should assure the parents that there is little likelihood that their son's problem is caused by an underlying physical abnormality.

5–D. The boy's symptoms suggest conduct disorder. The early onset of conduct disorder is associated with a more severe clinical course. The onset of conduct disorder is usually in late childhood, but in this case, the onset is much earlier. Severe symptoms of conduct disorder rarely start before 5 years of age. The presence of violent symptoms has not been associated with a more severe clinical course.

8

Childhood Anxiety

I. Childhood Anxiety Disorders

A. Overview

1. **Anxiety is common during child development;** it's nerve wracking being a child.
2. **Childhood anxiety is the centerpiece of many metapsychological theories** of child development.
3. Childhood anxiety disorders involve anxiety that is inappropriate in terms of focus or intensity.

B. Symptoms. The symptoms of childhood anxiety may present differently from those of adult anxiety.

1. **Physical complaints are often prominent.** Stomach aches and malaise are the most common complaints.
2. **Unrealistic fears** (e.g., monsters) and nightmares are common.
3. **Various phobias** are common, especially of animals or the dark.
4. The child may have **difficulty sleeping.**
5. **Self-mutilation** including scratching, nail biting, and hair pulling is common.

C. Specific types of anxiety are common at different ages and are developmentally appropriate.

1. **Stranger anxiety.** Fear of strangers in unfamiliar contexts is present from 8 months to approximately 2 years of age.
2. **Separation anxiety.** Fear of separation from the caregiver is present from approximately 1 to 3 years of age.
3. **Phobias.** Irrational fears are often present from approximately 3 to 6 years of age.

II. Separation Anxiety Disorder

A. Epidemiology

1. **Occurrence.** Separation anxiety disorder is present in **4% of school-age children.** Separation anxiety disorder is **more common in females.**

2. **Familial pattern.** There is a higher prevalence of separation anxiety disorder and panic disorder among relatives of individuals with separation anxiety disorder.

B. Etiology

1. Children with separation anxiety disorder often come from **close-knit families,** and this may cause more anxiety in the absence of family members.
2. **Undue parental anxiety about separation** may be copied by children.
3. **Exposure to traumatic separation** may play an etiologic role.

C. Diagnosis

1. **Diagnostic features** include excessive and persistent anxiety concerning separation from those to whom the child is attached. Separation anxiety disorder with early onset is a subtype of this disorder.
2. **Associated features and diagnoses** include:
   a. Fantastic worries about separation in younger children; older patients may deny a subjective sense of separation anxiety
   b. School refusal and academic difficulties
   c. Depressive disorders
   d. Family conflict over separation issues
3. **Differential diagnoses** include other anxiety disorders, autistic disorder, and developmentally appropriate levels of separation anxiety.

D. Clinical course

1. **Onset.** The onset is usually in early childhood and may be gradual or appear after a period of stress (especially stress related to the death of a relative or pet), illness, or immigration.
2. **Symptoms** may wax and wane, depending on environmental circumstances and emotional factors. Symptoms may persist into adolescence and adulthood.
3. The child's anxiety may be manifested by worry about harm befalling parents or being separated from them by fantastic circumstances.
4. The child's refusal to tolerate separation may lead to family discord; parents may become virtual prisoners.
5. Some parents may not recognize the excessive degree of the child's resistance to separation, and school problems may bring the disorder to clinical attention. School refusal is a common complication.
6. "Homesickness" is a common manifestation of separation anxiety, and children with this disorder have more somatic complaints.
7. To avoid separation, a child may unduly limit his range of social activities, which may adversely affect psychosocial development.

E. Treatment

1. **Behavioral psychotherapy**
   a. The **mainstay of effective treatment** involves a number of behavioral psychotherapeutic techniques, including **systematic desensitization** and **operant conditioning.**
   b. In essence, the use of behavioral psychotherapy involves teaching behavioral techniques to the parents.

2. Family therapy

a. It is often helpful to clarify to parents how their own attitudes and behaviors may contribute to the exacerbation or amelioration of the problem.

b. Intrafamilial emotional conflicts and ambiguities involving separation and independence of family members may need psychotherapeutic exploration and resolution.

c. Family routines and living arrangements may require modification.

3. Pharmacotherapy. In some cases, **benzodiazepines** or **imipramine** may have a limited role in decreasing the panic associated with separation.

III. Social Phobia in Childhood

A. Overview

1. Until recently, **social phobia with an onset in childhood was known as avoidant disorder of childhood.**
2. **Social phobia** in children may be **manifested by excessive shyness with strangers, but normal social involvement with familiar people.**

B. Clinical picture

1. **Stranger anxiety** is common up to 2 ½ years of age. If this anxiety persists, it may interfere with normal social development.
2. **Onset.** Social phobia is often first apparent during the first years of schooling, but may start earlier.
3. **Learning and communication disorders** may predispose a child to social phobia.
4. **Symptoms** include excessive shyness, embarrassment, timidity with strangers, and situational mutism.
5. Social phobia **interferes with normal psychosocial development,** including psychosexual development.
6. Children with social phobia often appear to lack self-confidence and have low self-esteem.
7. A major complication of social phobia is a **failure to form normal social bonds with nonfamily members,** leading to isolation, depression, and persistent social phobia and avoidant personality disorder in adulthood.

C. Treatment

1. **Behavioral psychotherapy** involving assertiveness training techniques is often indicated.
2. As with separation anxiety disorder, behavioral psychotherapy requires **considerable parental involvement.**

IV. Generalized Anxiety Disorder in Childhood

A. Overview

1. Until recently, **generalized anxiety disorder in childhood was known as overanxious disorder of childhood.**
2. Generalized anxiety disorder in children may be manifested by excessive or unrealistic anxiety about future events, past behaviors, and competence.

B. Clinical picture

1. **Predisposing factors** for generalized anxiety disorder in childhood include birth order (eldest), **a small family, an upper socioeconomic group,** and **a family that strongly emphasizes achievement.**

2. Children with generalized anxiety disorder often appear tense and suffer from many symptoms of childhood anxiety including worry, somatic complaints, insomnia, nervous habits, and phobias.

3. **A constant need for approval and reassurance** can result in perfectionism, excessive conformity, self-doubt, and depression.

4. The child may appear mature to adults, but have difficulty gaining peer acceptance.

5. The child may avoid activities that involve performance demands.

6. Symptoms have a variable onset, and generalized anxiety disorder may persist into adulthood, often with development of social phobia.

C. Treatment

1. **Psychotherapy.** Child patients may do well with **psychodynamic psychotherapy techniques,** in part, perhaps, because of their need to please.

2. **Pharmacotherapy. Benzodiazepines** are sometimes used for treatment.

Review Test

Directions: Each of the numbered items or incomplete statements in this section is followed by answers or by completions of the statement. Select the ONE lettered answer or completion that is BEST in each case.

1. A 6-year-old boy worries constantly about "bad men" coming into his house and abducting his mother while he is away at school. Recently, he has been refusing to get on the school bus in the morning. Which of the following is the most likely diagnosis?

(A) Generalized anxiety disorder
(B) Schizophrenia
(C) School phobia
(D) Separation anxiety disorder
(E) Social phobia

Questions 2–3

A 10-year-old boy without previous interpersonal problems refuses to attend a 2-week summer camp away from home with his peers, but he is forced by his parents to go. It is the first time he has been away from home. After his first day at the camp, a counselor calls the parents to inform them that their child stayed in his bunk all day complaining of stomach cramps and dizziness. The boy demands to be sent home.

2. Which of the following is the most likely diagnosis for this child?

(A) Elective mutism
(B) Generalized anxiety disorder
(C) Schizotypal personality disorder
(D) Separation anxiety disorder
(E) Social phobia

3. Which of the following is the most appropriate management for this case?

(A) Advise the parent neither to telephone the child nor return his phone calls, and have the counselor explain to the child that all boys feel upset when they leave home for the first time
(B) Advise the camp to send the child to the camp infirmary and explain to the child that he can return to camp when he feels better
(C) Advise the parents to give the camp permission to return the child home the next day
(D) Advise the parents to telephone the child and carefully explain to him that he must stay at camp for the entire 2-week period, reassuring him that he will begin to have fun later
(E) Advise the parents to telephone the child and tell him that he may return home at the end of the week, if he still wishes to do so at that time

4. A 2 ½ - year-old toddler who does not have other behavioral problems refuses to leave her mother's side at a birthday party and cries whenever she loses sight of her mother for even a few moments. Which of the following is the most likely explanation for her behavior?

(A) Autistic disorder
(B) Normal separation anxiety
(C) Normal stranger anxiety
(D) Separation anxiety disorder
(E) Social phobia

5. Two months after a 9-year-old girl begins attending a new school, her teacher informs her parents that she never raises her hand to answer questions in class and refuses to speak to anyone, even if she is called on. The girl interacts normally with others at home, but she often wakes up in the middle of the night crying. Which of the following is the most likely diagnosis?

(A) Generalized anxiety disorder
(B) Major depressive disorder
(C) School phobia
(D) Selective mutism
(E) Separation anxiety disorder

Answers and Explanations

1–D. The child's symptoms are most suggestive of separation anxiety disorder, which is characterized by excessive fears of separation from caregivers. In younger children, the fears are often unrealistic and very concrete. School refusal is a common associated symptom.

2–D. The most likely diagnosis is separation anxiety disorder. When separation is forced, children with this problem often develop physical complaints related to the anxiety. The common term for this problem is "homesickness." Elective mutism, generalized anxiety disorder, schizotypal personality disorder, and social phobia are less likely diagnoses because of the previous absence of interpersonal difficulties.

3–E. The best course of management for this case is parental reassurance and an offer to have the child sent home in a few days if he is not feeling better. Often, initial "homesickness" quickly resolves as the child becomes more secure in the new environment. If the child indeed returns home, in the future, shorter stays away from home may help gradually accustom him to longer separations. Forcing the child to stay at the camp or failing to return his phone calls may needlessly increase his anxiety. If he has no physical findings, there is no reason to send him to the infirmary.

4–B. This toddler fears separation from her mother, which is a normal emotion before 3 years of age. If the behavior persisted after 3 years of age, it may be diagnosed as separation anxiety disorder. Stranger anxiety is fear of other people encountered in unfamiliar contexts (e.g., a houseguest may inadvertently frighten a toddler). Stranger anxiety is normal before 2 ½ years of age. If the anxiety persists in sufficient intensity after 2 ½ years of age, social phobia may be diagnosed. There is little information in this case to suggest the presence of autistic disorder.

5–D. The child's symptoms are most suggestive of selective mutism. However, underlying this disorder are symptoms that also suggest social phobia, which is often associated with selective mutism. Major depressive disorder may be present, but there is little evidence of it in this girl.

9

Mental Disorders Due to a General Medical Condition or Substance

I. **Overview.** Many common and serious mental disorders are caused by general medical conditions and by substances (e.g., abused drugs, medications, toxins).

    A. Grouping disorders with known pathophysiology as organic mental disorders erroneously implies that other disorders are nonorganic.

    B. Before the DSM-IV, **organic mental disorders** denoted those disorders that were caused by general medical conditions or by substances.

        1. Currently, these disorders are grouped in DSM-IV with other disorders that present with similar syndromes.

        2. For example, what was formerly called an organic mood disorder and described in the DSM-III-R organic mental disorders section is now called mood disorder due to a general medical condition and is described in the mood disorder section of the DSM-IV.

    C. **Diagnosis of a mental disorder due to a general medical condition.** The following three conditions must be met to diagnose a mental disorder due to a general medical condition.

        1. There must be **evidence that the disturbance is a direct physiologic consequence of a medical condition.**

        2. The disturbance is not better accounted for by another mental disorder.

        3. The disturbance does not occur exclusively during the course of a delirium.

    D. **Diagnosis of a substance induced mental disorder.** The following three conditions must be applicable to diagnose a substance-induced mental disorder.

        1. There must be **evidence that the disturbance developed in association with substance use** and generally does not persist during extended periods of abstinence.

        2. The disturbance is not better accounted for by another mental disorder that is not substance induced.

        3. The disturbance does not occur exclusively during the course of a delirium.

II. General Medical Conditions that Commonly Cause Psychopathology

A. **Cardiovascular conditions** that can cause psychopathology include:

1. Carotid artery stenosis
2. Aortic arch syndrome
3. Insufficient cardiac output, which can be caused by arrhythmia, congestive heart failure, pulmonary embolus, or myocardial infarction
4. Hypotension, including systolic or orthostatic decreases, which can be caused by psychiatric or other medication
5. Hypovolemia, which can be caused by dehydration or blood loss

B. **Cerebrovascular conditions** that can cause psychopathology include:

1. Multi-infarct dementia
2. Arteriosclerosis
3. Stroke
4. Vertebral–basilar artery insufficiency
5. Transient ischemic episodes

C. **Cerebrospinal fluid flow disturbance,** including normal pressure hydrocephalus, can cause psychopathology.

D. **Electrolyte disturbances** that can cause psychopathology include:

1. **Hypercalcemia** associated with carcinoma, hyperparathyroidism, multiple myeloma, Paget disease, and thiazide administration
2. **Hypernatremia** associated with hyperosmolar state due to inadequate fluid intake, cerebral concussion, excessive sweating with insufficient water intake, and iatrogenic etiology (e.g., intravenous or intraperitoneal hypertonic saline, tube feeding of high-protein mixtures)
3. **Hyponatremia** associated with hyposmolar syndrome due to increased antidiuretic hormone secretion, bronchogenic carcinoma, cerebrovascular accident, skull fracture, and postoperative states

E. **Endocrine conditions** that can cause psychopathology include:

1. **Adrenal disease,** including Addison or Cushing disease
2. **Hyperthyroidism**
3. **Hypothyroidism**

F. **Head trauma,** including that caused by tissue injury, subdural hematoma, or cerebral concussion can cause psychopathology.

G. **Hematologic conditions** that can cause psychopathology include:

1. Anemia
2. Polycythemia
3. Thrombocytosis
4. Thrombocytopenia

H. **Hypoxia and anoxia** can cause psychopathology, including that associated with:

1. Chronic lung disease with hypoxia, hypercapnia, or both
2. Central nervous system (CNS) receptor depression
3. Neuromuscular disease affecting muscles of respiration

    4. Pulmonary obstruction

    5. Anemia

    6. Carbon monoxide poisoning

I. Infectious diseases can cause psychopathology through several mechanisms, including:

    1. Cerebral abscesses (e.g., tuberculosis, cysticercosis, syphilis)

    2. Encephalitis (e.g., herpesvirus)

    3. Other brain tissue infections (e.g., bacterial, parasitic, spirochetal, viral, prion, and fungal infections)

    4. Systemic infections that cause immunocompromise and secondary CNS opportunistic infections (e.g., HIV)

    5. Systemic infections that cause fever or metabolic disturbance

J. Metabolic disturbances that can cause psychopathology include:

    1. Hepatic failure associated with cirrhosis or hepatitis

    2. Hyperglycemia associated with ketoacidosis, lactic acidosis, or nonacidotic hyperosmolarity syndrome

    3. Hypoglycemia associated with insulinoma or starvation

    4. Uremia associated with nephritis, nephropathy, or obstructive uropathy

K. Neoplasms. Space-occupying CNS lesions (primary CNS malignancies and metastatic lesions) and paraneoplastic syndromes can cause psychopathology.

L. Neurodegenerative diseases that can cause psychopathology include:

    1. Alzheimer disease

    2. Huntington disease

    3. Parkinson disease

    4. Pick disease

    5. Wilson disease

M. Nutritional deficiencies that can cause psychopathology include:

    1. Ascorbic acid (vitamin C) deficiency (scurvy)

    2. Cobalamin (vitamin B_{12}) deficiency (pernicious anemia)

    3. Folate deficiency

    4. Niacin deficiency (pellagra)

    5. Thiamine deficiency (beriberi)

N. Other general medical conditions that can cause psychopathology include:

    1. Autoimmune, inflammatory, and other diseases of unknown etiology (e.g., multiple sclerosis, sarcoidosis, systemic lupus erythematosus)

    2. Errors of metabolism (e.g., lipid and glycogen storage diseases, aminoacidurias)

    3. Seizure disorders

Review Test

DIRECTIONS: Each of the numbered items or incomplete statements in this section is followed by answers or by completions of the statement. Select the ONE lettered answer or completion that is BEST in each case.

1. A 20-year-old woman has an onset of persecutory delusions and auditory hallucinations after heavily abusing amphetamines for several months. She is hospitalized, undergoes detoxification and rehabilitation, and claims abstinence for 2 months. A weekly urine screen to detect amphetamine use confirms her abstinence. However, she continues to suffer from persecutory delusions and auditory hallucinations. Which of the following is the most likely diagnosis?

(A) Schizophreniform disorder
(B) Schizophrenia
(C) Amphetamine-induced psychotic disorder
(D) Delusional disorder, persecutory type
(E) Acute psychotic episode

Questions 2–3

A 31-year-old man complains of a 6-month history of malaise, fatigue, depressive rumination, sleep disturbances, and weight loss. He also complains of having difficulty concentrating on tasks. He admits to occasional intravenous opioid abuse. Psychological testing reveals mild cognitive deficits.

2. Which of the following is the most appropriate next step for management of this patient?
(A) Initiate imipramine
(B) Initiate outpatient drug rehabilitation
(C) Initiate fluoxetine
(D) Obtain a blood specimen for HIV screening
(E) Obtain a urine specimen for a toxicology screen for opioids

3. Which of the following is the least likely cause of the patient's depressive symptoms?

(A) Adjustment disorder with depressed mood due to HIV infection
(B) HIV dementia
(C) Mood disorder due to HIV wasting syndrome
(D) Mood disorder due to central nervous system (CNS) lymphoma
(E) Mood disorder due to tuberculous meningitis

4. A 45-year-old man remains depressed and apathetic after recovering from a self-induced carbon monoxide poisoning during a suicide attempt he made 1 month ago. Psychological testing reveals significant cognitive deficits, and some gait unsteadiness remains. Which of the following would be the most appropriate treatment of his psychological condition?

(A) Cognitive psychotherapy without antidepressant medication
(B) Electroconvulsive therapy
(C) Administration of fluoxetine
(D) Psychodynamic psychotherapy
(E) Administration of tacrine

5. A 57-year-old man with a 5-year history of Parkinson disease begins to experience the onset of persecutory delusions and vivid hallucinations. He has a 2-year history of treatment with carbidopa, and he was recently started on trihexyphenidyl. Mental status examination shows agitation, disorientation to time and place, and intermittent somnolence. Physical examination shows a a temperature of 102°F, and laboratory studies show leukocytosis. Which of the following is the most likely cause of his abnormal psychological findings?

(A) Anticholinergic delirium due to trihexyphenidyl
(B) Carbidopa-induced delirium
(C) Delirium due to infection
(D) Delirium due to multiple etiologies
(E) Febrile delirium

Answers and Explanations

1–A. This case is suggestive of schizophreniform disorder, which is characterized by the onset of schizophrenia-like symptoms that last from 1 to 6 months. Although the disturbance began in association with amphetamine abuse, amphetamine-induced psychotic disorder is not diagnosed because there has been an extended period of abstinence from the substance. Acute psychotic episode is diagnosed only if symptoms last less than 1 month, and schizophrenia is diagnosed only if symptoms last more than 6 months. Delusional disorder is rarely accompanied by hallucinations.

2–D. This patient most likely has HIV, which can present with mental symptoms, especially mood disturbances and cognitive deficits. Intravenous substance abuse is a risk factor for HIV infection in this case. Before beginning definitive treatment, general medical conditions, including infections, must be ruled out as a cause for a mental disturbance. A urine screen for opioids would be of less value, given that the patient admits that he uses heroin. Drug rehabilitation may be indicated later, but the initial steps for management of this case should be for diagnostic purposes.

3–A. Adjustment disorder with depressed mood due to HIV is the least likely diagnosis, because the patient presumptively is not aware of having HIV. As with other infectious causes, HIV can cause mental symptoms through a variety of mechanisms, including direct infection of the central nervous system (CNS), effects from systemic illness, associated disorders (e.g., neoplastic disease), and opportunistic infections.

4–C. The patient may be suffering from a major depressive disorder, a mood disorder due to carbon monoxide–induced central nervous system (CNS) damage, or both. Mood disorders due to general medical conditions may respond well to antidepressant treatment, which should only be initiated after stabilization of the patient's underlying physiologic problem. Electroconvulsive therapy also may be considered as a treatment option, especially in consideration of the patient's history for suicide attempt; electroconvulsive therapy should be used cautiously due to the still incomplete cognitive recovery. With the exception of supportive psychotherapy, psychotherapy would likely be difficult considering the patient's cognitive problems and apathy. Tacrine has been shown to improve cognitive deficits only in Alzheimer disease.

5–D. The patient's symptoms are suggestive of delirium, which sometimes is caused by a combination of general medical conditions and use of substances. Delirium due to multiple causes is common in the elderly and in individuals suffering from an underlying central nervous system (CNS) disease. It may be impossible to isolate a single cause of this patient's altered mental status, and the diagnostic workup and treatment must be sufficiently comprehensive to address several concurrent disturbances.

10
Cognitive Disorders

I. Overview

A. General information. Cognitive disorders are characterized by the **syndromes of delirium, dementia,** and **amnesia,** which are caused by general medical conditions, substances, or both.

B. Disturbance of cognition. Cognitive disturbances include:

1. **Memory impairment**
2. **Aphasia,** which is the failure of language function (e.g., difficulties with articulation)
3. **Apraxia,** which is the failure of ability to execute complex motor behaviors (e.g., using a key or tying shoe laces)
4. **Agnosia,** which is the failure to recognize or identify people or objects
5. **Disturbance in executive function,** which include impairment in the ability to think abstractly and plan, initiate, sequence, monitor, and stop complex behavior. For example, an individual with this deficit may be unable to make a shopping list, go to the market, find and purchase food, and take the food home.

C. Distinguishing among cognitive disorders

1. **Delirium** is characterized by prominent disturbances in alertness, confusion, and a short and fluctuating course. It is often caused by acute metabolic problems or substance intoxication.
2. **Dementia** is characterized by prominent memory disturbances coupled with other cognitive disturbances. It is often caused by central nervous system (CNS) damage and is likely to have a protracted course.
3. **Amnestic disorders** are characterized by prominent memory impairment in the absence of disturbances in level of alertness or the other cognitive problems that are present with delirium or dementia.

D. Diagnostic clues

1. **Presenting complaints.** Difficulty with cognition or recall and personality change are common.
2. **History** often includes the presence of general medical conditions or substance use, recent CNS insults, and a late onset of psychopathology. The patient is often elderly.

3. **Mental status examination** may indicate problems with arousal or attention, disorientation, difficulty with thought processing, and impaired memory, language, motor, and executive functions (see Chapter 2). Standardized tests for detecting cognitive impairment such as the Folstein Mini-Mental Status Examination are sometimes used.

4. **Physical examination** may show evidence of general medical conditions, signs of substance abuse, focal neurologic deficits, and incoordination.

5. **Laboratory studies** may show abnormal serum electrolytes; abnormal cellular indices; abnormal liver, renal, and thyroid function tests; abnormal neuroimaging; abnormal electroencephalogram (EEG); and positive toxicologic findings.

II. Delirium

A. Epidemiology

1. **Occurrence.** Delirium is present in up to 25% of elderly, hospitalized patients.
2. Children and the elderly are more susceptible to delirium.
3. There is no familial pattern associated with delirium.

B. Etiology

1. **General medical conditions.** Systemic infections, metabolic disorders, hepatic and renal diseases, seizures, and head trauma can cause delirium.
2. **Substance-induced conditions.** High, sustained, or rapidly decreasing levels of many drugs can cause delirium, especially in predisposed individuals (e.g., the elderly and the severely ill).

C. Diagnosis

1. **Diagnostic features** include clouding of consciousness and impaired cognition, with a short and fluctuating course. The disturbance is caused by a general medical condition or is substance-induced. The symptoms are not better accounted for by dementia.
2. **Types of delirium** include:
   a. Delirium due to a general medical condition
   b. Substance-induced delirium
   c. Delirium due to multiple etiologies
3. **Associated features and diagnoses** include agitation, fear, emotional lability, hallucinations, delusions, and disturbed psychomotor activity. An EEG may show generalized slowing of activity or fast-wave activity.
4. **Differential diagnoses** include dementia, substance intoxication or withdrawal, and psychotic disorders.

D. Clinical course.
The onset of delirium is often abrupt. The condition usually has a short duration, often with fluctuating symptoms.

E. Treatment
of delirium includes:

1. Correction of physiologic problems
2. Placement of patient in a quiet, well-lit room
3. Frequent orientation

    4. Protective use of physical restraints for agitation

    5. High-potency antipsychotic medications, which decrease agitation

III. Dementia

A. Epidemiology

1. **Occurrence.** Dementia is present in **5% of the population over 65** years of age and in over **20% of the population over 85** years of age.

2. Some types of neurodegenerative dementias are heritable (e.g., Huntington disease).

B. Etiology

1. **Dementias due to general medical conditions** may be associated with:

    a. Alzheimer disease

    b. Cerebrovascular disease

    c. Other neurodegenerative diseases (e.g., Parkinson disease, Huntington disease, Pick disease, and Creutzfeldt-Jakob disease)

    d. Intracranial processes such as CNS infections (e.g., HIV), traumatic brain injuries, radiation, and tumors

    e. Seizure disorders

    f. Metabolic disorders (e.g., disease of protein, lipid, and carbohydrate metabolism; diseases of myelin; Wilson disease; and uremic encephalopathy)

    g. Endocrinopathies (e.g., hypothyroidism)

    h. Nutritional deficiencies [e.g., beriberi (thiamine deficiency), pellagra (niacin deficiency), pernicious anemia (cobalin deficiency)]

2. **Substance-induced persisting dementias** are associated with exposure to alcohol, inhalants, sedative–hypnotics, anxiolytics, anticonvulsants, heavy metals, insecticides, and solvents.

C. Diagnosis

1. **Diagnostic features** include impairments in cognition and memory that result from general medical conditions or are substance-induced. The disturbance does not occur exclusively during delirium.

2. **Types of dementia** include:

    a. Dementia due to a general medical condition

    b. Substance-induced persisting dementia

    c. Dementia due to multiple etiologies

3. **Cortical and subcortical dementing syndromes.** Some clinicians distinguish between cortical and subcortical dementing syndromes.

    a. Cortical dementia is characterized by an early appearance of aphasia and difficulties with memory and calculation. There are less prominent disturbances of speech and motor behavior.

    b. Subcortical dementia is characterized by an early appearance of dysarthria, motor symptoms, slowed cognition, and personality changes.

4. **Associated features and diagnoses** include disorientation, anxiety, depression, emotional lability, personality disturbances, hallucinations,

delusions, and abnormal findings from neuroimaging and neuropsychiatric testing.

5. **In children,** dementia may involve developmental delays rather than deterioration of function.

6. **In the elderly,** dementia must be distinguished from age-related, less severe cognitive decline.

7. **Differential diagnoses** include substance-induced impairments, mental retardation, major depressive disorder, and age-related cognitive decline.

D. **Clinical course.** Depending on the underlying etiology:

1. Onset may be sudden or gradual
2. Function may stabilize or deteriorate further
3. Social, occupational, and psychological problems may intensify

E. **Treatment** includes:

1. Correction or amelioration of underlying pathology
2. Avoidance of medication that further impairs cognition
3. Familiar surroundings, reassurance, and support for the patient

IV. Specific Dementias

A. **Dementia of the Alzheimer type (DAT)** is the most common type of dementia, accounting for 75% of dementias in individuals over 65 years of age.

1. **Epidemiology.** DAT is present in 4% of the population over 65 years of age and 20% of the population over 85 years of age. DAT seldom occurs before 50 years of age and is slightly more common in women. DAT occurs more often in relatives of individuals with DAT.

2. **Etiology**

   a. Presumptively, there is a **heritable component** to the illness, and genetic linkage studies implicate a variety of chromosomes, including chromosomes 21, 14, and 19.

   b. **Selective loss of cholinergic neurons,** amyloid plaques (composed of abnormal τ proteins), and neurofibrillary tangles are histopathologic findings in the brain.

   c. **Reduced brain volume,** especially in frontal and temporal lobes, is evident on gross morphologic examination.

3. **Differential diagnoses** includes other dementias and major depressive disorder.

4. **Clinical course**

   a. The **onset** of DAT is usually insidious and the course is usually slowly progressive. The duration from clinical onset to death is usually 8 to 10 years.

   b. **Early deficits** commonly involve recent memory and mood disturbance, emotional lability, and impulsivity.

   c. **Motor disturbances supervene** later in the disease.

5. **Treatment**

   a. **Goals** of treatment are to **reduce behavioral disturbances and psychosis, improve mood, maintain adequate nutrition,** and **help caregivers cope with the burden of the patient's illness.**

      b. Pharmacotherapy

         (1) Tacrine, a reversible acetylcholinesterase inhibitor, is effective in slowing cognitive decline in some cases.

         (2) Antipsychotic agents may be used to reduce agitation and psychosis.

      c. General measures. It is important to help the individual maintain adequate food intake and exercise.

B. Vascular dementia

    1. Epidemiology. Vascular dementia is less common than DAT and is slightly more common in men.

    2. Etiology. Vascular dementia is associated with CNS lesions caused by vascular insults.

    3. Associated features

      a. Evidence of focal CNS lesions and atrophy are often seen on imaging studies.

      b. Motor findings are common.

      c. Seizure foci may be detected by EEG.

      d. General medical conditions associated with vascular disease may be present.

    4. Differential diagnoses include other dementias.

    5. Clinical course. The overall course depends on the nature of the underlying vascular pathology, the location of lesions, and the effectiveness of treatment.

      a. The **onset** is often abrupt with an uneven progression of deficits.

      b. Deficits are often localized to certain mental functions.

    6. Treatment includes amelioration (and prevention) of underlying general medical conditions.

C. Dementia due to HIV disease. HIV directly destroys brain tissue, and the course of the dementia is gradually progressive.

D. Dementia due to head trauma occurs most often in young men. It is often accompanied by emotional lability and impulsivity and is usually nonprogressive.

E. Dementia due to Parkinson disease

    1. Overview. Parkinson disease is a common, progressive neurologic condition involving loss of nigrostriatal dopaminergic neurons. The disease is manifested by bradykinesia, resting tremor, and gait disturbances.

    2. Occurrence. Dementia accompanies Parkinson disease in approximately 40% of cases, is usually more evident in advanced disease, and must be distinguished from the depressive symptoms, which are also commonly present.

F. Dementia due to Huntington disease

    1. Overview. Huntington disease is a progressive neurodegenerative disease caused by a defect in an autosomal dominant gene on chromosome 4.

    2. Neuroanatomy. Structural changes are especially evident in the striatum.

3. The clinical **onset** is usually at approximately 40 years of age, and **symptoms include choreoathetosis and dementia.** Dementia often develops early in the course of Huntington disease.

G. **Dementia due to Pick disease**

1. **Overview.** Pick disease is a neurodegenerative disease of the frontal and temporal lobes.
2. **Clinical course.** Personality and language changes are usually first evident at approximately 50 years of age, followed by other symptoms of dementia.

H. **Dementia due to Creutzfeldt-Jakob disease.** This spongiform encephalopathy is caused by a slow virus (prion). The disease is characterized by a rapidly progressive dementia with myoclonus and EEG abnormalities (i.e., sharp, triphasic, synchronous discharges).

I. **Substance-induced persisting dementias.** The following substances are associated with persisting dementia:

1. **Drugs of abuse** such as alcohol, inhalants, sedatives, hypnotics, and anxiolytics
2. **Medications** such as anticonvulsants and antineoplastic agents
3. **Toxins** such as heavy metals, carbon monoxide, organophosphate insecticides, and industrial solvents

V. Amnestic Disorder

A. **Epidemiology.** There are no data regarding the prevalence of amnestic disorder, and there is no familial pattern.

B. **Etiology**

1. **Amnesia due to general medical conditions** are often associated with processes involving generally bilateral damage to diencephalic and mediotemporal structures (e.g., mammillary bodies, fornix, hippocampus). Such processes can be caused by thiamine deficiency associated with alcohol dependence, head trauma, cerebrovascular disease, hypoxia, local infection (e.g., herpes encephalitis), ablative surgical procedures, and seizures.
2. **Substance-induced persisting amnesia** can be caused by drugs of abuse, medications, and toxins. Alcohol-induced persisting amnesia is probably the most common type.

C. **Diagnosis**

1. **Diagnostic features** include impairment in memory with clear consciousness and relatively intact cognition.
2. **Types of amnestic disorder** include:
   a. Amnestic disorder due to a general medical condition
   b. Substance-induced persisting amnestic disorder
   c. Amnestic disorder due to multiple etiologies
3. **Associated features and diagnoses** include disorientation, confabulation, emotional blandness and apathy, and other mild cognitive impairments.

   4. **Differential diagnoses** include delirium, dementia, dissociative disorders, substance intoxication or withdrawal, and age-related cognitive decline.
D. **Clinical course.** The rapidity of onset and course depends on the underlying etiology, and the symptoms may be transient or chronic.
E. **Treatment.** When possible, correction of the underlying pathophysiology (e.g., administration of thiamine in alcohol-induced amnestic disorder) may be effective in reversing or slowing the progression of the illness.

Review Test

Directions: Each of the numbered items or incomplete statements in this section is followed by answers or by completions of the statement. Select the ONE lettered answer or completion that is BEST in each case.

1. A 33-year-old man being treated for pneumocystis carinii pneumonia becomes increasingly restless, disoriented, and combative during the second day of hospitalization. He is moderately hypoxic. The patient is receiving amitriptyline for depression and for pain due to a peripheral neuropathy. Friends of the patient report significant benzodiazepine and alcohol abuse before hospitalization. Which of the following is the most likely diagnosis?

(A) Alcohol withdrawal with delirium
(B) Delirium due to multiple etiologies
(C) Depressive disorder not otherwise specified
(D) HIV dementia with delirium
(E) Hypoxic encephalopathy

2. A 48-year-old woman has a 3-year history of gradually progressive writhing movements of her extremities, emotional lability, aggressive outbursts, and memory impairment. Mental status examination reveals a withdrawn and irritable woman who speaks only in monosyllables. Which of the following is the most appropriate pharmacologic intervention?

(A) Benztropine
(B) Carbamazepine
(C) Chlorpromazine
(D) Haloperidol
(E) Lorazepam

3. A 54-year-old man is completely disoriented after stabilization for complications of alcohol withdrawal and alcoholic cirrhosis. The patient is alert, friendly, loquacious, and interactive. Although he has no obvious cognitive impairment, he is unable to give his current home address, has no knowledge of current events, and cannot accurately describe his activities during the last several years. Which of the following is the most likely diagnosis?

(A) Alcohol withdrawal with delirium
(B) Alcohol-induced persisting amnestic disorder
(C) Alcohol-induced persisting dementia
(D) Alcohol-induced psychotic disorder
(E) Hepatic encephalopathy

Questions 4–5

A 65-year-old woman is found by the police in a filthy apartment following a phone call by neighbors complaining about an unpleasant odor. In the apartment, there is long-spoiled food in the kitchen, clogged sinks and toilets, and severe infestation of cockroaches. The woman angrily refuses to leave with the police officers, claiming that her neighbors have threatened to attack her and that they will rob her apartment in her absence. During emergency room assessment, mental status examination shows an alert but very frail and unkempt woman who is completely alert and attentive. She believes it is 10 years earlier than it actually is, and she seems confused about her current finances and social contacts. She is unable to give the current addresses or phone numbers of her children and cannot find her phone book or purse.

4. Which of the following disturbances is the most likely diagnosis?

(A) Agoraphobia
(B) Amnestic disorder
(C) Anorexia nervosa
(D) Delirium
(E) Dementia

The patient's daughter, who lives in another city, states that her mother has become increasingly irritable and reclusive over the last 4 years, telling her children that she believes they are plotting to steal her savings and ultimately forbidding them to visit. Recently, the patient has been alluding to speaking with friends and relatives who died years ago. According to the daughter, the mother has no known serious general medical conditions. The mother also has no history of alcohol abuse or emotional difficulties.

5. Which of the following is the most likely etiology for the patient's disturbance?

(A) Alzheimer disease
(B) Cerebrovascular disease
(C) Pick disease
(D) Thiamine deficiency
(E) Unconscious fear and hostility

Answers and Explanations

1–B. The history of a rapid onset of confusion and disorganized behavior in a severely ill individual is most suggestive of delirium. For these patients, the delirium is often the result of multiple factors. Alcohol and benzodiazepine withdrawal, central nervous system HIV infection, hypoxia, and the anticholinergic effects of amitriptyline are all likely to play an etiologic role. Although depression may present with apathy and slowing of cognitive function, it is unlikely to account for disorientation and combativeness.

2–D. The woman's clinical presentation is suggestive of Huntington dementia, which is characterized by the onset of choreoathetoid movements and dementia during middle age. A high-potency antipsychotic medication, such as haloperidol, may both diminish the motor symptoms and decrease agitated outbursts, preserving some quality of life for a longer period of time. Chlorpromazine and lorazepam are less useful for this patient because of their more significant interference with cognitive function. Neither benztropine nor carbamazepine are useful for this patient.

3–B. The patient presents with memory impairment in the absence of other cognitive disturbances and delirium. This clinical presentation is most suggestive of amnestic disorder, and alcohol is the most likely cause. Sometimes called Korsakoff psychosis, this amnestic disorder may be related to thiamine deficiency, which sometimes occurs during chronic alcohol abuse. Individuals with amnestic disorders may confabulate (e.g., make up events that occurred during periods of amnesia), but actual hallucinations or delusions are less common.

4–E. The woman presents with evidence of memory disturbance and severe problems managing her activities. This presentation is most consistent with dementia, which is characterized by memory impairment and other cognitive deficits. Delirium is characterized by problems with arousal and attention in addition to cognitive disturbances. Amnestic disorder is a less likely diagnosis because no cognitive disturbances other than memory impairment are present in this patient. Although the woman is apparently reclusive, there is little evidence that it is caused by fear of being in a situation in which escape is difficult (i.e., agoraphobia). The woman is frail, but there is no evidence that she suffers from anorexia nervosa.

5–A. Alzheimer disease is the most common cause of dementia in elderly individuals. The gradual onset of impairment over several years also suggests this etiology. Although cerebrovascular disease is also a fairly common cause of dementia in this age group, it is often characterized by an uneven course, motor deficits, and other evidence of cardiovascular pathology. Pick disease is a neurodegenerative dementia that might present with these symptoms, but it is much less common than Alzheimer disease. Thiamine deficiency can cause memory impairment and dementia, but it usually is associated with a history of alcoholism or geographic areas where malnutrition is endemic. Although unconscious fear and hostility may lead to the patient's suspiciousness, it is an unlikely explanation for her change of behavior.

11
Substance Abuse

I. Overview of Substance-Related Disorders

A. Types. There are two types of substance-related disorders:

1. **Substance use disorders,** which include **substance dependence** and **substance abuse**

   a. Substance use disorders often lead to substance-induced disorders.

   b. Substance dependence and abuse are both characterized by **continued use of substances despite significant cognitive and behavioral problems.**

   (1) Unlike substance abuse, substance dependence also implies the **presence of tolerance, withdrawal,** or **compulsive use.**

   (2) Substance use disorders **usually start in adolescence** and may have a lasting impact on social, occupational, and emotional functioning.

2. **Substance-induced disorders,** including intoxication, withdrawal, substance-induced delirium, substance-induced psychosis, and substance-induced mood disorders (see Chapter 12)

B. Affected population. Substance use disorders affect a large number of people.

1. Alcohol abuse affects 14 million people in the United States.
2. Drug abuse affects 3 million people in the United States.

II. Definitions

A. Substance use. Recreational substance use does not necessarily imply psychopathology, but it may represent:

1. Experimentation with drugs, especially in adolescence
2. A symptom of other emotional problems
3. The presence of substance abuse or dependence

B. Substance abuse suggests a maladaptive pattern of substance use with adverse consequences that fall short of complete dependence.

C. Substance dependence suggests the presence of several substance-related symptoms.

1. **Loss of control.** The individual uses more of the substance than intended for longer periods of time.
2. **Monopolization of time.** The individual spends the majority of his time obtaining and using drugs, recovering from drug use, and discussing drugs.
3. **Presence of adverse medical, social, or emotional consequences** often are accompanied by physiologic changes associated with:
   a. **Tolerance,** which is characterized by the need for larger amounts of a substance to produce the same degree of intoxication
   b. **Withdrawal,** which is characterized by a substance-specific syndrome that occurs because of decreased use of the substance

III. Epidemiology

A. **Overview.** It is difficult to obtain reliable epidemiologic data for substance-related disorders. Periodic surveys of high school seniors are used to help gauge the relative magnitude of abuse for various drugs.

B. **General findings**
   1. A majority of adolescents experiment with alcohol and nicotine.
   2. Fifty percent of adolescents experiment with illicit drugs at some point.
   3. The highest prevalence of substance abuse is between 18 and 22 years of age.
   4. The greatest risk for substance abuse occurs when onset of use is before 15 years of age and other psychopathology is present.
   5. Negative outcomes of substance use are more likely in disadvantaged groups.

C. **Trends.** The epidemiology of abuse for specific drugs varies widely by culture and gender; however, there are some general trends.
   1. Illicit drug use is rising.
   2. Use of alcohol and tobacco remains high.
   3. Substance abuse is becoming endemic in some adolescent subgroups.
   4. Substance use is starting at an earlier age.
   5. Currently, substance abusers who present for treatment have fewer financial and social resources than those who sought treatment in the past.
   6. **Media depictions** of substance abuse have become less glamorous, which may help decrease substance use.

IV. Commonly Abused Substances

A. **Gateway drugs**
   1. Adolescent use of these substances is associated with future abuse of cocaine and opioids.
   2. Gateway drugs include **nicotine, alcohol, marijuana,** and **inhalants.**

B. **Nicotine**
   1. Approximately 25% of the United States population uses nicotine regularly.

2. Patterns of use provide a model for studies of substance abuse prevention in various segments of the population.

C. **Alcohol** is the most commonly abused substance in the United States.

1. **Epidemiology**

   a. There is a 14% lifetime prevalence of alcohol abuse.
   b. Studies indicate that one third of high school seniors drink heavily.
   c. Over 5% of the general population have severe alcohol abuse problems, and the rate is greatest in young adults.

2. **Contributing factors**

   a. Alcohol may be initially used to decrease social anxiety.
   b. Alcohol may be used to potentiate or alleviate effects of other drugs.

3. **Types**

   a. In adolescents, beer and wine are the alcoholic beverages of choice.
   b. In adults, the use of distilled spirits is more common.

D. **Marijuana (cannabis)**

1. Marijuana is the **most frequently used illicit drug.**
2. Compulsive use of marijuana is associated with poor adaptation skills.

E. **Cocaine**

1. **Cocaine use peaked in mid-1980s,** partly owing to its glamorous image in popular media, but has since declined.
2. **Crack cocaine**

   a. Use of this type of cocaine has become endemic in some inner-city populations.
   b. The decreasing price of crack and the less severe penalties for juvenile use may contribute to its use by increasingly younger populations.

3. **Complications.** Unlike marijuana, severe physical and psychological complications are commonly associated with cocaine.

   a. Intravenous cocaine abuse is associated with blood-borne infections (e.g., HIV, hepatitis B).
   b. Significant withdrawal symptoms occur, and this may strongly contribute to compulsive use.
   c. Intermittent psychosis, panic, and violence are common findings in heavy users.

4. Cocaine is often adulterated with many other chemicals, including amphetamines and phencyclidine (PCP).

F. **Amphetamines**

1. Amphetamines are generally used for their **euphorigenic** properties.
2. Some occupational groups, especially those that require prolonged alertness (e.g., truck drivers), are at risk for amphetamine abuse.
3. **Methamphetamine** ("crystal," or "ice") is usually the amphetamine of choice. It can be administered intranasally or intravenously.
4. The usual pattern of abuse is by bingeing, and alcohol is often used to lessen the distress of withdrawal.

    5. Tolerance develops quickly.

    6. Amphetamines are both diverted from legal distribution and manufactured in illicit laboratories.

G. Opioids

    1. Heroin is the opioid of choice for most abusers.

    2. Opioid abusers often develop **markedly antisocial and otherwise deviant behavior,** isolating themselves from nonusers.

    3. Withdrawal

        a. A protracted abstinence syndrome following withdrawal, characterized by anxiety and depression, may contribute to associated psychopathology.

        b. Avoidance of opioid withdrawal often leads quickly to daily use and the need for money to support the habit.

H. Inhalants

    1. Inhalants include **gasoline, glues, paint thinners, solvents,** and **nitrous oxide.**

    2. Because inhalants are cheap and accessible, they are often the gateway drugs for younger and poorer populations.

    3. Some inhalants may be associated with significant cognitive decline early in the course of abuse.

I. PCP

    1. Heavy use of PCP has declined.

    2. Violence and psychosis during PCP intoxication is fairly common.

J. Hallucinogens and "designer drugs"

    1. Hallucinogenic drugs

        a. These drugs include **lysergic acid diethylamide** (LSD; "acid"), **mescaline** (peyote), **psilocybin** (mushrooms) as well as some "designer drugs."

        b. Experimentation with hallucinogens is reportedly increasing in adolescents.

        c. Use of hallucinogens is usually intermittent, and rare cases of heavy use are associated with severe psychopathology.

    2. "Designer drugs" (controlled substance analogues)

        a. These drugs are produced in illicit laboratories and are transiently popular among small groups (e.g., those who frequent nightclubs, some college students).

        b. New "designer drugs" are developed regularly and older ones become passe. Many of these drugs are methoxylated amphetamines, including 3,4-methylenedioxymethamphetamine (MDMA), which is known as "XTC," or "ecstasy" and N,N-dimethyltryptamine (DMT).

K. Benzodiazepines and other sedative–hypnotics

    1. Benzodiazepines may be supplied unwittingly by physicians for adult abusers; adolescent abusers usually obtain them illicitly.

    2. Patterns of use are variable. Older persons may be at special risk because of problems with insomnia.

    3. Tolerance and withdrawal are common.

L. Anabolic steroids

1. Approximately 5% of adolescents, predominantly males, have used anabolic steroids.

2. **Reasons for use**

   a. Anabolic steroids are most often used in athletic subcultures (e.g., bodybuilding).

   b. They are also used for perceived athletic prowess and physical beauty.

3. **Complications**

   a. Some anabolic steroids may have psychoactive effects ("roid rage") and withdrawal effects.

   b. Anabolic steroids are commonly associated with other substance abuse.

M. Over-the-counter (OTC) drugs

1. OTC (nonprescription) drugs include **antihistamines, decongestants, caffeine,** and **dextromethorphan.**

2. Patterns of use are highly variable.

3. These drugs are attractive to adolescents because of availability and affordability.

V. Risk Factors

A. Genetics. Heritable traits may predispose an individual to substance abuse.

1. Studies indicate that **children of alcoholics are more likely to develop alcoholism** than children of nonalcoholics.

2. Individuals who are innately tolerant to alcohol may be more likely to develop alcohol abuse than those with less tolerance.

3. Some subtypes of alcoholism may have a **genetic component,** as suggested by family studies.

   a. Several biologic markers for risk of alcoholism have been suggested, including the A1 allele of the dopamine D^2 receptor.

   b. There are few data on genetic factors related to abuse of substances other than alcohol.

B. Family dynamics associated with an increased risk for development of substance abuse include:

1. General family stress
2. Parenting problems
3. Permissive attitudes toward substance abuse
4. History of physical or sexual abuse

C. Environmental conditions that may foster substance abuse include:

1. Peer drug use
2. Social isolation
3. Academic difficulties
4. Involvement in drug trafficking
5. Economic disadvantage

6. Exposure to drug use through mass media (e.g., promotion by advertising)
7. Membership in an occupational group with increased access to drugs (e.g., physicians, nurses, pharamacists)

D. **Other psychopathology** may increase the likelihood of substance abuse.

1. **Conduct disturbances** in adolescents are associated with substance abuse.
2. **Low self-esteem and depression** are often associated with substance abuse.
3. **Self-medication hypotheses.** Some clinicians believe that individuals with certain psychological problems may abuse substances in an effort to alleviate symptoms (e.g., a person suffering from an anxiety disorder uses alcohol to decrease innate anxiety).

VI. Course

A. **Early experimentation**

1. Experimentation with gateway drugs may start as early as preadolescence.
2. Experimentation often involves substance use for perceived status in social situations.

B. **Substance abuse**

1. Increasing use of substances on a regular basis may occur, often to relieve stress.
2. Often, new substances or combinations of substances are used.
3. As the user becomes preoccupied with drugs, there is a narrowing of other interests.
4. Abuse may lead to social and occupational consequences.

C. **Substance dependence**

1. A **loss of control of drug use** develops.
2. Serious social, psychological, and physical consequences result.
3. **Tolerance and withdrawal** often become evident.

VII. Prognosis

A. **Most substance users do not progress to substance abuse.**
B. **Abusers are at high risk** for psychological and physical complications as well as dependence.
C. **Predictive factors for progression** to substance dependence are **unclear.**

VIII. Complications

A. **Substance-induced mental disorders** (see Chapter 12)
B. **General medical conditions**

1. **Physical trauma** from accidents and from suicide attempts is common.
2. **Central nervous system (CNS) pathology.** Direct CNS damage may occur with use of inhalants, alcohol, and possibly other drugs.

C. Developmental pathology. The use of drugs in adolescence may interfere with successful mastery of developmental milestones.

D. Social pathology involves social deviancy and isolation.

E. Emotional pathology

1. Low self-esteem, dysphoria, and anxiety are common in substance abusers.
2. Substance abuse is a major risk factor for suicide.

IX. Assessment

A. General guidelines. When assessing substance abuse in an individual, a clinician should:

1. Maintain an index of suspicion
2. Expect denial from abusers and their families
3. Attempt to obtain additional history from other significant family members or friends, maintaining appropriate respect of the patient's independence and privacy

B. Clinical interview

1. The clinical interview should include questions about:
   a. Family functioning
   b. School and occupational performance
   c. Interactions with friends and acquaintances
2. The substance use history should include questions about:
   a. Types of substances used
   b. Dosages
   c. Substance effects and reactions
   d. Circumstances of use

C. Common screening instruments. Although screening instruments may be useful, many clinicians believe that a less structured interview is more productive.

1. **CAGE.** Affirmative answers to any of the following questions are suggestive of alcohol abuse:
   a. Have you ever felt that you should **cut** down your drinking?
   b. Have you ever felt **annoyed** by others who have criticized your drinking?
   c. Have you ever felt **guilty** about your drinking?
   d. Have you ever had a morning drink (**eye-opener**) to steady your nerves or alleviate a hangover?
2. **Michigan Alcohol Screening Test (MAST)** is a common questionnaire used to detect alcohol abuse.

D. History from parents or peers. Other individuals close to the patient may be able to provide information concerning recent behavioral changes, the quality of school or job performance, changes in peer groups, and episodes of intoxication.

E. Physical examination. In addition to a general physical examination, the clinician should look for signs of:

1. Poor hygiene
2. Poor nutrition
3. Cough
4. Physical signs of drug use, including burns, needle marks, and skin infections
5. Evidence of self-inflicted injuries or accidents
6. Substance intoxication
7. Substance withdrawal

F. **Laboratory studies**

1. **Blood and urine drug screens** and other studies may be used for:

   a. Identifying the abused substance
   b. Identifying medical complications of substance abuse
   c. Monitoring the presence of substance abstinence
   d. Deterring substance use by increasing an abuser's concern about discovery

2. **Enzyme testing.** A number of enzymes may be fairly sensitive indicators of alcohol abuse, including SGGT (serum gamma-glutamyl transpeptidase), SGOT (serum glutamic-oxaloacetic transaminase), SGPT (serum glutamic-pyruvic transaminase), and LDH (lactate dehydrogenase).

3. **Other tests**

   a. **HIV testing** is indicated for intravenous substance users.
   b. Few other specific laboratory tests have clear diagnostic utility in the management of substance abuse.

G. **Assessment of other mental disorders**

1. **Comorbidity**

   a. Significant comorbidity exists for substance abuse and other psychiatric diagnoses; however, actual statistics are controversial.
   b. Studies suggest that 50% of substance abusers have other psychopathology.

2. **Dual diagnosis** is a term used to denote the **presence of both a substance use disorder and another mental disorder.**

3. **Emotional problems** that present with oppositional defiant symptoms, poor school performance, mood and interpersonal disturbances, and unconventional behavior may be mistaken for signs of substance abuse; however, they often occur as additional problems.

X. **Treatment.** Substance abuse treatment involves four distinct phases: **prevention, detoxification, rehabilitation,** and **relapse prevention.**

A. **Prevention**

1. The **most effective prevention programs teach resistance to social pressures** to use drugs and enhance other social and personal skills.

2. Changing **drug regulatory and taxing policies** (e.g., cigarette and alcohol taxes) has also been effective.

3. Parental groups, mass media drug prevention campaigns, and drug interdiction programs have had a less clear impact.

4. Providing factual information about drugs, moral instruction, and alternative activities have not proved to effectively decrease substance abuse.

B. Detoxification

1. Detoxification is **substance-specific** but generally involves calming support, reassurance, occasional adjunctive pharmacology, and diagnosis and treatment of medical complications. Adolescent substance abusers rarely require medical detoxification.

2. **Prolonged withdrawal syndromes.** Recent clinical literature suggests that what is often considered emerging underlying psychopathology may actually be a consequence of substance withdrawal.

C. Rehabilitation

1. **Components** of drug rehabilitation include:

    a. Cessation of drug use
    b. Development of new coping skills, social competencies, and environments, making relapse less likely
    c. Development of new sources of personal satisfaction and reward

2. **Outpatient rehabilitation** is the **most common mode of treatment,** and it may vary in intensity.

    a. **Types.** Outpatient rehabilitation may have individual, group, family, social, educational, vocational, and recreational components.
    b. **Indications** for outpatient treatment include high patient motivation, family support and involvement, and minimal additional psychopathology.

3. **Inpatient/residential rehabilitation**

    a. **Therapeutic community model.** This model includes **peer support, substance abuse education, social skills training,** and **family therapy.** Drug searches and urine screens may be conducted.
    b. **Successful programs** encourage openness, self-expression, independent decision making, and extended postcare participation.
    c. **Staff.** Inpatient programs often have both experienced staff counselors and volunteers who help solve concrete problems.
    d. **Psychotherapy** in these programs often uses cognitive and behavioral approaches as well as relaxation techniques.
    e. **Indications** for inpatient/residential rehabilitation include:

        (1) Inability to function in school, work, or home environment
        (2) Inability to maintain abstinence in outpatient treatment
        (3) Low motivation to stop substance abuse
        (4) The presence of additional severe psychopathology, especially depression and suicidal thoughts or intent
        (5) Forensic considerations (e.g., courts may mandate inpatient rehabilitation)

4. **Self-help groups**

   a. Self-help groups are often modeled after the 12-step program of Alcoholics Anonymous and have been the most effective treatment available for many adult substance abusers, both for rehabilitation and relapse prevention.

   b. The 12-step model provides **close and prolonged peer support** through a series of stages during which the individual admits her problems with substance abuse and her own powerlessness to cure herself without help (e.g., from God or others), develops the determination to overcome her problem, makes amends to those she has hurt, and helps others overcome abuse.

   c. **Family treatment.** The spouse and other family members may focus on family interactions that perpetuate substance abuse (e.g., codependency issues). This treatment may be helpful to both the abuser and the family.

D. **Relapse prevention**

   1. **Occurrence**

      a. **Relapse is common,** but less likely with ongoing treatment.

      b. **Relapse in adolescents** appears more **related to peer pressure** than to personal distress.

   2. **Self-help groups are especially effective** and may require a lifetime commitment.

   3. **Monitoring drug use** is critical when patient motivation is low and treatment is externally imposed by the criminal justice system.

   4. **Structured living settings** may be especially useful for substance abusers from adverse environments.

   5. **Pharmacologic interventions**

      a. **Disulfiram** is an aldehyde dehydrogenase inhibitor. Regular use causes an unpleasant reaction when alcohol is ingested.

      b. **Naltrexone** is an opioid antagonist. Regular use blocks the pleasurable effects of opioids and alcohol.

      c. **Methadone** is an opioid agonist. Regular use decreases the chance of recurrence of severe heroin dependence.

E. **Overall efficacy**

   1. The best predictor of successful treatment outcome is time spent in treatment.

   2. Approximately 50% of patients who stay in treatment have good outcomes, but only a minority stay in treatment longer than 6 months.

   3. Substance abusers who do not receive treatment have worse outcomes than those who are treated.

Review Test

Directions: Each of the numbered items or incomplete statements in this section is followed by answers or by completions of the statement. Select the ONE lettered answer or completion that is BEST in each case.

1. A 15-year-old boy is brought in by his parents after they find marijuana in his room. Which of the following is the best initial intervention?

(A) Determine the exact circumstances in which the marijuana was discovered and notify civil authorities if the parents have not already done so
(B) Inform the parents that marijuana is a gateway drug and that drug rehabilitation is necessary to avoid the likelihood of future substance dependence
(C) Inform the parents that although marijuana use is unlikely to progress to substance dependence, any recent changes in peer relationships or a decline in school performance may indicate more serious problems
(D) Inform the parents that experimentation with illegal drugs is a normal part of adolescence and should not be the focus of family arguments
(E) Warn the boy that marijuana use can cause serious physical and emotional problems and suggest outpatient counseling

2. A 28-year-old woman is brought to the emergency room after a heroin overdose and is stabilized with naloxone. Which of the following nonemergent laboratory studies is most urgently indicated?

(A) Bone marrow biopsy
(B) Echocardiogram
(C) Electroencephalogram
(D) HIV antibody test
(E) Serial plasma liver enzymes

3. A 29-year-old man is brought to a physician by his spouse, who demands that he receives treatment for heroin addiction. She threatens to leave the marriage if he does not begin treatment. Which of the following factors is most suggestive of heroin dependence in this case?

(A) He has a family history of substance abuse
(B) He has been arrested many times for heroin possession
(C) He vehemently denies that his heroin use causes any problems and says that his wife is manipulating him
(D) He spends most of his time trying to obtain heroin, and he cannot stop himself from using it
(E) He says that he genuinely wants treatment for his addiction

4. A 30-year-old man with heroin dependence enrolls in outpatient drug rehabilitation but fails to maintain abstinence. He despondently says that all of his friends use drugs and that he is unable to stay away from them. He says that he desperately wants to stop using heroin. Which of the following is the best intervention?

(A) Administration of naltrexone
(B) Methadone maintenance
(C) Enrollment in a therapeutic community
(D) Suggest that he moves to a new neighborhood, makes new friends, and re-enrolls in outpatient drug rehabilitation
(E) Suggest that he seeks religious guidance

5. A 32-year-old man seeks treatment for severe, recurrent depression. His most recent depressive episode lasted for several months. He is moderately intoxicated when he presents, and he admits to a 10-year history of daily alcohol use. He denies any suicidal intent. Physical examination and routine laboratory studies show no remarkable findings except for mild elevation of plasma liver enzyme levels. Which of the following is the best initial treatment?

(A) Begin administration of chlordiazepoxide, tapering the dose for several days before administering fluoxetine
(B) Begin administration of disulfiram and refer the patient to counseling
(C) Begin administration of fluoxetine and refer the patient to Alcoholics Anonymous
(D) Inform him that because of the drug interactions that occur from combined use of antidepressants and alcohol, he can receive treatment for depression only after he achieves sobriety
(E) Refer the patient to Alcoholics Anonymous and suggest that he returns for additional treatment if his depression continues after he has achieved sobriety

Answers and Explanations

1–C. The majority of adolescents experiment with illegal substances, but this experimentation is not likely to progress to substance dependence. However, accompanying changes in the adolescent's social or educational performance suggest that more serious emotional problems, substance abuse, or both may be present. When these circumstances exist, therapeutic intervention should be attempted. Warnings have not proved to decrease drug use in adolescents.

2–D. Heroin abuse is strongly associated with HIV infection, and testing is essential. Without evidence of additional pathology, bone marrow biopsy, echocardiogram, electroencephalogram, and serial plasma liver enzymes are not as urgently indicated.

3–D. Substance dependence is characterized by a group of symptoms that suggest compulsive substance use, monopolization of time by substance-related activities, social and occupational consequences, and physiologic changes, including tolerance and withdrawal. A family history of substance abuse, arrests for substance possession, denial of substance-related problems, and a desire for treatment all may occur in individuals with substance dependence, but no factor occurring exclusively is diagnostic.

4–C. Therapeutic communities are composed of recovered addicts who live together and support each other's abstinence. These communities are indicated for individuals who are highly motivated but for whom outpatient treatment has failed. Naltrexone is useful for decreasing binge use of opioids, but this individual's social network is likely to defeat such strategies. Methadone maintenance decreases the morbidity associated with heroin abuse; however, it is unlikely to stop the abuse. Religious guidance may be helpful, but without additional intervention, it is unlikely to cure substance dependence. It is unrealistic to expect individuals to start a new life (i.e., move to a new neighborhood and make new friends) as a prelude to treatment.

5–C. Concurrent morbidity resulting from substance abuse and mood disorders is common, and both conditions should be treated simultaneously. The presence of both a mood disorder and alcohol abuse is likely in this individual; therefore, use of an antidepressant and referral to Alcoholics Anonymous is indicated. Witholding selective antidepressant treatment until sobriety is maintained may indefinitely prolong his symptoms. Treatment with chlordiazepoxide is not currently indicated, because there is no evidence of withdrawai. Disulfiram causes severe discomfort if alcohol is consumed; therefore, it is indicated only for relapse prevention in some cases if the individual has achieved sobriety.

12

Substance-Induced Disorders

I. Overview

  A. **Definition.** Substance-induced mental disorders are **disturbances that are a direct physiologic result of a substance.**

  B. **Effects.** The capacity of a substance to induce a mental disorder depends on the nature of the substance, route of administration, dosage, the psychological and physical state of the individual, and the social context in which the substance is used.

  C. **Substances** that can induce mental disorders include:

  1. Recreational drugs, both legal and illicit
  2. Therapeutic medications, both prescription and nonprescription
  3. Environmental toxins

II. Substance-Induced Disorders

  A. **Substance intoxication** is a reversible, substance-specific syndrome caused by the recent ingestion of or exposure to a substance (DSM-IV).

  B. **Substance withdrawal** is a substance-specific, maladaptive behavioral change, with physiologic and cognitive concomitants, caused by the cessation of or reduction in heavy and prolonged substance use (DSM-IV).

  C. **Other substance-induced disorders** are categorized and described in the DSM-IV according to the presenting cluster of symptoms (Table 12–1). Onset for these disorders is described as occurring during intoxication or withdrawal or persisting after withdrawal symptoms have resolved (Table 12–2).

III. Diagnosis and Treatment. Substance-induced disorders are often associated with substance dependence and abuse (see Chapter 11).

  A. **Diagnostic assessment** of individuals who may have substance-induced disorders includes:

  1. **History of substance use,** including the substances used, dosages, effects, and duration and social context of use
  2. **Medical history,** including complications of substance abuse and the presence of painful conditions

Table 12–1. DSM-IV References for Substance-Induced Disorders

Disorder	DSM-IV Section
Intoxication delirium	Cognitive disorders
Withdrawal delirium	Cognitive disorders
Substance-induced dementia	Cognitive disorders
Substance-induced amnestic disorder	Cognitive disorders
Substance-induced psychotic disorder	Psychotic disorders
Substance-induced mood disorder	Mood disorders
Substance-induced anxiety disorder	Anxiety disorders
Substance-induced sexual disorder	Sexual disorders
Substance-induced sleep disorder	Sleep disorders

DSM-IV-Diagnostic and Statistical Manual of Mental Disorders, 4th ed.

Table 12–2. Other Substance-Induced Disorders (DSM-IV)

Substance	Onset During Intoxication	Onset During Withdrawal	Persisting
Alcohol	Delirium, psychotic disorder, mood disorder, anxiety disorder, sexual dysfunction, sleep disorder	Delirium, psychotic disorder, mood disorder, anxiety disorder, sleep disorder	Dementia, amnestic disorder
Amphetamines and similar substances	Delirium, psychotic disorder, mood disorder, anxiety disorder, sexual dysfunction, sleep disorder	Mood disorder, sleep disorder	***
Cannabis	Delirium, psychotic disorder, anxiety disorder	***	***
Cocaine	Delirium, psychotic disorder, mood disorder, anxiety disorder, sexual dysfunction, sleep disorder	Mood disorder, anxiety disorder, sleep disorder	***
Hallucinogens	Delirium, psychotic disorder, mood disorder, anxiety disorder	***	Perception disorder
Inhalants	Delirium, psychotic disorder, mood disorder, anxiety disorder	***	Dementia
Opioids	Delirium, psychotic disorder, mood disorder, sexual dysfunction, sleep disorder	Sleep disorder	***
Phencyclidine	Delirium, psychotic disorder, mood disorder, anxiety disorder	***	***
Sedatives, hypnotics, and anxiolytics	Delirium, psychotic disorder, mood disorder, sexual dysfunction, sleep disorder	Delirium, psychotic disorder, mood disorder, anxiety disorder, sleep disorder	Dementia, amnestic disorder

DSM-IV = Diagnostic and Statistical Manual of Mental Disorders, 4th ed.

3. **Psychiatric history,** including other primary psychiatric diagnoses and past treatments
4. **Social history,** including peer groups and support systems
5. **Mental status examination,** including signs of substance-induced disorders
6. **Physical examination,** including signs of substance use
7. **Toxicologic examination,** including types of substances and concentrations
8. **Other laboratory studies,** including evidence of systemic damage from substance use

B. **Diagnostic clues.** Diagnosing a substance-induced disorder may depend on clinical judgment, but clues include:

1. The temporal association between substance ingestion and the mental disturbance
2. The known likelihood of a substance to cause a particular disturbance

C. **Diagnostic difficulties**

1. There is a higher incidence of other mental disorders in individuals who abuse substances, which complicates diagnosis.
2. When polysubstance use has occurred, accurate diagnosis of the presenting substance-induced disorder may be particularly challenging.

D. **Treatment** includes correction of physiologic complications resulting from substance use, emotional reassurance, a structured and secure environment, and pharmacologic intervention to ameliorate psychological or physical symptoms.

IV. Review of Substance-Induced Disorders

A. **Alcohol**

1. **Overview**
   a. **Common preparations** include beer, wine, fortified wines, and distilled liquor.
   b. **Route of administration** is oral ingestion.
   c. **Environmental context.** With the exception of youthful experimentation, alcohol-induced disorders are usually associated with alcohol abuse or dependence.
   d. **Laboratory evaluation.** Alcohol levels are obtained from breath or from blood or urine samples.

2. **Intoxication.** Blood alcohol levels are usually greater than 0.10 mg%, and an odor of alcohol is present on the individual's breath.
   a. **Psychological and behavioral changes** include euphoria, inappropriate sexual or aggressive behavior, mood lability, and impaired judgment.
   b. **Other signs** associated with alcohol intoxication include slurred speech, incoordination, unsteady gait, nystagmus, impairment in attention or memory, stupor, and coma.
   c. **Course.** The duration of alcohol intoxication is variable but usually lasts several hours.

    d. Treatment includes physiologic support for hepatic and metabolic complications, emotional reassurance, and a structured and secure environment.

  3. Withdrawal

    a. Symptoms. Alcohol withdrawal is associated with autonomic hyperactivity, tremor, insomnia, nausea and vomiting, transient hallucinations, agitation, anxiety, and seizures. Few individuals develop severe symptoms.

    b. Course

      (1) The course of withdrawal may last from **several hours to several days,** and the most severe symptoms occur approximately 24–48 hours after cessation of drinking.

      (2) A **protracted withdrawal syndrome,** including anxiety and insomnia, may persist for weeks.

      (3) The **presence of delirium** may indicate the presence of additional general medical conditions, such as acute thiamine deficiency (Wernicke syndrome), hepatic failure, head trauma, and seizures.

    c. Treatment includes **metabolic support** and the tapering use of **benzodiazepines** to decrease both cognitive and physical distress.

      (1) Thiamine, folate, magnesium, and other vitamin supplements are often given prophylactically.

      (2) Occasionally, **anticonvulsants** are used prophylactically.

  4. Other alcohol-induced disorders (see Table 12–2)

B. Amphetamines and similar substances

  1. Overview

    a. Common substances include methamphetamine (e.g., Desoxyn, "crystal," "ice"), amphetamine (e.g., Benzedrine, "speed"), dextroamphetamine (Dexedrine), methylphenidate (Ritalin), and other anorectic agents (e.g., diet pills).

    b. Routes of administration are oral ingestion, intranasal application ("snorting"), intramuscular injection ("skin popping"), and intravenous injection ("shooting").

    c. Environmental context. Amphetamine-induced disorders are usually associated with amphetamine abuse.

    d. Laboratory evaluation. Urinalysis is positive for 1–3 days.

  2. Intoxication

    a. Psychological and behavioral changes include euphoria, affective blunting, social expansiveness or withdrawal, emotional lability, hypervigilance, impaired judgment, and anger.

    b. Other signs associated with amphetamine intoxication include tachycardia or bradycardia, pupillary dilation, changes in blood pressure, nausea and vomiting, perspiration or chills, and psychomotor agitation or retardation.

      (1) Muscular weakness, respiratory depression, chest pain, and cardiac arrhythmias may be noted.

      (2) Confusion, seizures, dyskinesia, dystonia, and coma may occur.

    c. Course. The duration of intoxication is usually from several hours to approximately 1 day.

    d. Treatment includes physiologic support for cardiac and central nervous system (CNS) complications, emotional reassurance, and a structured and secure environment. **Pharmacologic intervention** includes the judicious use of benzodiazepines and antipsychotic medications to control agitation and anxiety.

  3. Withdrawal

    a. Symptoms. Amphetamine withdrawal is associated with dysphoric mood, fatigue, disturbing dreams, insomnia or hypersomnia, increased appetite, and psychomotor retardation or agitation.

    b. Course. The duration of withdrawal is usually from several days to several weeks.

    c. Treatment includes emotional reassurance and a structured and secure environment. **Pharmacologic intervention** includes the judicious use of benzodiazepines for insomnia and agitation and, occasionally, antidepressants for protracted dysphoria.

  4. Other amphetamine-induced disorders (see Table 12–2)

C. Cannabis

  1. Overview

    a. Common substances include marijuana ("weed") and hashish ("hash").

    b. Routes of administration are inhalation of smoke or, more rarely, oral ingestion.

    c. Environmental context. Cannabis-induced disorders are often associated with social contexts or with an individual's ignorance of the potency of a preparation.

    d. Laboratory evaluation. Urinalysis for cannabinoids is positive for 1–4 weeks.

  2. Intoxication

    a. Psychological and behavioral changes include impaired motor coordination, euphoria, anxiety, sensation of slowed time, impaired judgment, and social withdrawal.

    b. Other signs associated with cannabis intoxication include conjunctival injection, increased appetite, dry mouth, and tachycardia.

    c. Course. The duration of cannabis intoxication is usually several hours.

    d. Treatment includes emotional reassurance and a structured and secure environment.

  3. Withdrawal. Although a cannabis withdrawal syndrome characterized by irritability has been described, it is not recognized universally.

  4. Other cannabis-induced disorders (see Table 12–2)

D. Cocaine

  1. Overview

    a. Common preparations include cocaine hydrochloride ("coke") and cocaine alkaloid ("crack," "rock").

    b. Routes of administration. Cocaine hydrochloride is inhaled or intravenously injected. Cocaine alkaloid is vaporized in pipes and then inhaled.

    c. Environmental context. Cocaine-induced disorders may be associated with experimentation or abuse.

    d. Laboratory evaluation. Urinalysis is positive for benzoylecgonine, a metabolite of cocaine, for 1–12 days.

2. Intoxication

    a. Signs and symptoms of cocaine intoxication are almost identical to those of amphetamine intoxication (see IV B 2 a–b).

    b. Course. The duration of cocaine intoxication is brief, usually lasting a few minutes to 1 hour.

    c. Treatment is the same as that for amphetamine intoxication (see IV B 2 d).

3. Withdrawal

    a. Signs and symptoms of cocaine withdrawal are almost identical to those of amphetamine withdrawal (see IV B 3 a).

    b. The **onset** of cocaine withdrawal is usually faster than that for amphetamines, often within minutes after intoxication ceases. The duration of withdrawal is from several hours to several days.

    c. Extreme dysphoria should be carefully observed; it may lead to suicidal behavior.

    d. Treatment is the same as that for amphetamine withdrawal (see IV B 3 c).

4. Other cocaine-induced disorders (see Table 12–2)

E. Hallucinogens

1. Overview

    a. Common specific substances include:

        (1) Indolealkylamines, such as lysergic acid diethylamide (LSD), psilocybin, and N,N-dimethyltryptamine (DMT)

        (2) Phenylalkylamines, such as mescaline, 2,5-dimethoxy-4-methylamphctamine (STP), and 3,4-methylenedioxymethamphetamine (MDMA), or "ecstasy"

    b. Route of administration is usually oral ingestion.

    c. Environmental context. Hallucinogen-induced disorders are often associated with experimental or social use.

    d. Laboratory evaluation. Clinical assays for hallucinogens are rarely available.

2. Intoxication

    a. Psychological and behavioral changes include euphoria, hyperarousal, anxiety, depression, ideas of reference, persecutory ideation, and impaired judgment.

    b. Perceptual changes include vivid perceptions, depersonalization, derealization, illusions, hallucinations, and synesthesias (i.e., experiencing sounds as colors).

    c. Other signs of hallucinogen intoxication include pupillary dilation, tachycardia, sweating, palpitations, blurred vision, tremors, and incoordination.

d. Course. The duration of intoxication with LSD is approximately 1 day. Other hallucinogens may produce intoxication for several hours.

e. Treatment includes emotional reassurance and a structured and secure environment. Occasionally, benzodiazepines are used to decrease anxiety.

3. Hallucinogen persisting perception disorder (flashbacks)

a. Some individuals who have used hallucinogens reexperience some of the perceptual symptoms, usually visual images, originally experienced during intoxication. These flashbacks may be induced by stress, fatigue, or visual difficulties, such as those encountered in low-light situations or fog.

b. Course. The course is extremely variable, and symptoms may recur for several years. Episodes may last for seconds, minutes, or hours. There is no specific treatment.

4. Other hallucinogen-induced disorders (see Table 12-2)

F. Inhalants

1. Overview

a. Common substances include gasoline, paint and paint thinners, and glue.

b. Route of administration is usually inhalation of fumes.

c. Environmental context. Inhalant-induced disorders are usually associated with inhalant abuse.

d. Laboratory evaluation. No direct assay is available for inhalants.

2. Intoxication

a. Psychological and behavioral changes include euphoria, belligerence, apathy, and impaired judgment.

b. Other signs associated with inhalant intoxication include dizziness, nystagmus, incoordination, slurred speech, unsteady gait, lethargy, depressed reflexes, psychomotor retardation, tremor, muscle weakness, blurred vision (diplopia), stupor, and coma.

c. Course. The **onset** of intoxication is usually rapid, and its duration is brief, lasting a few hours.

d. Treatment includes physiologic support for hepatic and cardiovascular complications, emotional reassurance, and a structured and secure environment.

3. Other inhalant-induced disorders (see Table 12–2)

G. Nicotine

1. Overview

a. Common preparations include smoking products (e.g., cigarettes, cigars, pipes), chewing tobacco, and powdered tobacco ("snuff").

b. Routes of administration are inhalation of smoke and absorption through oral mucosa.

c. Environmental context. Intoxication is usually associated with experimentation, and withdrawal is usually associated with cessation after long-term use.

    d. Laboratory evaluation. There are no clinical applications for measurement of nicotine and cotinine, a nicotine metabolite, in body fluids.

  2. Intoxication

    a. Although there is no disorder associated with nicotine intoxication, **signs** of intoxication include a sense of well-being, nausea, headache, and dizziness.

    b. Tolerance to physical effects of nicotine intoxication **develops rapidly.**

  3. Withdrawal

    a. Nicotine withdrawal is associated with dysphoria, insomnia, irritability, anxiety, difficulty concentrating, restlessness, decreased heart rate, and increased appetite or weight gain.

    b. Course. The duration of withdrawal is several days or more.

    c. Treatment involves emotional support and may include tapering doses of nicotine through the use of nicotine chewing gum or transdermal patches.

H. Opioids

  1. Overview

    a. Common substances include natural opioid (e.g., opium, morphine), semisynthetic opioid (e.g., heroin), and synthetic opioid [e.g., codeine, methadone, meperidine (Demerol), fentanyl, pentazocine (Talwin)].

    b. Routes of administration are oral ingestion and intravenous and intramuscular injection. Rarely, opioids are inhaled.

    c. Environmental context. Opioid-induced disorders are usually associated with opioid abuse and may be associated with medicinal use (e.g., for analgesia).

    d. Laboratory evaluation. Urinalysis for opioids is positive for 1–2 days.

  2. Intoxication

    a. Psychological and behavioral changes include initial euphoria, apathy, dysphoria, psychomotor agitation or retardation, and impaired judgment.

    b. Other signs of intoxication include pupillary constriction, drowsiness or coma, slurred speech, and impairment in attention or memory.

    c. Course. The **onset** and **duration** depend on the mode of administration, but intoxication usually lasts a few hours.

    d. Treatment includes physiologic support for respiratory and CNS complications, emotional reassurance, and a structured and secure environment. **Pharmacologic intervention** occasionally includes opioid antagonists such as naloxone, which is used to counter respiratory depression.

  3. Withdrawal

    a. Opioid withdrawal is associated with dysphoric mood, nausea, muscle aches, lacrimation, rhinorrhea, pupillary dilation, piloerection, sweating, diarrhea, yawning, fever, and insomnia.

    b. Course. The **onset** is variable and may be precipitated by administration of an opioid antagonist.

    c. Treatment includes physiologic support for gastrointestinal and metabolic complications, emotional reassurance, and a structured and secure environment. **Pharmacologic intervention** involves tapering doses of opioids, usually methadone, for several days; administration of clonidine to ameliorate gastrointestinal symptoms and sweating; and administration of benzodiazepines to decrease severe insomnia.

  4. Other opioid-induced disorders (see Table 12–2)

I. Phencyclidine (PCP)

  1. Overview

    a. Route of administration is inhalation of smoke from cigarettes laced with PCP.

    b. Environmental context. PCP-induced disorders are usually associated with PCP abuse.

    c. Laboratory evaluation. Urinalysis may be positive for several weeks.

  2. Intoxication

    a. Psychological and behavioral changes include euphoria, dissociation, body image distortion, hallucinations, impulsiveness, belligerence, and impaired judgment.

    b. Other signs of intoxication include vertical and horizontal nystagmus, hypertension, tachycardia, hyperacusis, numbness and anesthesia, ataxia, dysarthria, muscle rigidity, seizures, and coma.

    c. Course. The **onset** of intoxication is usually rapid, and the duration is several hours.

    d. Treatment includes physiologic support for cardiovascular complications, emotional reassurance, and a structured and secure environment. **Pharmacologic intervention** includes the careful administration of antipsychotic medication to decrease severe agitation.

  3. Other phencyclidine-induced disorders (see Table 12–2)

J. Sedatives, hypnotics, and anxiolytics

  1. Overview

    a. Common substances include benzodiazepines and barbiturates.

    b. Route of administration is almost always oral ingestion.

    c. Environmental context. Sedative-, hypnotic-, and anxiolytic-induced disorders are associated with dependence.

    d. Laboratory evaluation. Quantitative blood and urine test results are positive for several days.

  2. Intoxication

    a. Signs and symptoms of sedative, hypnotic, and anxiolytic intoxication are almost identical to those of alcohol intoxication, but seizures are more common (see IV A 2 a–b).

    b. Course. The duration of intoxication is usually several hours, depending on the substance.

    c. Treatment includes physiologic support for CNS complications, emotional reassurance, and a structured and secure environment.

3. **Withdrawal**
   a. **Signs and symptoms** of sedative, hypnotic, and anxiolytic withdrawal are almost identical to those of alcohol withdrawal, but seizures are more common (see IV A 3 a). Anxiety and insomnia can persist for several weeks.
   b. **Course.** The **onset** and **duration** depend on the half-life of the specific substance.
   c. **Treatment** includes physiologic support for CNS complications, emotional reassurance, and a structured and secure environment. **Pharmacologic intervention** includes tapering doses of benzodiazepines and barbiturates. Anticonvulsants are occasionally used prophylactically.

4. **Other sedative-, hypnotic-, and anxiolytic-induced disorders** (see Table 12–2)

Review Test

Directions: Each of the numbered items or incomplete statements in this section is followed by answers or by completions of the statement. Select the ONE lettered answer or completion that is BEST in each case.

1. A 14-year-old boy is brought to the emergency room by his parents because of confusion and ataxia since he returned home 1 hour ago. Mental status examination shows lethargy and apathy. Physical examination shows slurred speech, incoordination, diplopia, and depressed reflexes. There is no odor of alcohol on his breath. Which of the following substances is most likely responsible for this clinical presentation?

(A) Cocaine
(B) Codeine
(C) Gasoline
(D) Marijuana
(E) Phencyclidine (PCP)

2. A 19-year-old man is brought to the emergency room by the police. He was picked up for belligerence toward strangers. His speech is incoherent. Mental status examination shows disorientation and anxiety and that he is having visual hallucinations and persecutory delusions. Physical examination shows agitation, a blood pressure of 170/110, nystagmus, slurred speech, and insensitivity to pain. Which of the following substances is most likely responsible for this clinical presentation?

(A) Alcohol
(B) Amphetamine
(C) Lysergic acid diethylamide (LSD)
(D) Phencyclidine (PCP)
(E) Psilocybin

3. A 30-year-old man presents to the emergency room complaining of muscle aches, nausea, and vomiting. He also complains that he has been sweating for several hours. Physical examination shows a fever of 100.5°F, pupillary dilation, and rhinorrhea. Which of the following substances is most likely responsible for this clinical presentation?

(A) Alcohol
(B) Cocaine
(C) Diazepam
(D) Heroin
(E) Phencyclidine (PCP)

4. A 34-year-old woman who is involuntarily admitted to a smoking-restricted psychiatric unit because of depression and suicidal threat complains of severe craving for cigarettes. She is irritable and has difficulty concentrating. Which of the following is the best intervention for immediately alleviating her symptoms?

(A) Chewing tobacco
(B) Clonidine
(C) Emotional reassurance
(D) Moderate doses of benzodiazepines
(E) Nicotine chewing gum

5. Twenty-four hours after elective hospitalization for a hysterectomy, a 46-year-old woman develops anxiety, restlessness, and tremulousness. She has a temperature of 100°F and a pulse of 125 beats/min. Her liver enzymes are moderately elevated. Withdrawal from which of the following substances is most likely responsible for this clinical presentation?

(A) Alprazolam
(B) Cocaine
(C) Heroin
(D) Methamphetamine
(E) Phencyclidine (PCP)

Answers and Explanations

1–C. This clinical presentation is most suggestive of gasoline intoxication. Inhalant intoxication is characterized by euphoria, belligerence, apathy, impaired judgment, dizziness, nystagmus, incoordination, slurred speech, unsteady gait, lethargy, depressed reflexes, psychomotor retardation, tremor, muscle weakness, and blurred vision (diplopia). Stupor and coma may occur.

2–D. This clinical presentation is most suggestive of phencyclidine (PCP) intoxication. PCP intoxication is characterized by euphoria, dissociation, body image distortion, hallucinations, impulsiveness, belligerence, impaired judgment, vertical and horizontal nystagmus, hypertension, tachycardia, hyperacusis, numbness, anesthesia, ataxia, and dysarthria. Muscle rigidity, seizures, and coma may occur.

3–D. This clinical presentation is most suggestive of opioid, in this case heroin, withdrawal. Opioid withdrawal is characterized by dysphoric mood, nausea, muscle aches, lacrimation, rhinorrhea, pupillary dilation, piloerection, sweating, diarrhea, yawning, fever, and insomnia. Treatment involves stabilizing the patient with the use of tapering doses of methadone, clonidine, and benzodiazepines.

4–E. This clinical presentation is most suggestive of nicotine withdrawal, which is characterized by difficulty concentrating, insomnia, dysphoria, and irritability. Immediate treatment often includes the use of chewing gum. Nicotine transdermal patches are also available. Emotional reassurance and biofeedback are useful components of a smoking cessation program; however, this individual does not indicate a desire to stop smoking. Clonidine and benzodiazepines are not useful for treatment of nicotine withdrawal.

5–A. This clinical presentation is most suggestive of alprazolam withdrawal. Benzodiazepine withdrawal is characterized by autonomic hyperactivity, tremor, insomnia, agitation, anxiety, nausea, and vomiting. Transient hallucinations and seizures may occur. It is likely that this woman was taking alprazolam until her hospitalization and is now experiencing withdrawal.

13
Psychotic Disorders

I. Overview

A. **Definition.** Psychosis is a syndrome characterized by **gross impairments in the ability to assess reality and behave coherently.**

B. **General information**

1. Because of its often **striking presentation** and **links to creativity**, psychosis can both fascinate and frighten observers.
2. **Attitudes** toward psychotic individuals have varied throughout history; sufferers have been deified, killed, and neglected.
3. **Psychosis is observed in all cultures;** it is not merely a "sane reaction to an insane environment."
4. **Psychosis is never a normal phenomenon;** it is always an indication of a psychiatric disorder (see III).
5. **The presence of psychosis has critical diagnostic importance;** it is accounted for by relatively few psychiatric disorders.

II. Clinical Features of Psychosis. Psychosis is diagnosed if one or more of the following symptoms are present.

A. **Hallucinations** are sensory impressions that occur without external stimulation of the relevant sensory organ.
B. **Delusions** are false beliefs based on incorrect inferences about external reality. These beliefs are firmly sustained despite the beliefs of almost all others and despite incontrovertible and obvious proof or evidence to the contrary (DSM-IV).
C. **Disorganized speech** is characterized by incoherence or rambling (e.g., intermittently muttering and shouting unintelligible statements and monologues).
D. **Disorganized behavior** is characterized by aimless, bizarre, agitated, or grossly inappropriate behavior (e.g., wandering alone in the streets dressed inappropriately).
E. **Disorganized motor behavior (catatonia)** is characterized by marked motor anomalies including immobility, excessive motor activity, extreme negativism, mutism, posturing, stereotyped movements, echolalia, and echopraxia. (DSM-IV)

III. Psychiatric Disorders that Account for Psychosis

A. **Cognitive disorders.** Psychosis may occur in delirium and dementia.

B. **Mood disorders**

1. Psychosis may be present in major depressive disorder and bipolar disorders.

2. If psychosis is present in a mood disorder, it only occurs during depressive or manic episodes, and not during periods of normal mood.

3. Psychosis in a mood disorder is described as either **mood congruent** or **mood incongruent.**

   a. **Mood congruent.** The content of psychotic thought is characterized by themes of guilt, suffering, worthlessness, or death during depressive episodes and themes of grandiosity or power during manic episodes.

   b. **Mood incongruent.** The content of psychotic thought during depressive or manic episodes may involve paranoia, bizarre ideation, or catatonia.

C. **Autistic disorder,** a pervasive developmental disorder of childhood onset, may present with disorganized speech or behavior that suggests psychosis.

D. **Psychotic disorders** (see V–XII)

IV. Diagnostic Clues of Psychosis

A. **Presenting complaints** may include auditory or visual hallucinations, bizarre beliefs, unusual suspiciousness, change in social behavior, marked decrease in motivation or self-care, and peculiar behavior or mannerisms.

B. **History** may include past episodes of psychosis, past psychiatric hospitalization or treatment with antipsychotic medication, marked decline from previous level of function, and family history of psychotic disorders.

C. **Mental status examination** may show hallucinations, delusions, disorganized speech or behavior, peculiar psychomotor activity, and peculiar mood or affect.

D. **Physical examination** is usually unremarkable but may reveal findings consistent with general medical conditions that may cause psychosis.

E. **Laboratory studies** may show positive toxicology for substances that may induce psychosis and metabolic disturbances and imaging findings consistent with general medical conditions that may cause psychosis.

V. Schizophrenia

A. **Overview.** Schizophrenia is a common and devastating psychiatric illness characterized by **psychosis** and **disintegration of abilities to think logically** and maintain normal social behavior.

1. **History**

   a. Schizophrenia may be synonymous with historical psychiatric descriptions of "madness." The exact nature of symptoms necessary for diagnosis of schizophrenia has been debated up to the present.

   b. Schizophrenia was formally described by Kraepelin in the late nineteenth century as **dementia praecox.** Bleuler introduced the term **schizophrenia** at the turn of the century.

2. **Symptoms.** Often, symptoms of schizophrenia are classified as either positive or negative.

   a. **Positive symptoms** include hallucinations and delusions.
   b. **Negative symptoms** include affectual blunting, avolition (i.e., lack of motivation), alogia (i.e., poverty of speech), disinterest, and social withdrawal.

3. **Psychological changes** in schizophrenia involve disturbances in:

   a. **Content and form of thought.** The individual's thoughts may be about bizarre subjects and may be illogical.
   b. **Perception.** The individual's perception of the environment may be influenced by hallucinations and delusions.
   c. **Affect.** The individual's affect may be inappropriate or blunted.
   d. **Sense of self.** There may be identity confusion.
   e. **Volition.** The individual may have an extreme lack of initiative or motivation.
   f. **Relationship to the external world.** The individual may have marked difficulty adapting to the demands of the environment.
   g. **Psychomotor behavior.** The individual's behavior may be repetitive, aimless, or inappropriate.

4. **Psychosis during the active phase of schizophrenia** may include:

   a. Specific types of bizarre delusions and prominent hallucinations
   b. Marked loosening of associations
   c. Catatonic behavior

5. **Prodromal and residual phases** of schizophrenia are characterized by attenuated symptoms of the active phase, including social withdrawal, impairment in role functioning, peculiar behavior, neglect of hygiene and grooming, blunted or inappropriate affect, bizarre speech or ideation, unusual perceptual experiences, and apathy.

6. **Increased concern for preserving the civil liberties** of patients with schizophrenia is warranted; the symptoms that make treatment so important may also render patients unable to give fully informed consent.

B. **Epidemiology**

1. **Occurrence.** Schizophrenia occurs at a **1 : 1 male to female ratio**; however, females may have a later onset, more associated mood symptoms, and a better prognosis. There is a 1% lifetime prevalence of schizophrenia.
2. **Familial pattern.** There is a 10% prevalence in first degree biologic relatives and a greater than 50% concordance in monozygotic twins.
3. The content of delusions and hallucinations in schizophrenia may vary by culture.

C. **Etiology**

1. **Genetic factors.** The etiologic role of genetics is indicated by adoptive studies, which show a greater prevalence of schizophrenia in biologic relatives but no greater prevalence in adoptive families.

2. **Environmental factors** are present, as indicated by the discordance rate in monozygotic twins (10%—50%).
3. Various etiologic abnormalities of central nervous system (CNS) biochemistry and morphology have been hypothesized in individuals with schizophrenia; however, no consensus has emerged.
4. Psychodynamic and behavioral etiologic theories of schizophrenia have been largely discredited.

D. **Diagnosis**

1. **Diagnostic features** include:

   a. **Total duration of at least 6 months,** including prodromal, active, and residual phases
   b. **An active phase of at least 1 month** (less if treated) characterized by some of the following:
      (1) Delusions
      (2) Hallucinations
      (3) Disorganized speech
      (4) Grossly disorganized or catatonic behavior, including:
         (a) Disorganized behavior, which includes neglect of self-care and deterioration of ability to function
         (b) Catatonic behavior, which includes psychomotor abnormalities such as decreased reactivity to the environment, bizarre posturing, muscular rigidity, purposeless activity, and passive resistance (negativism)
      (5) Negative symptoms
   c. Symptoms that are not better explained as part of a mood disorder, schizoaffective disorder, or psychosis due to a general medical condition or substance

2. **Subtypes.** Schizophrenia is often classified by a subtype based on the predominant symptoms. Subtypes may be suggestive of a particular treatment or prognosis.

   a. **Catatonic.** The active phase of the illness has catatonic features. Benzodiazepines may be indicated.
   b. **Disorganized.** The active phase has disorganized features but there are no catatonic symptoms. Special protection for patients may be necessary.
   c. **Paranoid.** Hallucinations or delusions are present, but there are no catatonic or disorganized symptoms. Prognosis may be more benign.
   d. **Undifferentiated.** The active phase does not appear as catatonic, disorganized, or paranoid.
   e. **Residual.** No active phase criteria are present.

3. **Associated features and diagnoses**

   a. **Inappropriate or bizarre emotions and affect**, such as silliness, shallowness, and depressive symptoms, may be present.
   b. **Suicide attempts** are more common.
   c. **Sleep disturbances** are often present.
   d. **Cognitive problems.** Difficulty with concentration and memory may be present.

      e. Motor abnormalities. Rocking, pacing, and stereotypy may be present.

      f. Substance abuse, especially alcohol and stimulant abuse, is common.

      g. Associated laboratory findings. Several abnormalities are reported to be more common in patients with schizophrenia.

         (1) Gross brain morphology. Reported findings include increased ventricular size and prominent sulci, decreased cerebral mass, decreased hippocampal and temporal mass, and increased basal ganglia mass.

         (2) Functional imaging (photon emission tomography) may show decreased activity in the prefrontal cortex.

         (3) Neuropsychological studies may show abnormalities of attention and concept formation.

         (4) Neurophysiologic studies may show abnormal eye-tracking and sensory gating.

      h. Associated physical examination findings and general medical conditions include more minor physical abnormalities and more perceptual–motor problems.

    4. Differential diagnoses include brief psychotic disorder, psychotic disorder due to general medical conditions, substance-induced psychotic disorders, mood disorders with psychotic features, schizoaffective disorders, delusional disorder, autism, and obsessive-compulsive disorder.

E. Clinical course

    1. Onset is often in adolescence or early adulthood, and it may be sudden or insidious. The course of schizophrenia is characterized by a **progressive deterioration of function** for at least the first few years.

    3. Many individuals with schizophrenia have a course characterized by exacerbations and partial remissions. Positive symptoms are often prominent during exacerbations, and negative symptoms may persist during remissions.

    4. Schizophrenia is often devastating in terms of social and occupational function; social withdrawal, depression, and substance abuse often supervene.

    5. Prognosis (Table 13-1)

F. Treatment

    1. Antipsychotic medication is often highly effective during the active phase of illness and useful in preventing relapse.

    2. Social and family therapy appears to ameliorate the degree of disability during residual phases.

VI. Schizophreniform Disorder

A. Overview

    1. Definition. Schizophreniform disorder, essentially a clinical picture of schizophrenia with a duration of 1 to 6 months, is a **separate diagnosis because of its unpredictable clinical course.** Schizophreniform disorder replaces the term **acute schizophrenia.**

Table 13-1. Features Weighting toward Good to Poor Prognosis in Schizophrenia

Good Prognosis	Poor Prognosis
Late onset	Young onset
Obvious precipitating factors	No precipitating factors
Acute onset	Insidious onset
Good premorbid social, sexual, and work histories	Poor premorbid social, sexual, and work histories
Mood disorder symptoms (especially depressive disorders)	Withdrawn, autistic behavior
Married	Single, divorced, or widowed
Family history of mood disorders	Family history of schizophrenia
Good support systems	Poor support systems
Positive symptoms	Negative symptoms
	Neurological signs and symptoms
	History of perinatal trauma
	No remissions in three years
	Many relapses
	History of assaultiveness

Reprinted with permission from Kaplan HI, Sadock BJ, Grebb JA: *Synopsis of Psychiatry*, 7th ed. Baltimore, Williams & Wilkins, 1994, p. 472.

   2. Formerly, a distinction was made between acute and chronic schizophrenia, because only 50% of patients with acute schizophrenia developed a chronic psychosis.

B. Epidemiology (see V B)

C. Diagnosis

   1. **Diagnostic features** are almost identical to those of schizophrenia; however, the duration of schizophreniform disorder is 1 to 6 months.

   2. **Subtypes**

      a. Schizophreniform disorder has two subtypes, **good** and **poor prognosis,** because there is evidence that schizophrenia with a rapid onset has a less pernicious course than schizophrenia with an insidious onset.

      b. Good prognostic features include rapid onset of psychosis, subjective sense of confusion, good premorbid functioning, and normal affect.

   3. **Associated features and diagnoses** (see V D 3)

D. Clinical course. One third to one half of patients with schizophreniform disorder develop schizophrenia.

VII. Schizoaffective Disorder

A. Overview

   1. **General information**

      a. Distinguishing between schizophrenia with prominent mood disturbances and mood disorder with psychotic features has always been difficult.

      b. Based on clinical course and response to treatment, there is evidence that a third type of disorder, schizoaffective disorder, may also present with both psychosis and mood disturbances.

2. Criteria for diagnosis of schizoaffective disorder are designed to distinguish it from both schizophrenia and mood disorders with psychosis.

    a. These distinctions are made on the basis of clinical course.

    b. The diagnosis is based on the temporal relationship between psychotic and mood symptoms.

B. Epidemiology

  1. Occurrence. There is little data, but this disorder is probably less common than schizophrenia. Schizoaffective disorder may be more common in females, and schizoaffective disorder, depressive type may be more common in the elderly.

  2. Schizophrenia and mood disorders are more common among relatives of individuals with schizoaffective disorder.

C. Etiology. Presumptively, genetic factors play a role.

D. Diagnosis

  1. Diagnostic features

    a. During any uninterrupted period of illness, both a mood episode and the psychotic features of schizophrenia must be present simultaneously.

    b. During the same uninterrupted period of illness, there must be at least 2 weeks of hallucinations or delusions in the absence of a mood episode.

    c. Significant mood symptoms must be present during a substantial portion of the overall course of the illness.

    d. The symptoms are not better accounted for by other psychotic disorders and not due to a general medical condition or substance-induced.

  2. Subtypes

    a. Bipolar type. Manic or mixed episodes must be present at some point during the clinical course.

    b. Depressive type. Only depressive episodes are present during the clinical course.

  3. Associated features and diagnoses

    a. Many of the features associated with both schizophrenia and mood disorders may be present (e.g., social impairment, difficulties with self-care, suicide).

    b. Substance-related disorders may also be more common.

  4. Differential diagnoses include other psychotic disorders and mood disorders with psychotic features.

E. Clinical course

  1. The onset may occur at any time and may be preceded by personality pathology.

  2. The course of schizoaffective disorder may be less severe than schizophrenia but more severe than the course for mood disorders. The course for bipolar type may be less severe than the course for depressive type.

  3. Patients diagnosed with schizoaffective disorder are sometimes rediagnosed as having schizophrenia or a mood disorder on the basis of subsequent clinical course.

F. Treatment. Antidepressants, mood-stabilizing medication (e.g., lithium, anticonvulsants), and antipsychotic medication may be used for the treatment of this disorder. Sometimes, electroconvulsive therapy is necessary.

VIII. Delusional Disorder

A. Overview

1. **Delusional disorder,** formerly called paranoia, **is characterized by delusions about plausible events,** such as being persecuted, having a serious illness, or having a secret relationship with another person.
2. Unlike patients with schizophrenia, paranoid type, individuals with delusional disorder are not overtly bizarre, and their thoughts are generally organized.
3. These patients usually present to clinical attention as a result of:
   a. Their anxiety about their delusions
   b. The discovery of their delusions during the course of medical examination for other problems
   c. Threats or illegal activities resulting from their delusions
4. Because the onset is often in middle age or later, examination for psychosis due to a general medical condition and substance-induced psychotic disorder is extremely important.

B. Epidemiology

1. **Occurrence.** Delusional disorder occurs at a **1:1 male to female ratio**. There is a 0.05% lifetime prevalence of this disorder.
2. The content of delusions vary by culture.
3. There is some evidence that schizophrenia may be more common in relatives of individuals with delusional disorder.

C. Diagnosis

1. **Diagnostic features**
   a. Plausible delusions without otherwise markedly abnormal behavior or serious mood symptoms are present.
   b. There is no previous period in which other symptoms of schizophrenia were present, and the disorder is not due to a general medical condition or substance-induced.

2. **Subtypes**
   a. **Erotomanic type,** characterized by delusions of having a special relationship with another person, often a famous person
   b. **Grandiose type,** characterized by delusions of power, wealth, or other inflated status
   c. **Jealous type,** characterized by delusions of infidelity of a sexual partner
   c. **Persecutory type**, characterized by delusions of being persecuted in some way
   d. **Somatic type,** characterized by delusions of having a physical problem or condition
   e. **Mixed type,** characterized by delusions of more than one subtype

      3. **Associated features and diagnoses** may include:

         a. Irritability and dysphoria

         b. Social and occupational problems resulting from delusional beliefs

         c. Litigious behavior and other legal difficulties resulting from delusional beliefs

         d. Occasional violence

         e. A premorbid paranoid personality disorder

         f. An association with hearing impairment and psychosocial stressors

      4. **Differential diagnoses** include dementia with delusions; psychosis due to a general medical condition; substance-induced psychosis; schizophrenia, paranoid type; and mood disorders with psychotic features.

D. Clinical course

      1. The premorbid individual may have long-standing paranoid traits and relative social isolation.

      2. The onset is during middle age or later.

      3. Severe social and occupational dysfunction may occur during the course of the illness.

      4. The course is often chronic, but the degree of delusional preoccupation may fluctuate.

E. Treatment

      1. **Antipsychotic medication** may be effective in ameliorating delusions in some cases, but patients are not always compliant.

      2. **Anxiolytic medication** may be effective in alleviating the anxiety resulting from the delusional preoccupation.

      3. **Supportive and cognitive psychotherapies** may be helpful in lessening the patient's delusional preoccupation and improving functioning.

IX. Brief Psychotic Disorder

A. Overview. Brief psychotic disorder is characterized by the **sudden onset of brief psychotic episodes.**

      1. The onset may occur in **response to severe stress, during the postpartum period,** or it **may occur without obvious relationship to environmental events.**

      2. Episodes may resolve within 1 month, warranting this diagnosis. If the episode persists, the diagnosis is often changed to schizophreniform disorder, schizoaffective disorder, or a mood disorder with psychotic features.

      3. Physicians may encounter this disorder in the context of severe general medical conditions (**"ICU psychosis"**).

B. Epidemiology. The occurrence of brief psychotic disorder is apparently rare. Some culturally sanctioned response patterns may resemble brief psychotic disorder.

C. Etiology

      1. **Severe stress** may play an etiologic role in the development of some brief psychotic episodes.

2. **Neuroendocrine changes** have been postulated as etiologic in some cases of postpartum psychosis.

D. **Diagnosis**

1. The **diagnostic feature** is the presence of psychosis for more than 1 day but less than 1 month and subsequent complete return to normal functioning. The disorder is not better accounted for by other psychotic disorders and not due to a general medical condition or substance-induced.

2. **Subtypes** include:

   a. With marked stressors
   b. Without marked stressors
   c. With postpartum onset

3. **Associated features and diagnoses** include:

   a. Severe agitation and confusion
   b. Self-destructive behavior and suicide attempts
   c. Preexisting personality pathology
   b. Bizarre behavior, transient hallucinations and delusions, and apparent memory impairment

4. **Differential diagnoses** include delirium; psychosis due to a general medical condition; substance-induced psychosis; and onset or exacerbations of other psychotic disorders, such as schizophrenia, factious disorder, and malingering.

E. **Clinical course**

1. Premorbid personality disorders may predispose an individual to brief psychotic disorder.

2. The onset is usually sudden and is often in response to stress.

3. The degree of agitation, confusion, and impairment is often severe, and precautions must be taken to prevent harm to the patient or others.

4. The diagnosis is provisional until the disorder resolves. By definition, complete return to normal functioning occurs within 1 month, or the diagnosis is changed.

F. **Treatment**

1. **A careful search for responsible underlying general medical conditions** or substances is essential.

2. Protection of the patient from harm resulting from agitation or self-destructive behavior is important.

3. **Frequent reassurance and orientation** are helpful.

4. **Antipsychotic medication** is often used to decrease agitation.

X. Shared Psychotic Disorder

A. **Overview**

1. This disorder, formerly called **folie a deux,** usually **develops slowly in an individual who is under the influence of a person with psychotic delusions (i.e., the primary inducer).**

   a. The pair (or, rarely, more than two persons) usually live in social isolation.

b. Because of this isolation, shared psychotic disorder often does not present in clinical settings.

c. Such pairs may withdraw from social contact and move from place to place to escape a delusional predicament.

2. The delusions often involve persecution by others and may be bizarre.

B. Epidemiology. This disorder may be more common in women.

C. Diagnosis

1. The **diagnostic feature** is the development of delusions in the context of a close relationship with a person who already has similar delusions. The disturbance is not better accounted for by another psychotic disorder.

2. **Associated features and diagnoses.** There is little abnormality other than the shared delusions.

3. The **differential diagnosis** includes other psychotic disorders.

D. Clinical course

1. The age of onset is variable, and the development of delusions is usually gradual.

2. The disorder usually remits when the relationship between the patient and the individual with the primary disorder is terminated.

E. Treatment

1. Successful treatment of the individual with the primary disorder usually resolves the symptoms of shared psychotic disorder.

2. Modification of the relationship with the primary inducer and decrease in social isolation may be necessary.

XI. Psychosis Due to a General Medical Condition

A. Overview

1. Many general medical conditions may cause a variety of psychotic symptoms (see XI C 3).

2. **Pathogenesis**

a. The pathogenesis of the psychotic symptoms may be direct insults to the CNS caused by head trauma, cerebrovascular disease, infection, or seizures.

b. The pathogenesis of the psychotic symptoms may have an indirect effect on the CNS, which can occur in systemic infection, metabolic disturbances, or endocrinopathies.

B. Presumptively, the **etiology** is alterations in CNS function caused by the underlying disease process.

C. Diagnosis of this disorder is made if a general medical condition causes psychosis in the absence of delirium or dementia. Psychotic symptoms that occur only during the course of delirium or dementia do not need additional diagnoses to explain their presence.

1. **Diagnostic features** include prominent hallucinations or delusions and evidence that the disturbance is a direct physiologic consequence of a medical condition. The disturbance is not better accounted for by another mental disorder.

2. **Subtypes** include:

   a. With delusions

   b. With hallucinations

3. **Associated medical conditions** include:

   a. **Neurodegenerative conditions**, including Parkinson disease and Huntington disease

   b. **Cerebrovascular conditions**, including stroke and vascular insufficiency

   c. **CNS lesions** caused by head trauma, tumor, radiation, and infections

   d. **Metabolic conditions**, including electrolyte disturbances, hypoglycemia, hypoxia, and hypercarbia

   e. **Vitamin deficiencies** (e.g., thiamine, vitamin B_{12})

   f. **Endocrine conditions**, including thyroid, parathyroid, and adrenal pathologies

   g. **Autoimmune conditions with CNS involvement**, including systemic lupus erythematosus

   h. **Neoplasms** of the CNS and possibly other sites (e.g., paraneoplastic syndromes)

4. **Differential diagnoses** include delirium, dementia with psychotic features, and other psychotic disorders.

D. **Clinical course**. The onset and course depend on the etiology.

E. **Treatment** includes correction of underlying pathophysiology, antipsychotic medications, and reassurance.

XII. Substance-Induced Psychosis

A. **Overview**. A variety of abused and prescribed medications can cause psychotic symptoms (see Chapter 12).

   1. The psychosis may have an onset during intoxication, or within 1 month of withdrawal.

   2. Patients with substance-related disorders, patients being treated with a wide variety of medications, and elderly patients are at greater risk for development of substance-induced psychosis than the general population.

B. The **epidemiology** of this disorder is closely associated with patterns of substance abuse.

C. Presumptively, the **etiology** is alterations in CNS function caused by the substance.

D. **Diagnosis**

   1. **Diagnostic features**

      a. Prominent psychotic symptoms that develop as a direct result of intoxication or withdrawal from a drug of abuse, medication, or a toxin are present.

      b. The disturbance is not better accounted for by another mental disorder that is not substance-induced, and it does not occur exclusively during the course of a delirium.

2. **Subtypes.** Substance-induced psychotic disorder may be subclassified by the predominant psychotic symptoms (e.g., hallucinations or delusions) or by the time of onset (e.g., during intoxication or withdrawal).

3. **Associated substances**

   a. Onset can occur during intoxication with alcohol, amphetamines, cannabis, cocaine, hallucinogens, inhalants, opioids, phencyclidine, sedatives, hypnotics, anxiolytics, digitalis, cimetidine, amantadine, steroids, and many other medications.

   b. Onset can occur during withdrawal from alcohol, sedatives, hypnotics, and anxiolytics.

4. **Differential diagnoses** include delirium, dementia with psychotic features, and other psychotic disorders.

E. **Clinical course.** The onset and clinical course depend on the substance.

F. **Treatment** includes:

1. Discontinuation of the responsible substance when possible
2. Treatment of drug withdrawal when indicated
3. Time-limited symptomatic treatment with antipsychotic medication when indicated

Review Test

Directions: Each of the numbered items or incomplete statements in this section is followed by answers or by completions of the statement. Select the ONE lettered answer or completion that is BEST in each case.

1. A 16-year-old boy has a 2-year history of gradual onset of social withdrawal and decreased emotional responsiveness. Recently, he believes that his food is being poisoned and he will choke unless his food is pureed. He has lost weight, and he has started to neglect personal hygiene. He sleeps poorly and insists on chanting before eating. He has no history of significant substance abuse or general medical conditions. Which of the following is the most likely diagnosis?

(A) Anorexia nervosa
(B) Delusional disorder
(C) Schizoaffective disorder
(D) Schizophreniform psychosis
(E) Schizophrenia

2. A 25-year-old female college student has the sudden onset of disturbing auditory hallucinations in which voices utter derogatory statements to her. These hallucinations have persisted for 6 weeks. She is perplexed and frightened, and she seeks constant reassurance from her friends and family. Which of the following statements about her case is most accurate?

(A) Antipsychotic medication should be avoided because she has maintained social contact
(B) Her symptoms suggest a better prognosis
(C) She has a 75% likelihood of developing schizophrenia
(D) She is likely to have abnormal cerebral morphology
(E) She should receive intensive exploratory psychotherapy to uncover and resolve unconscious conflicts

3. A 42-year-old car salesman is arrested for breaking into the home of a popular television actress. He insists that he has been involved in a romantic relationship with the actress and that she has betrayed him by being photographed kissing a male costar. The actress, who called the police, has never met the intruder. If this patient has a delusional disorder, which of the following subtypes is most likely present?

(A) Erotomanic type
(B) Grandiose type
(C) Jealous type
(D) Persecutory type
(E) Somatic type

4. A 54-year-old man who has been hospitalized in a state mental institution for many years spends hours sitting almost motionlessly; refuses to make eye contact; and passively resists attempts to get him to stand up, walk, or participate in activities. He has a history of violently attacking strangers and claiming that demons are pursuing him. Which of the following is the most likely diagnosis?

(A) Schizophrenia, catatonic type
(B) Schizophrenia, disorganized type
(C) Schizophrenia, paranoid type
(D) Schizophrenia, residual type
(E) Schizophrenia, disorganized type

5. A 60-year-old secretary becomes convinced that her coworkers are stealing papers from her desk and misfiling them. She angrily accuses them of sabotaging her work, and she is detained at her workplace by security police and taken to an emergency room. Mental status examination reveals markedly impaired memory for recent events, slowed mentation, and difficulty describing common objects. Which of the following is the most likely diagnosis?

(A) Delusional disorder, persecutory type
(B) Dementia
(C) Major depressive disorder with mood congruent psychosis
(D) Major depressive disorder with mood incongruent psychosis
(E) Psychosis due to a general medical condition

Answers and Explanations

1–E. The boy's 2-year history of social withdrawal and neglect of personal hygiene suggest negative symptoms of schizophrenia. His peculiar beliefs and behaviors suggest delusions, which are positive symptoms that are prominent in the active phase of schizophrenia. If the boy had a morbid fear of obesity and a distorted body image, anorexia nervosa may be considered as the diagnosis. Delusional disorder is a less likely diagnosis because of the presence of his bizarre behavior. Schizoaffective disorder is a less likely diagnosis because the boy does not have prominent mood symptoms. Schizophreniform disorder is a likely diagnosis if the duration of the patient's symptoms were less than 6 months.

2–B. The woman's symptoms are most suggestive of schizophreniform disorder, which is characterized by symptoms of schizophrenia that persist for 1—6 months. A better prognosis is suggested by the sudden onset, her feelings of confusion, and her maintenance of social contact. Additional features of a better prognosis are her gender and the later onset of the illness. Several long-term studies suggest that the early initiation of antipsychotic medication is associated with a better prognosis in schizophrenia. There is 30%—50% likelihood of an ultimate diagnosis of schizophrenia for individuals with schizophreniform disorder. Abnormal cerebral morphology, particularly a decreased cerebral mass, enlarged ventricles, and prominent sulci, is more often associated with individuals who have an insidious onset of schizophrenic symptoms, including social withdrawal and emotional blunting. Psychotherapy for individuals with schizophrenia should not be centered on anxiety-arousing intrapsychic exploration, because it often leads to exacerbation of symptoms.

3–A. The individual has a delusional belief that he has a special relationship with another person, which is characteristic of delusional disorder, erotomanic type. Grandiose type is characterized by delusions of power or influence. Jealous type is characterized by delusions about infidelity of a sexual partner. Persecutory type is characterized by delusions of persecution. Somatic type is characterized by delusions about physical problems.

4–A. The patient's symptoms are most suggestive of catatonia, which is characterized by motor anomalies that may include immobility, excessive motor activity, extreme negativism, mutism, posturing, stereotyped movements, echolalia, and echopraxia. Schizophrenia, catatonic type, is diagnosed when catatonic symptoms are present during the course of schizophrenia. Schizophrenia, disorganized type, is diagnosed when disorganized speech or behavior is present in the absence of catatonic symptoms. Schizophrenia, paranoid type, is diagnosed when hallucinations or delusions are present in the absence of catatonic or disorganized symptoms. Schizophrenia, residual type, is diagnosed when active symptoms are attenuated. Schizophrenia, undifferentiated type, is diagnosed when there are no patterns of the other subtypes.

5–B. The presence of memory impairment and other cognitive deficits are suggestive of dementia. Psychotic symptoms, particularly persecutory delusions, are commonly present with dementia. Delusional disorder is not diagnosed if demential is present. There is little evidence of mood symptoms that would characterize major depressive disorder. Psychosis due to a general medical condition is not diagnosed if symptoms of delirium or dementia are present in addition to psychotic symptoms.

14

Mood Disorders

I. Overview: Depression and Mania

A. Depression

1. **Definition.** Unhappiness is one of the most common psychiatric complaints and often signifies the presence of depression. The syndrome of depression is not a disorder in itself; however, it may be associated with many psychiatric problems, and it is the primary complaint in several mood disorders.

2. **Theory**

   a. According to **psychodynamic theory**, depression is associated with loss of relationships or other attachments. When individuals cannot adequately recover from losing something of value, they may become pathologically depressed.

   b. **Behavioral theory** associates depression with "learned helplessness." Individuals become depressed when their life experiences suggest that they can do little to improve their situation or ameliorate their suffering.

   c. **Cognitive theory** associates depression with "faulty cognitive frameworks": Individuals may learn to interpret the environment in a way that creates unhappiness. Depression results from demoralizing ideas about self, the world, and the future.

3. The **syndrome of depression** is characterized by the following:

   a. **Change in mood.** The individual may be either dysphoric (i.e., sad, unhappy) or anhedonic (i.e., showing markedly diminished interest or pleasure in almost all activities).

   b. **Change in activity and appetite** (vegetative symptoms), including insomnia or hypersomnia, psychomotor agitation or retardation, fatigue or diminished energy, and decrease or increase in appetite

   c. **Change in thinking,** including a diminished ability to think or concentrate, indecisiveness, recurrent thoughts of death or suicide, and feelings of worthlessness or guilt

B. Mania

1. **Definition.** Mania, a state of elevated mood and activity, may appear as the converse of depression. The syndrome of mania is present in some mood disorders.

2. **Theory**

   a. Because mania is sometimes associated with depression in mood disorders, **psychodynamic theorists** postulate that mania may be an individual's attempt to overcompensate for feelings of loss and depression.

   b. **Biologic theories** about mania have involved various neurochemical abnormalities; however, no consensus exists.

3. The **syndrome of mania** is characterized by the following:

   a. **Change in mood,** including elevated, euphoric, expansive, and irritable moods

   b. **Change in activity and appetite**, including a markedly decreased need for sleep, increased goal-directed activity or psychomotor agitation, hypersexuality, aggressiveness, and excessive involvement in high-risk activities

   c. **Change in thinking,** including grandiosity or increased self-esteem, racing thoughts, increased speech, distractibility, and poor judgement

II. Mood episodes are characterized by episodes of severe mood disturbance. Mood disorders are distinguished from each other by the presence of different types of mood episodes.

A. Types

1. A **major depressive episode** is characterized by a depressive syndrome that is present for at least 2 weeks. The episode is not caused by a general medical condition, is not substance-induced, is not caused by bereavement, and is not mixed with manic symptoms.

2. A **manic episode** is characterized by a manic syndrome that is present for at least 1 week, or less than 1 week if psychosis is present. The episode is not caused by a general medical condition, is not substance-induced, and is not mixed with predominantly depressive symptoms for more than 1 week.

3. A **mixed episode** is characterized by the presence of both manic and depressive symptoms for at least 1 week. The episode is neither caused by a general medical condition nor is it substance-induced.

4. A **hypomanic episode** is a marked change in functioning that is characterized by milder symptoms of mania, which usually do not cause the same level of impairment. Psychosis is not present, and the episode is neither caused by a general medical condition nor is it substance-induced.

B. Subtypes

1. **Mood episodes with psychosis.** Psychosis may be present during the mood episodes in mood disorders, but it is absent between episodes. The psychosis may be mood congruent (i.e., self-condemnatory or accusatory

hallucinations) or mood incongruent (i.e., delusions or hallucinations without obvious depressive content).

2. **Mood episodes with catatonic features.** Bizarre motor behaviors may be present during the episode, including immobility, negativism, agitation, peculiar mannerisms, and posturing.

3. **Mood episodes with melancholic features.** A distinctive cluster of symptoms are present, including loss of ability to react to any pleasurable stimuli, marked anorexia, psychomotor retardation or agitation, excessive guilt, and early morning awakening with depressive symptoms that are worse in the morning.

4. **Mood episodes with atypical features. Mood reactivity** (i.e., mood improves or worsens in response to events) is present. Also, hypersomnia, weight gain, severe lassitude (i.e., feeling of heaviness in extremities), and sensitivity to rejection by others may be present.

5. **Mood episodes with postpartum onset** occur within 1 month postpartum.

C. **Features of the clinical course of mood episodes**

1. **With or without full interepisode recovery.** The course of mood disorders is most often characterized by normal mood between episodes; however, residual symptoms may be present.

2. **Seasonal pattern.** Some individuals with a mood disorder have episodes during specific times of the year. For example, the most notable seasonal pattern is major depressive episodes during winter and is sometimes called seasonal affective disorder.

3. **Rapid cycling.** Some individuals with bipolar disorder have four or more mood episodes yearly.

III. Conditions in which mood pathology may be evident

A. **Bereavement** is the depressive reaction to the death of a loved one. Other losses in life trigger the syndrome of depression.

B. **Adjustment disorder with depressed mood.** Adjustment disorder is probably the most common cause of the syndrome of depression (see Chapter 23).

C. **Psychotic disorders**

1. **Schizoaffective disorder.** Both manic and depressive episodes can be present in schizoaffective disorder. Psychosis must also be present during some period when mood symptoms are absent (see Chapter 13).

2. **Schizophrenia.** Depression is often present in the residual phase of schizophrenia.

D. **Mood disorders**

1. **General features.** Mood disorders are characterized by single or recurrent mood episodes. Each mood disorder is characterized by a different set of mood episodes during the course of the illness and is further classified by the features of the most recent mood episode (see II A). It is still unclear whether the various subtypes of mood disorders represent different disorders or variants of one or more disorders.

2. **Depressive disorders**

   a. **Major depressive disorder** is characterized by one or more episodes of depression that do not occur in the context of schizophrenia, schizoaffective disorder, or bipolar disorder.

   b. **Dysthymic disorder** is characterized by chronic depressive symptoms without clear-cut mood episodes.

3. **Bipolar disorders**

   a. **Bipolar I disorder** is characterized by one or more episodes of mania.

   b. **Bipolar II disorder** is characterized by one or more episodes of hypomania and one or more major depressive episodes.

   c. **Cyclothymic disorder** is characterized by episodes of hypomania and depressive symptoms without a full major depressive episode.

4. **Mood disorder due to general medical condition**
5. **Substance-induced mood disorder**

IV. Diagnostic Clues

A. **Presenting complaint**

   1. In **depressive disorders,** presenting complaints include demoralization, sadness, fatigue, sleep disturbance, weight loss, feelings of guilt, difficulty in concentrating, multiple somatic complaints, and suicidal thoughts and behaviors.

   2. In **bipolar disorders**, presenting complaints include erratic behavior and grandiosity or depressive symptoms.

B. **History**

   1. In **depressive disorders,** there may be a history of sad or listless periods or suicide attempts.

   2. In **bipolar disorders**, there may be a history of episodes of behavior markedly out of character, with grandiosity, poor judgement, sleeplessness, and foolish or impulsive behavior. There also may be a history of depressive episodes.

C. **Mental status**

   1. **Depressive episodes** may present with psychomotor retardation or agitation, sad facial expression, slow and soft speech, lack of response to humor, depressive rumination, trouble concentrating, and suicidal ideation.

   2. **Manic episodes** may present with increased psychomotor activity, euphoria, expansiveness, grandiosity, irritability, pressured speech, flight-of-ideas, impaired judgement, and impulsivity.

D. **Physical examination** may show evidence of suicide gestures or attempts (e.g., wrist cuts, scars), weight loss or neglect of self-care, and general medical conditions that may cause mood disturbances.

E. **Laboratory findings** may include evidence of general medical conditions or use of substances that may cause mood disturbances.

V. Major Depressive Disorder

A. Epidemiology

1. Major depressive disorder occurs at a **1:2 male to female ratio**. The **prevalence** is 5% of the population, with a 20% lifetime prevalence.
2. Depressive mood disorders and alcohol dependence are more common in relatives of individuals with major depressive disorder.
3. Major depressive disorder is less common in the elderly.

B. Etiology

1. **Psychodynamic, behavioral, and cognitive theories** (see I A 2)
2. **Biologic theories** (catecholamine hypothesis). Depression is a result of abnormal function of neurotransmitters, particularly serotonin and norepinephrine.

C. Diagnosis

1. The **diagnostic feature** of this disorder is one or more major depressive episodes without a history of manic or hypomanic episodes. If psychosis is present, it is not better accounted for by schizoaffective disorder or other psychotic disorders with mood symptoms.
2. **Subtypes** include:

    a. **Single episode, or recurrent.** About 50% of individuals who develop a single depressive episode will have additional episodes.

    b. Major depressive disorder may be further classified by the features of the depressive episode, including psychosis, melancholia, catatonia, and atypical features (see II B).

3. **Associated features**

    a. **Predisposing factors** include chronic physical illness, alcohol and cocaine dependence, psychosocial stressors, and childbirth.

    b. **Suicide attempts** are associated with major depressive disorder, and there is a 15% lifetime mortality by suicide. Morbidity and mortality from other concurrent medical conditions (e.g., end-stage renal disease) is greater in individuals with major depressive disorder.

    c. Dysthymia, which may be pre-existing, substance-related disorders, anxiety disorders, eating disorders, and some personality disorders are more common in patients with major depressive disorder.

    d. **Associated laboratory findings**. Numerous abnormal laboratory findings are reported in patients with major depressive disorder, most of which are found only during major depressive episodes.

    (1) **Polysomnographic changes** include decreased rapid eye movement (REM) latency, increased REM sleep time relative to non-REM sleep time, and intermittent wakefulness. These findings may persist in some individuals between depressive episodes.

    (2) **Changes in neurotransmitter levels** in blood and cerebrospinal fluid (CSF) are reported. The most consistent finding is decreased levels of serotonin, especially in individuals who have committed violent suicide.

(3) **Neuroendocrine changes,** such as relative dexamethasone nonsuppression, are fairly consistent findings; however, they are nonspecific.

4. **Differential diagnoses** include mood disorder due to general medical conditions, substance-induced mood disorders, dysthymic disorder, dementia, adjustment disorder with depressed mood, schizoaffective disorder and other psychotic disorders, and bereavement.

D. **Clinical course**

1. **Onset** can occur at any age, but it is often in the third decade. It may be sudden or gradual, and it may be associated with precipitating factors (e.g., stress).
2. **Prodromal symptoms** of anxiety, brooding, or hypochondriasis may occur.
3. During **depressive episodes**, individuals may be tearful, agitated, and dysphoric, or they may be withdrawn and anhedonic. These episodes usually last about 6 months without treatment. Major depressive episodes are usually interspersed with long periods of normal function, but depressive symptoms may occasionally persist much longer (see II C 1)
4. Depressive episodes in children with this disorder are more frequently characterized by somatic complaints, irritability, and social withdrawal. Cognitive symptoms may be more prominent in elderly patients.
5. **Complications** of major depressive disorder include suicide and substance abuse.

E. **Treatment.** The goals of treatment are to relieve depressive episodes and to prevent future episodes, suicide, and other disabilities.

1. **Antidepressants** are almost always indicated during depressive episodes.
2. **Lethality** must be carefully and continuously assessed, and hospitalization should be considered if there is risk of suicide.
3. According to some authorities, **cognitive psychotherapies** are especially effective for treating depression.
4. **Electroconvulsive therapy (ECT)** may be indicated if:

   a. The patient is unresponsive to adequate trials of antidepressants or there are contraindications to use of these agents
   b. The patient's immediate risk for suicide is too great to wait for response to antidepressants
   c. There is a history of good response to ECT during past episodes

VI. Dysthymic Disorder

A. **Epidemiology**

1. This disorder occurs at a **1:2 male to female ratio. The prevalence** is 3% of the population, with a 6% lifetime prevalence.
2. There is more irritability and poor social skills in children.
3. Major depressive episodes are more common in relatives of individuals with dysthymic disorder.

B. Etiology. Some of the causes of this disorder may be the same as those of major depressive disorder and may also involve predisposing personality traits.

C. Diagnosis

  1. **Diagnostic features**

    a. There is **almost continuous depressed mood for at least 2 years,** but there is no history of the full features of a major depressive episode.

    b. **Depressive symptoms** include appetite and sleep disturbances, fatigue, low self-esteem, difficulty in focusing thinking, and feelings of hopelessness.

    c. There is **no history of manic, mixed, or hypomanic episodes.** The symptoms are neither superimposed on a chronic psychotic disorder nor part of cyclothymic disorder. Also, it is neither caused by a general medical condition nor is it substance-induced.

  2. **Subtypes** include:

    a. Early onset (before 21 years of age)

    b. Late onset (after 21 years of age)

    c. Dysthmic disorder with atypical features

  3. **Associated features**

    a. Individuals have a significantly higher risk of subsequently developing major depressive disorder. Also, personality disorders, interpersonal problems, and substance dependence are more common in these individuals.

    b. In children, attention deficit hyperactivity disorder (ADHD), conduct disorder, anxiety disorders, learning disorders, and mental retardation are more common.

    c. About 50% of patients with dysthymic disorder have laboratory findings similar to those with major depressive disorder (see V C 3 d).

  4. **Differential diagnoses** include major depressive disorder in partial remission, mood disorder due to a general medical condition, substance-induced mood disorder, and normal mood fluctuations.

D. Clinical course

  1. People with dysthymic disorder are often depressed for many years, but may not seek treatment unless a major depressive episode supervenes.

  2. Children with dysthymic disorder may have irritability and poor social skills.

  3. There is usually no clear precipitant for the disorder, but **predisposing factors** include childhood psychiatric illness, chronic psychosocial stressors, and a family history of major depressive disorder.

  4. **Morbidity** is created by the chronicity of the illness. There are often insidious effects on an individual's social and occupational function and self-esteem.

  5. The relationship of dysthymic disorder to other psychiatric and medical problems is not always clear, and distinguishing between dysthymic disorder and major depressive disorder may be very difficult.

E. Treatment. Long term psychotherapies and antidepressants may be useful.

VII. Bipolar I Disorder

A. Epidemiology

1. This disorder occurs at a **1:1 male to female ratio.** The **prevalence** is approximately 1% of the population.
2. There is a strong familial component to bipolar I disorder, and there are also familial associations with other mood disorders.

B. Etiology.
Several studies have implicated specific genetic foci; however, the exact nature of the biochemical defects are unclear.

C. Diagnosis

1. **Diagnostic features.** There is a history of one or more manic or mixed episodes, and the disorder is not better accounted for by schizoaffective disorder or another psychotic disorder.
2. **Subtypes.** Bipolar I Disorder is classified by the **nature of the last episode**: whether it was a manic, mixed, hypomanic, or depressive episode. It is also classified by the various features of the most recent episode (e.g., with psychotic or catatonic features) and the clinical course (see II C).
3. **Associated features**

   a. There is a 10%–15% mortality rate by suicide.
   b. Violence and social and interpersonal problems often occur. Injuries from fighting, accidents caused by impulsive behavior, encounters with law enforcement, and marital conflict are common.

4. **Differential diagnoses** include other mood disorders, psychotic disorders with mood symptoms, mood disorder due to a general medical condition, and substance-induced mood disorder.

D. Clinical course

1. The **onset** may be during adolescence or adulthood.
2. **Episodes.** Individuals are likely to have both manic and major depressive episodes during the course of this disorder.

   a. **Manic episodes** usually develop over days, lasting about 3 months without treatment.

      (1) Ninety percent of individuals with an initial manic episode will develop more mood episodes.
      (2) Men are more likely to have initial manic episodes, whereas women are more likely to have initial major depressive episodes.

   b. **Major depressive episodes** in bipolar disorder are clinically indistinguishable from those in major depressive disorder.
   c. **Mixed episodes** are more common during adolescence.
   d. Some individuals may develop psychosis during mood episodes, but psychosis is absent between episodes.
   e. The **time period between episodes** is usually a couple of years, but it may shorten as the patient ages. Some individuals have very rapid cycling between episodes (see II C 3). Changes in the sleep–

wake cycle may precipitate episodes. Episodes are more likely to occur during the postpartum period.

  f. Most individuals recover fully between episodes; however, some individuals continue to have symptoms of mood lability and social difficulties.

E. **Treatment**. The goals of treatment are to relieve mood episodes, to prevent future episodes, suicide, and other disabilities, and to heal damaged relationships.

  1. **Lithium** is the mood-stabilizing medication of choice for bipolar I disorder (see Chapter 29).
  2. **Valproate** and **carbamazepine** are also used to treat this disorder when lithium is ineffective or contraindicated. Other anticonvulsants may also have some efficacy in treating this disorder.
  3. **Antidepressants** may be used to treat the major depressive episodes in this disorder; however, this medication can precipitate a manic episode. Therefore, treatment response must be carefully assessed and mood stabilizing medication is used concurrently.
  4. **Antipsychotic agents** may be used to treat psychosis in bipolar I disorder.

VIII. Bipolar II Disorder

A. **Epidemiology**

  1. This disorder is **more common in women**, and the postpartum period may increase risk of mood episodes. There is 0.5% lifetime prevalence for this disorder.
  2. Mood disorders are more common in relatives of individuals with bipolar II disorder.

B. **Diagnosis**

  1. **Diagnostic features**

    a. There is a history of one or more major depressive episodes and one or more hypomanic episodes.
    b. The individual has never had a manic or mixed episode.
    c. The disturbance is not better accounted for by schizoaffective disorder or another psychotic disorder.

  2. **Subtypes** are based on the nature of the most recent episode and its longitudinal course.
  3. **Associated features**

    a. Individuals with this disorder have a significant risk for suicide.
    b. Social and interpersonal problems are common.
    c. Substance-related disorders, anxiety disorders, and borderline personality disorder are more common.

  4. **Differential diagnoses** include other mood disorders and psychotic disorders with mood symptoms.

C. **Clinical course**

  1. **Hypomanic episodes** often occur soon before or soon after major depressive episodes.

      a. The **intervals between mood episodes shorten** as the patient ages, and some patients have rapid cycling of episodes.

      b. Most patients are asymptomatic between episodes, but some will have mood lability or social difficulties.

   2. Changes in the sleep—wake cycle may precipitate mood episodes.

   3. Some patients with bipolar II disorder will ultimately have a manic episode; their diagnosis changes to bipolar I disorder.

   4. Psychosis may be present during major depressive episodes.

   5. Between episodes, some individuals continue to have mood lability and social difficulties.

D. Treatment goals and methods are similar to those for bipolar I disorder (see VII E).

IX. Cyclothymic Disorder

A. Epidemiology

   1. This disorder occurs at a **1:1 male to female ratio**. There is a 0.5% lifetime prevalence of this disorder.

   2. Mood disorders and substance-related disorders are more common in relatives of individuals with cyclothymic disorder.

B. Diagnosis

   1. Diagnostic features

      a. Numerous, closely spaced periods of hypomanic symptoms and numerous periods of depressive symptoms occur for at least 2 years, but there is no full major depressive episode.

      b. The symptoms not better accounted for by other mood disorders nor are they superimposed on psychotic disorders.

   2. Associated diagnoses include substance-related disorders and sleep disorders.

   3. Differential diagnoses include other mood disorders, particularly rapid cycling bipolar disorders, and borderline personality disorder.

C. Clinical course

   1. Onset is usually during adolescence or early adulthood.

   2. These symptoms are often interpreted as a temperament problem. Individuals may be perceived as moody and unpredictable, and social and occupational problems develop.

   3. There is risk of subsequent development of a bipolar disorder.

D. Treatment

   1. Group and individual psychotherapy may be useful for dealing with interpersonal problems and negative self-perceptions that develop because of the underlying mood swings.

   2. Some data suggests that **mood-stabilizing medications** (e.g., lithium, anticonvulsants) may be useful.

X. Mood Disorder Due to a General Medical Condition

A. **Epidemiology.** This disorder occurs at a **1:1 male to female ratio**. It is common in the course of some medical conditions, particularly neurodegenerative disease. There is no familial pattern.

B. Presumptively, the **etiology** is alterations in central nervous system (CNS) function that are the result of the underlying disease process.

C. **Diagnosis**

1. The **diagnostic feature** is a prominent and persistent mood disturbance that is a direct physiologic effect of a general medical condition. The symptoms are not superimposed on delirium or dementia.

2. **Subtypes** include:

   a. With depressive features
   b. With major depressive-like episode
   c. With manic features
   d. With mixed features

3. **Associated general medical conditions** include:

   a. **Neurodegenerative conditions,** such as Parkinson and Huntington diseases
   b. **Cerebrovascular conditions,** such as cerebral infarcts
   c. **Metabolic and nutritional conditions,** such as electrolyte disturbances and vitamin deficiencies
   d. **Endocrine conditions,** such as hyperthyroidism (e.g., Graves disease), hypothyroidism, hyperparathyroidism, hypoparathyroidism, adrenocortical hyperactivity (e.g., Cushing syndrome), and adrenal insufficiency (e.g., Addison disease)
   e. **Autoimmune conditions,** such as systemic lupus erythematosus and other vasculitides
   f. **Infections,** such as neurosyphilis, hepatitis, mononucleosis, and HIV
   g. **Neoplasms,** such as pancreatic cancer
   h. Epilepsy
   I. Head trauma

4. **Differential diagnoses** include delirium, some dementias with depressive symptoms (e.g., dementia of the Alzheimer type and vascular dementia), substance-induced mood disorder, and other mood disorders.

D. The **clinical course** depends on the underlying disease process.

E. **Treatment**

1. The underlying disease process must be treated if possible.

2. **Antidepressant and mood-stabilizing** medications may be indicated in certain cases (e.g., mood disorder due to left cerebral infarction)

XI. Substance-Induced Mood Disorder

A. **Epidemiology** is determined by the substance involved. This disorder is commonly diagnosed.

B. Presumptively, the **etiology** is alterations in CNS function caused by the substance.

C. Diagnosis

1. The **diagnostic feature** is a persistent and prominent mood disturbance that develops as a direct result, and within 1 month, of intoxication or withdrawal from a drug of abuse, medication, or toxin. The mood disturbance is more severe than that expected with uncomplicated intoxication or withdrawal.

2. **Subtypes** include substance-induced mood disorder with depressive features, with manic features, or with mixed features. This disorder is further classified by the time of onset (i.e., if it occurs during intoxication or withdrawal).

3. **Associated substances**. A wide variety of abused drugs and prescribed medications can cause mood symptoms.

   a. **Drugs of abuse** that cause mood symptoms include alcohol, psychostimulants, anxiolytics, sedative—hypnotics, hallucinogens, and inhalants.

   b. **Prescribed drugs** that frequently cause depressive moods include antihypertensive medications and steroids.

4. **Differential diagnoses** include substance intoxication or withdrawal, delirium, and other mood disorders.

D. The **clinical course** is determined by the substance involved; however, the disorder usually resolves when administration of the substance ceases.

E. **Treatment** includes:

1. Discontinuation of use of the responsible substance when possible
2. Time-limited symptomatic treatment with antidepressant or mood-stabilizing medication when indicated

Review Test

Directions: Each of the numbered items or incomplete statements in this section is followed by answers or by completions of the statement. Select the ONE lettered answer or completion that is BEST in each case.

1. A 26-year-old man becomes intensely depressed and suicidal on the third day of an amphetamine binge. Which of the following is the most likely diagnosis?

(A) Amphetamine intoxication
(B) Amphetamine withdrawal
(C) Amphetamine-induced mood disorder with depressive features and with onset during intoxication
(D) Amphetamine-induced mood disorder with depressive features and with onset during withdrawal
(E) Major depressive disorder, single episode

2. A 27-year-old woman with systemic lupus erythematosus has become increasingly emotionally labile. She has frequent episodes of crying, disinhibition and grandiosity, and anger and irritability. She has been taking prednisone for 2 weeks for an acute flare-up. Which of the following is the best initial treatment for her mood lability?

(A) Initiate cognitive therapy
(B) Administer lithium
(C) Administer maprotiline
(D) Administer valproate
(E) Taper the prednisone to the lowest effective dose

3. A 29-year-old woman seeks guidance about becoming pregnant. At 22 years of age, she had a 2-month episode of sleeplessness, grandiosity, and behavioral indiscretions. She was briefly hospitalized in a psychiatric unit, and she took a 6-month course of lithium. Since that time, she has not had any similar episodes. Which of the following is the most accurate information about her psychopathology and the implications of pregnancy?

(A) It is likely that pregnancy will precipitate further psychopathology
(B) It is unlikely that pregnancy will increase her risk for further psychiatric symptoms
(C) She should seek spiritual guidance
(D) She should begin a prophylactic course of lithium before becoming pregnant
(E) She should avoid pregnancy

4. A 33-year-old woman complains of being persistently unhappy with her life for the past several years. She often ruminates about her poor career choices and her inability to use her time and talents effectively. She describes periods of malaise, self-doubt, and low self-esteem. She also experiences moderate anxiety. She has had no previous psychiatric treatment, and she has managed to work steadily and raise two children. Which of the following would be the best initial course of treatment?

(A) Cognitive psychotherapy
(B) Administration of diazepam
(C) Administration of fluoxetine
(D) Administration of lithium
(E) Supportive psychotherapy

5. A 68-year-old man suffers a left-sided cerebrovascular stroke and has residual right hemiparesis, gait difficulties, slowing of mentation, and a mild aphasia. Two months after his stroke, he shows little interest in physical rehabilitation, refuses to speak with friends, and is often tearful. Which of the following is the most appropriate management for this case?

(A) Initiate cognitive psychotherapy
(B) Initiate increasing levels of exercise, but avoid psychotherapy
(C) Administer sertraline
(D) Administer tacrine
(E) Withhold antidepressant medications and initiate supportive psychotherapy

Answers and Explanations

1–C. This presentation is most consistent with amphetamine-induced disorder with depressive features and with onset during intoxication. His depressive symptoms are too severe to be ascribed to intoxication alone. Treatment would likely involve detoxification from amphetamine, careful monitoring of the course of his depressive symptoms, and use of antidepressants if his depression does not remit quickly.

2–E. This presentation is most suggestive of a prednisone-induced mood disorder with mixed features; symptoms of both depression and mania are present. It is likely that the prednisone plays an etiologic role; however, the psychological stress of her illness may also contribute. The first intervention should be lowering her dose of prednisone, because mood symptoms that prednisone commonly cause are often dose-related. If continued lupus symptoms preclude lowering her dose of prednisone, mood stabilizers (e.g., lithium, valproate) should be considered. Use of an antidepressant alone may exacerbate her manic symptoms. Cognitive psychotherapy may be helpful, but it is unlikely to resolve a substance-induced mood disorder.

3–A. The woman's history suggests that she had a manic episode. Ninety percent of individuals who have a manic episode will eventually have additional mood episodes. The postpartum period is strongly associated with an increased risk for mood episodes in individuals with a bipolar disorder. Although spiritual guidance may be useful, it does not address her request for medical expertise in making a decision about pregnancy. Prophylactic use of lithium during pregnancy is contraindicated because of its teratogenic effects. Avoiding pregnancy may deprive the woman of a life experience that is important to her. She should be closely monitored during the postpartum period, and if she becomes symptomatic, appropriate medication should be initiated rapidly.

4–A. This presentation is most suggestive of dysthymic disorder, which is characterized by a persistently depressed mood for at least 2 years, without any complete depressive episodes or manic symptoms. Moderate anxiety is a commonly associated symptom. Cognitive psychotherapy is often a highly effective treatment for this disorder. Antidepressants, such as fluoxetine, may also be effective but only in a minority of cases. In practice, cognitive therapy and a trial of antidepressants are often combined Diazepam or other benzodiazepines alone are not effective antidepressants. Lithium is not useful in the treatment of dysthymia. Supportive psychotherapy alone has not proved to be as effective as other interventions.

5–C. This patient's symptoms are suggestive of a mood disorder due to cerebrovascular disease, with a major depressive-like episode. This mood pathology is particularly common following a left-sided cerebrovascular stroke and often responds well to antidepressant medications, such as sertraline. Cognitive psychotherapy is often useful in treating depression; however, it may be too demanding and frustrating for an individual with slowed mentation and aphasia. Exercise is often a useful adjunct for treating depressive symptom; however, it is unlikely to be useful as treatment alone, particularly in an individual with new physical limitations. Tacrine may ameliorate cognitive impairments in Alzheimer dementia; however, it is unlikely to be useful in treating cognitive deficits caused by vascular pathology. Supportive therapy alone may be useful; however, there is little reason to withhold antidepressant medication.

15

Anxiety Disorders

I. Overview. Anxiety is one of the most common psychiatric complaint.

    A. Freudian theory. Freud based much of his metapsychology on anxiety management. He believed that the subjective experience of anxiety occurs when instinctual drives are thwarted.

        1. He suggested that the goal of most higher mental functions is to decrease this anxiety by modulating satisfaction of instinctual drives, based on a perception of external realities, and that psychopathology is caused by a failure to manage anxiety appropriately.

        2. Freud described conscious and unconscious anxiety as being central to almost all psychopathology, making it more difficult to discuss discrete primary anxiety disorders.

    B. Behavioral and biologic theories describe anxiety in physiologic terms, closely associating it with autonomic arousal.

    C. The advent of specific therapies for specific types of anxiety created the need for a rigorous diagnostic framework.

II. Diagnostic Clues

    A. Chief complaints and **history** include excessive nervousness, fears, a sense of impending doom, irrational avoidance of objects or situations, and anxiety attacks.

    B. Mental status examination may show hyperarousal, exaggerated startle responses, timidity, and excessive worries.

    C. Physical examination may show evidence of autonomic arousal, motor restlessness, or general medical conditions that cause anxiety.

    D. Laboratory studies may show evidence of general medical conditions or substances that cause anxiety disorders.

III. Anxiety as a Syndrome. Anxiety can be conceptualized as a syndrome with both psychological and physiologic components.

    A. Psychological components include:

        1. Worry that is difficult to control

        2. Hypervigilance and restlessness

   3. Difficulty concentrating
   4. Sleep disturbance

B. Physiologic components include:

   1. Autonomic hyperactivity
   2. Motor tension

C. The specific **symptom complex** of anxiety may vary among individuals and may present with characteristic variations.

   1. Generalized anxiety is excessive worry about several issues.
   2. Panic attacks are attacks of intense anxiety that often include marked physical symptoms, such as tachycardia, hyperventilation, dizziness, and sweating.
   3. Obsessive-compulsive symptoms are anxiety-provoking, intrusive thoughts (i.e., obsessions) or repetitive, often peculiar behaviors that reduce anxiety (i.e., compulsions).

   a. Common obsessions are about contamination, doubt, guilt, aggression, and sex.
   b. Common compulsions are hand washing, organizing, checking, counting, and praying.

   4. Phobic symptoms are unreasonable fears and avoidance of objects or situations.

IV. Disorders in which the syndrome of anxiety occurs

A. Normal anxiety. Although it may feel uncomfortable, the syndrome of anxiety is ubiquitous and probably essential in mentally stable people.

B. Mental disorders. Anxiety is a commonly associated symptom of many mental disorders.

   1. Components of anxiety may be the presenting feature in adjustment disorders (see Chapter 23).
   2. Symptoms of anxiety and avoidance are the major features of anxiety disorders, and these symptoms are not simply the result of other psychiatric disorders. The main anxiety disorders are **panic disorder, phobic disorders, obsessive-compulsive disorder, posttraumatic stress disorder, generalized anxiety disorder, anxiety due to a general medical condition,** and **substance-induced anxiety disorder.**

V. Panic Disorder

A. Epidemiology

   1. This disorder occurs at a **1:2 male to female ratio.** The **prevalence** is 2% of the population; there is a lifetime prevalence of 3%.
   2. There are some culture-specific syndromes that may be associated with this disorder, such as **ataque de nervious,** which is seen in Latin American cultures.
   3. Panic disorder is more common in relatives of individuals with the disorder.

B. Etiology

1. Panic disorder may be associated with separations during childhood and interpersonal loss in adulthood.
2. This disorder may be associated with mitral valve prolapse and abnormal neurophysiology. Some studies suggest that individuals with panic disorder, unlike other individuals, have panic symptoms in response to lactate infusion.
3. Twin studies suggest a genetic component.

C. The major **diagnostic feature** is recurrent, unexpected panic attacks.

1. **Types** include panic disorder with agoraphobia and panic disorder without agoraphobia.
2. **Associated features.** Panic attacks usually last a few minutes. Agoraphobia, depression, generalized anxiety, and substance abuse are commonly present.
3. **Differential diagnoses** include anxiety disorder due to a general medical condition, substance-induced anxiety disorder, and other anxiety disorders.

D. Clinical course. The onset is often during the third decade. The severity of symptoms may wax and wane and may be associated with intercurrent stressors.

E. Treatment

1. Treatment **goals** are to reduce the frequency, duration, and intensity of panic attacks and to decrease the anxiety associated with anticipating attacks.
2. **Pharmacologic interventions** include benzodiazepines, particularly alprazolam and clonazepam, tricyclic antidepressants (e.g., imipramine), selective serotonin reuptake inhibitors (e.g., fluoxetine) and monoamine oxidase inhibitors (e.g., phenelzine).
3. **Psychotherapeutic** interventions include relaxation training for panic attacks and systematic desensitization for agoraphobic symptoms (see Chapter 30).

VI. Phobic Disorders

A. A **phobia** has three components.

1. There is fear and avoidance of an object or situation.
2. Exposure to the feared stimulus produces anxiety.
3. Except in children, the individual recognizes the fear as excessive.

B. Agoraphobia

1. **Epidemiology**

   a. Agoraphobia is **more common in women** and may be misdiagnosed in cultures that restrict public access to certain groups or genders.
   b. **Prevalence.** Agoraphobia in the absence of panic disorder is rare; less than 5% of individuals with agoraphobia do not have panic disorder.

2. The major **diagnostic feature** is fear or avoidance of places from which escape would be difficult or help could not be obtained in event of panic symptoms; the individual has never had panic disorder.

    a. Associated features. Agoraphobia is usually associated with panic-like symptoms.

       (1) Agoraphobia usually involves fear and avoidance of public places, being outside alone, public transportation, crowds, and bridges.

       (2) It often leads to severe restrictions on the individual's travel and daily activities, and the individual may become completely housebound.

    b. Differential diagnoses include panic disorder with agoraphobia, social phobia, specific phobia, major depressive disorder, and realistic fears.

  3. The **clinical course** is chronic, and severe restriction of activities leads to an isolated existence.

  4. Treatment includes **behavioral therapy** (e.g., systematic desensitization) and use of **antidepressants**.

C. Specific phobia

  1. Epidemiology

    a. This disorder occurs predominantly in women and is common in children. The **prevalence** is 9% of the population.

    b. Specific phobia, particularly blood-injection-injury phobia, is more common in relatives of individuals with a specific phobia.

  2. Etiology. Specific causal factors are unknown, and there is little evidence for a symbolic significance of phobic stimuli.

  3. The **diagnostic feature** is the presence of phobias involving objects or situations other than agoraphobia or social phobia. (see VI A, D)

    a. Subtypes include animal type, natural environment type, blood-injection-injury type, and situational type.

    b. Associated features. The individual may have a restricted lifestyle, another anxiety disorder, or a history of fainting.

    c. Differential diagnoses include other phobic disorders, PTSD, obsessive-compulsive disorder, hypochondriasis, and psychotic disorders.

  4. Clinical course

    a. Onset of animal phobias commonly occurs during childhood; blood-injection-injury phobia often starts during adolescence; and other phobias often emerge in the third decade.

    b. With **adult onset**, the course tends to be chronic but may cause little impairment.

  5. Treatment includes behavioral therapies.

    a. Systematic desensitization. An individual with blood-injection-injury phobia may be gradually exposed to hypodermic needles at an ever-increasing distance, coupled with relaxation exercises.

    b. Flooding. An individual with animal phobia may be taken to a zoo, and his anxiety may decrease with a few hours of exposure.

D. Social phobia

1. Epidemiology

  a. Social phobia is more common in women. The **prevalence** is 2% of population; there is a lifetime prevalence of 10%.

  b. In some cultures, social avoidance is associated with a fear of offending someone rather than a fear of embarrassment.

  c. Social phobia is more common in relatives of individuals with the disorder.

2. Etiology. Although there is limited data, social phobia may result from avoidant personality traits.

3. The major **diagnostic feature** is a fear of circumscribed or general social situations.

  a. Subtypes. Social phobia, generalized type, describes individuals who avoid most situations.

  b. Associated features and diagnoses

  (1) Individuals often have fears of public speaking, speaking in classrooms, eating or writing in public, urinating in public restrooms, and attending social events.

  (2) They may socially isolate themselves and have low self-esteem. There is often a concurrent diagnosis of avoidant personality disorder, and other anxiety disorders also may be present.

  c. Differential diagnoses include other anxiety disorders, particularly panic disorder and agoraphobia, and schizoid and avoidant personality disorders.

4. Clinical course

  a. Onset is often during childhood or adolescence, and it is often preceded by avoidant personality symptoms.

  b. The severity of symptoms may wax and wane, and patients may conceal their disabilities.

  c. Concomitant drug abuse is common.

5. Treatment

  a. Cognitive and behavioral therapies are used, particularly assertiveness training (see Chapter 30).

  b. Some **anxiolytic medications** may be useful, including benzodiazepines and buspirone. Phenelzine, a monoamine oxidase inhibitor, is also used.

VII. Obsessive-Compulsive Disorder

A. Epidemiology. This disorder occurs at a **1:1 male to female ratio.** The **prevalence** is 2% of population; there is a lifetime prevalence of 2.5%. There is some evidence of heritability.

B. Etiology. This disorder may be associated with abnormalities of serotonin metabolism.

C. The major **diagnostic feature** is recurrent obsessions or compulsions, which are recognized by the individual as unreasonable, and are sufficiently severe to cause marked distress or interference with functioning.

1. Obsessive-compulsive disorder with poor insight is a variant and is characterized by lack of insight into the unreasonable nature of the behavior.
2. **Associated features** include depression, anxiety, hypochondriasis, feelings of guilt, phobic avoidance, Tourette disorder, and social and occupational problems.
3. **Differential diagnoses** include other compulsions, (e.g., eating disorders, paraphilias, pathologic gambling, substance abuse), specific phobias, hypochondriasis, and delusional disorder.

D. **Clinical course.** Insidious onset occurs during childhood, adolescence, or early adulthood. The symptoms usually wax and wane, and intercurrent depression and substance abuse are common.

E. **Treatment.** Behavioral psychotherapy and selective serotonin reuptake inhibitors (e.g., clomipramine, fluoxetine, fluvoxamine) are used.

VIII. Posttraumatic Stress Disorder

A. **Epidemiology.** PTSD is more common during times or in places characterized by natural or man-made traumatic events. There is little information about the prevalence and heritability of this disorder.

B. **Etiology.** Traumatic events precipitate PTSD in some individuals. The role of other premorbid factors, such as personality traits, is unknown.

C. **Diagnostic features**

1. Symptoms follow a threatening event (e.g., threat of death, physical injury) that the DSM-IV describes as causing intense fear, horror, or helplessness and last for more than 1 month.
2. The disorder is characterized by a triad of symptom groups:
   a. Reexperiencing of the traumatic event in dreams, flashbacks, or intrusive recollections
   b. Avoidance of stimuli associated with the trauma or numbing of general responsiveness
   c. Increased arousal that is manifested by anxiety, sleep disturbances, hypervigilance
3. There are three **subtypes: acute**, in which the disorder lasts for less than 3 months; **chronic**; and **delayed onset**, in which symptoms begin at least 6 months following the traumatic event. A separate diagnosis, acute stress disorder, is given if the symptoms last less than 1 month.
4. **Associated features** include anxiety and depression, impulsivity, difficulties concentrating, emotional lability, and feelings of guilt.
5. **Differential diagnoses** include adjustment disorders, other anxiety disorders, and dissociative disorders.

D. **Clinical course**

1. **Onset** may occur at any age. The **duration** is extremely variable, but about 50% of cases resolve within 3 months.
2. **Symptoms** usually begin immediately following trauma; however, symptoms may begin following a latency period of months or years.
3. The disorder is often complicated by phobic avoidance, impaired interpersonal relationships, emotional lability, feelings of guilt ("survivor guilt"), self-destructive behavior, and substance abuse.

E. **Treatment** goals are to relieve the patient from intrusive recollections, to decrease symptoms of anxiety, and to improve the patient's social relations and capacity for enjoyment.

1. **Group psychotherapy** is often the treatment modality of choice.
2. **Pharmacotherapy.** Symptomatic treatment with antidepressants and anxiolytics may be helpful; however there is a significant risk for substance abuse in patients with this disorder.
3. **Prevention.** Some clinicians believe that immediate counseling following a stressful event may prevent PTSD from developing.

IX. Generalized Anxiety Disorder

A. **Epidemiology.** Generalized anxiety disorder occurs at a **2 : 3 male to female ratio**.

1. The **prevalence** is approximately 5% of the population.
2. Children often have more concrete worries, and they often worry about competence.

B. **Etiology.** There may be a genetic predisposition for an anxiety trait.
C. The **diagnostic feature** is excessive, poorly controlled anxiety about life circumstances that continues for more than 6 months.

1. **Associated features and diagnoses.** This disorder is often associated with depression, concern with somatic symptoms, and substance abuse.
2. **Differential diagnoses** include other anxiety disorders (e.g., anxiety disorder due to a general medical condition) and adjustment disorders.

D. **Clinical course**

1. **Onset** is often during childhood but can occur during adulthood.
2. Children often have more concrete worries, and they often worry about competence.
3. The course is usually **chronic**, but symptoms worsen during stressful times.

E. **Treatment.** Benzodiazepines, buspirone, and some forms of behavioral psychotherapy (e.g., biofeedback) are helpful.

X. Anxiety Due to a General Medical Condition

A. Presumptively, the **etiology** is alterations in central nervous system (CNS) function as a result of the underlying disease process.
B. The **diagnostic feature** is significant anxiety in the absence of delirium that develops as a direct physiologic effect of a general medical condition.

1. **Subtypes** include:
    a. With generalized anxiety
    b. With panic attacks
    c. With obsessive-compulsive symptoms
2. **Associated general medical conditions** include:

    a. **Endocrine disorders,** including hyperthyroidism, pheochromocytoma, and hypoglycemia
    b. **Cardiovascular disorders,** including congestive heart failure, pulmonary, and tachyarrhythmias

        c. Respiratory disorders, including chronic obstructive pulmonary disease and hyperventilation

        d. Metabolic disorders, including electrolyte disturbances and hypoglycemia

        e. Neurologic disorders, including encephalitis and vestibular dysfunction

    3. Differential diagnoses include delirium, substance-induced anxiety disorder, and other anxiety disorders.

C. Treatment includes:

    1. Treatment of the underlying disease process

    2. Use of anxiolytic medication in some cases

XI. Substance-Induced Anxiety Disorder

A. Presumptively, the **etiology** is alterations in CNS function as a result of the substance.

B. The **diagnostic feature** is significant anxiety that develops as a direct result and within 1 month of intoxication or withdrawal from a substance of abuse, medication, or toxin.

    1. Subtypes include substance-induced anxiety disorder with generalized anxiety, with panic attacks, with obsessive-compulsive symptoms, and with phobic symptoms. This disorder is further classified by the time of onset (i.e., if it occurs during intoxication or withdrawal).

    2. Associated substances

        a. Stimulants, hallucinogens, marijuana, inhalants, and phencyclidine are associated with an onset during intoxication.

        b. Alcohol, sedative—hypnotics, anxiolytics, and cocaine are associated with an onset during withdrawal.

    3. Differential diagnoses include delirium, anxiety due to a general medical condition, and other anxiety disorders.

C. Clinical course. The onset must be within 1 month of intoxication or withdrawal from the substance, but the course differs depending on the substance.

D. Treatment includes:

    1. Discontinuation of the responsible substance when possible

    2. Time-limited symptomatic treatment with anxiolytic medication when indicated

Review Test

Directions: Each of the numbered items or incomplete statements in this section is followed by answers or by completions of the statement. Select the ONE lettered answer or completion that is BEST in each case.

1. A 26-year-old woman complains of being lonely. She says that she longs to have a close circle of friends and to attend social events, but she feels terrified in social situations and avoids social invitations from coworkers. She worries that other people notice her withdrawal and talk about her. Which of the following is the most likely diagnosis?

(A) Dependent personality disorder
(B) Generalized anxiety disorder
(C) Schizoid personality disorder
(D) Schizophrenia, paranoid type
(E) Social phobia

2. A 31-year-old local politician has a sudden onset of extreme anxiety, tremulousness, and diaphoresis immediately before his first scheduled appearance on national television, and he is unable to go on the air. For the next week, he is paralyzed by fear each time he faces an audience, and he cancels all of his scheduled public appearances. Which of the following is the most likely diagnosis?

(A) Acute stress disorder
(B) Adjustment disorder with anxious mood
(C) Panic disorder
(D) Social phobia
(E) Specific phobia

3. A 20-year-old man complains of difficulty controlling anxiety in almost all situations. He is teased by coworkers because of his nervousness and exaggerated startle responses. He describes frequent stress-related stomach cramps and insomnia. His wife says that he grinds his teeth in his sleep. Which of the following medications is most likely useful for the treatment of his disorder?

(A) Buspirone
(B) Imipramine
(C) Propranolol
(D) Thioridazine
(E) Valproate

4. A 24-year-old mother who has no previous psychiatric complaints reports that she has a recurrent and disturbing thought that she should smother her infant daughter. She is terrified that she may carry out this plan and that she is losing her sanity. She emphatically denies any history of abusing her daughter in any way and says that she loves her daughter dearly. Which of the following is the best initial management for this case?

(A) Remove the daughter immediately from the household
(B) Suggest to the mother that it is unlikely that she will harm her daughter and that antidepressant medication may be beneficial
(C) Admit the mother to a psychiatric hospital or unit and begin administration of antipsychotic medication
(D) Suggest to the mother to place her daughter in the care of others and begin psychotherapy to resolve the underlying hostility she may be experiencing
(E) Have the mother continue to care for her daughter, but advise that the mother should not be left alone with the daughter at any time

5. A 51-year-old female secretary who has no history of psychiatric problems is acutely anxious when she learns that her company is being relocated. The company will be moved from the first floor to the third floor of a small office complex. She has worked in her current job for 22 years and has always enjoyed it. She is especially concerned about traversing through an outside passageway to get to her office, despite the heavy protective railing on the passageway. She recognizes her fear as unreasonable. Nevertheless, when the elevator opens to the third floor, she can barely step out to the passageway and quickly returns to the elevator in a panic. Which of the following is the best treatment?

(A) She should begin practicing guided imagery at work, learning to imagine a calming scene when she feels anxious
(B) She should begin a course of hypnotherapy designed to build her self-esteem and confidence about working on the third floor
(C) She should threaten her employer with a lawsuit if she is forced to move to the third floor
(D) Accompanied by a friend, she should attempt daily to gradually walk a few feet farther on the passageway
(E) She should begin a course of lorazepam several days before the office moves and gradually increase the dosage as necessary to allow her to stay in the office

6. A 52-year-old woman is brought to the emergency room. Paramedics were called to a department store when the woman complained of severe shortness of breath, dizziness, tremulousness, and diaphoresis. Medical records indicate that in the last few weeks, the woman has presented to the emergency room on several occasions for similar symptoms. Physical examination, routine laboratory studies, cardiac enzymes, and electrocardiogram show unremarkable findings. The patient states that she is becoming increasingly concerned about these episodes, and that she is hesitant to travel alone. Which of the following is the most likely diagnosis?

(A) Factitious disorder
(B) Generalized anxiety disorder
(C) Panic disorder
(D) Social phobia
(E) Specific phobia

Answers and Explanations

1–E. This woman most likely has social phobia, which is characterized by fear and avoidance of social situations, despite a genuine desire for human contact. Low-self esteem is often present. Avoidant personality also is often present and is manifested by avoidance of social contact, loneliness, and low self-esteem. Schizoid personality disorder is characterized by social withdrawal, but loneliness is not symptom. Dependent personality disorder is characterized by poorly controlled anxiety about many problems. Schizophrenia is characterized by psychotic symptoms. Although the woman has some persecutory ideation, it is not of delusional intensity.

2–D This presentation is most suggestive of social phobia. In this case, exposure to public speaking precipitated a panic attack. Panic disorder is also characterized by panic attacks; however, there is no clear precipitant. Specific phobia, situations type, is a less likely diagnosis, because there is no specific cause of the fear other than social exposure. Acute stress disorder is characterized by the presence of intrusive recollections and emotional numbing that follow a severely stressful event Adjustment disorder with anxious mood is characterized by an adaptation problem that follows a psychological stressor, of which there is no evidence in this case.

3–A This case is most suggestive of generalized anxiety disorder, which is characterized by excessive and poorly controlled anxiety. Buspirone is indicated for treatment of this disorder. It does not have sedative effects nor does it cause cognitive impairment.

4–B The mother is suffering from a disturbing obsession, and she most likely has obsessive-compulsive disorder. These obsessions, which an individual rarely acts on, are commonly accompanied by feelings of guilt or shame. Treatment consists of reassurance about the patient's personal integrity and initiation of a serotonin agonist (e.g., fluoxetine, fluvoxamine, clomipramine). Behavioral techniques, such as thought stopping, are also useful. Separating the mother from the daughter may cause serious damage to the parent–child relationship, without offering any significantly increased security for the daughter.

5–D The woman suffers from acrophobia, which is a fear of heights or ledges. This phobia is a specific phobia, situational type. The best treatment for specific phobias is systematic desensitization, a behavioral technique that combines gradual exposure to the feared stimulus with calming activities. In this case, walking a few steps farther on the passageway each day, with the support of a friend, is likely to enable the woman to develop the ability to traverse the passageway within 1 month. Using benzodiazepines is unlikely to decrease phobic avoidance and may cause intolerable cognitive impairment while she is at work. Guided imagery and hypnotherapy are useful techniques for relaxation training and building confidence; however, these techniques are not substitutes for desensitization. This woman's job is a central part of her life; litigation is a stressful undertaking that may destroy her job situation.

6–C This woman's symptoms are most suggestive of panic attacks. Her attacks do not appear to be caused by general medical conditions or substances. She most likely has panic disorder; her attacks are frequent and she is concerned about them. Agoraphobic symptoms commonly develop in individuals with this disorder.

16

Somatoform Disorders

I. Overview

A. Psychosomatic theory. The relationship between psychological events and physical health has been recognized for a long time, but the precise nature of this relationship is unclear.

1. **Early psychodynamic theories** describe **psychosomatic illnesses**, in which specific psychological conflicts in childhood cause specific physical illnesses in adulthood. These illnesses include hypertension, peptic ulcer, colitis, asthma, migraine headaches, and rheumatoid arthritis.

2. **Later psychosomatic theories** de-emphasize relationships between specific conflicts and specific physical diseases and focus on the general relationship between psychological stress and physical symptoms.

3. Aspects of psychosomatic theory remain controversial, including the definitions of psychological stress, the nature of the psychological pathogenesis of physical illness, and the specificity of therapeutic interventions.

B. Several diagnostic groups in the DSM-IV are characterized by psychological problems that cause physical symptoms.

1. **Psychological factors affecting a general medical condition.** Psychological factors (e.g., mental disorders, psychological symptoms, personality traits, behaviors, responses to stress) are temporally associated with the initiation or exacerbation of a general medical condition.

2. **Somatoform disorders** are mental disorders characterized by physical symptoms. These symptoms suggest, but are not fully explained by, general medical conditions. The symptoms are not intentionally produced. Somatoform disorders include:

   a. Somatization disorder (see III)
   b. Undifferentiated somatoform disorder (see IV)
   c. Conversion disorder (see V)
   d. Pain disorder (see VI)
   e. Hypochondriasis (see VII)
   f. Body dysmorphic disorder (see VIII)

3. **Malingering** is the intentional production of false or grossly exaggerated physical or psychological symptoms and is motivated by external incentives. For example, the individual may malinger for financial compensation, to spend time away from work, or to avoid undesired activities (see Chapter 17).

4. **Factitious disorder** involves the intentional production or feigning of physical or psychological symptoms based primarily on a desire to assume a sick role, not as a response to external incentives. (see Chapter 17).

II. Diagnostic Clues to Somatoform Disorders

A. **Presenting complaints** may include dramatic, multiple, and peculiar medical complaints, extreme anxiety about relatively minor medical complaints, peculiar lack of anxiety about serious medical complaints, and medical complaints in the presence of significant psychological issues.

B. **History** may include vague and complex medical problems, multiple past medical workups with inconclusive findings, past or current treatment by many physicians, and extreme anxiety about medical symptoms.

C. **Mental status examination** may show anxiety or peculiar indifference to significant medical complaints.

D. **Physical examination and laboratory studies.** Findings may be inconsistent with medical complaints or known physiologic mechanisms.

III. Somatization Disorder. In this disorder, the individual has a long history of recurrent and multiple medical complaints, starting before 30 years of age, for which medical attention has been sought and that are apparently not fully explained by a general medical condition.

A. **Epidemiology**

1. This disorder **occurs predominantly in women** in most cultures, and the nature of medical complaints may differ by culture.

2. **Prevalence.** Estimates vary widely, but the prevalence is approximately 1% in the general population and 15% in primary care clinics.

3. Somatization disorder and antisocial personality disorder are more common in relatives of individuals with somatization disorder.

B. **Etiology.** This disorder may be associated with early experiences with illness in the patient or the patient's family and abusive childhood experiences.

C. **Diagnosis**

1. **Diagnostic features**

a. The **physical complaints** must include at least four different pain symptoms, two gastrointestinal symptoms, one sexual symptom, and one pseudoneurologic (i.e., motor, sensory, or psychiatric) symptom.

b. The symptoms are not intentionally produced.

2. **Associated features and diagnoses**

    a. The individual often has **numerous and confusing complaints.** Individuals may complain of pain in multiple organ systems. Common complaints include pain, nausea, diarrhea, constipation, sexual dysfunction, motor weakness, dysesthesias, anxiety, and depression.

    b. **Personality pathology**, particularly borderline and antisocial personality traits, is often present and is associated with chronic interpersonal problems and substance abuse.

3. **Differential diagnoses** include general medical conditions with multisystem pathology, schizophrenia with somatic delusions, mood and anxiety disorders with physical complaints, other somatoform disorders, factitious disorder, and malingering.

D. Clinical course

1. The **onset** is usually during adolescence or early adulthood, and the severity of symptoms waxes and wanes, without clear remissions.

2. The course is often complicated by social and occupational problems, difficulties with health care providers, substance abuse, iatrogenic conditions caused by invasive diagnostic procedures, and the misuse of analgesics and sedative—hypnotics.

E. Treatment

1. Careful documentation of the presence of this disorder following adequate medical and psychiatric consultation is essential.

2. Ongoing interactions with clinicians should focus on the psychological distress associated with the symptoms rather than on additional medical workups or treatment.

3. Clinicians should use extreme caution when prescribing medication, particularly analgesics, anxiolytics, and hypnotics.

IV. Undifferentiated Somatoform Disorder. In this disorder, medical complaints are present that are not fully explained by a general medical condition. This disorder is differentiated from somatization disorder by fewer complaints or by complaints that do not follow the pattern of somatization disorder.

A. Epidemiology. Although the prevalence of this disorder is probably high, there is limited data.

B. The **etiology** may involve worry or stress.

C. Diagnosis

1. **Diagnostic features** include the presence of one or more physical complaints that last for at least 6 months and are not fully explained by a general medical condition.

    a. The symptoms are not better accounted for by somatization disorder, other somatoform disorders, or other mental disorders.

    b. The symptoms are not intentionally produced.

2. **Associated features and diagnoses**

    a. Complaints often involve chronic fatigue, appetite loss, vaguely localized pain, and urinary problems.

    b. A significant degree of anxiety or depression may be present.

3. **Differential diagnoses** include other somatization disorders, major depressive disorder, anxiety disorders, adjustment disorders, factitious disorder, and malingering.

D. The **clinical course** is variable. In some individuals, medical complaints are chronic; in others, medical complaints are acutely associated with stress.

E. **Treatment** (see III E)

V. Conversion Disorder

V. Conversion Disorder. In this disorder, the individual has sensory or motor symptoms that suggest a general medical condition; however, the symptoms are related to stress or conflict.

A. **Epidemiology**

1. This disorder occurs at a **1:5 male to female ratio**. The prevalence of this disorder may be about 0.3% of the population, but data is unreliable.
2. Conversion disorder is more common in nonindustrial societies.
3. Conversion disorder is more common in relatives of individuals with this disorder.

B. **Etiology**

1. The postulated psychodynamic theory, which describes the conversion of psychological conflicts into symbolic physical symptoms, is no longer a fully accepted etiology. However, psychological stress is believed to play an important role in this disorder.
2. Some studies suggest there are various abnormalities of central nervous system (CNS) function during conversion episodes.

C. **Diagnosis**

1. **Diagnostic features** include paralysis, sensory symptoms that include more than pain, or seizure-like symptoms that are not fully explained known pathophysiology or cultural behavior.

   a. Symptoms are temporally related to psychological conflicts.
   b. Symptoms are not intentionally produced.

2. **Subtypes** include:

   a. With motor symptoms
   b. With sensory symptoms
   c. With seizures or convulsions
   d. With mixed presentation

3. **Associated features**

   a. Personality pathology, particularly histrionic, antisocial, and dependent personality disorders; major depressive disorder; and dissociative disorder are common in individuals with conversion disorder.
   b. Peculiar mood and affect may be noted, and it may present as inappropriate blandness ("la belle indifférence") or histrionics.
   c. Conversion disorder may occur in the presence of genuine medical conditions.

4. **Differential diagnoses** include general medical conditions, particularly occult neurologic disease (e.g., multiple sclerosis), factitious disorder, and malingering.

D. **Clinical course**

1. The **onset** is usually sudden, occurs during adolescence or early adulthood, and is associated with psychological stress.
2. **Motor symptoms** include paralysis of the extremities, and **sensory symptoms** usually involve anesthesia or visual disturbances.
3. The **duration** is usually less than 2 weeks, and recurrence is common.

E. **Treatment.** It is critical to rule out general medical conditions that may be responsible for symptoms.

1. **Suggestion and relaxation techniques** are sometimes used to restore motor or sensory function during acute episodes. Adjunctive use of barbiturates (e.g., amobarbital sodium) is no longer commonly employed; however, benzodiazepines may be prescribed if there are prominent anxiety symptoms.
2. **Long-term treatment** may include **psychotherapy** directed at resolving associated psychological conflicts.

VI. **Pain Disorder.** In this disorder, an individual has complaints of pain that are strongly influenced by psychological factors.

A. **Epidemiology**

1. This disorder is common in clinic populations, but estimates of the prevalence vary widely.
2. Depressive disorders, substance-related disorders, and pain disorders are more common in relatives of individual with pain disorder.

B. **Etiology.** It has been postulated that assuming a sick role helps the individual manage psychological conflicts.

C. **Diagnosis**

1. **Diagnostic features.** The individual has significant pain that is influenced by psychological factors regarding its onset, severity, exacerbation, or maintenance. The symptoms are not intentionally produced.
2. **Subtypes** include pain disorder associated with psychological factors and pain disorder associated with both psychological factors and a general medical condition. This disorder is also classified as either acute or chronic.
3. **Associated features and diagnoses**

   a. **General medical conditions** that are most commonly present include musculoskeletal conditions, neuropathies, and malignancies.
   b. Substance-related disorders and depressive mood disorders are common.
4. **Differential diagnoses** include somatization disorder, factitious disorder, and malingering.

D. Clinical course

1. The **onset, course,** and **recovery** are variable.
2. Interpersonal pathology and social and occupational problems often develop because of limitations of activity caused by the complaints of pain.
3. Substance abuse and dependence often supervene.

E. Treatment includes:

1. Detoxification from analgesic and other drugs if necessary
2. Pain management training
3. Resumption of normal activities
4. Psychotherapy directed at resolving underlying psychological conflicts

VII. Hypochondriasis. In this disorder, an individual is preoccupied with the fear of having a serious illness. The fear is based on the individual's misinterpretation of physical signs or symptoms, and the individual is not relieved by a physician's reassurance following a thorough evaluation.

A. Epidemiology. This disorder occurs at **a 1:1 male to female ratio.** The **prevalence** in the general population is unknown; however, in general medical practice, the prevalence is 5%.

B. Etiology. Displaced anxiety is a common psychodynamic explanation for this disorder.

C. Diagnosis

1. **Diagnostic features.** The preoccupation lasts for at least 6 months and is not of delusional intensity.
2. A **subtype** of this disorder is hypochondriasis with poor insight, in which the individual's belief about the reality of his physical problem has a delusional intensity.
3. **Associated features**

   a. Comorbid anxiety and depressive disorders are common.
   b. The individual may have had a serious childhood illness. Or, a family member may have had a serious illness during the individual's childhood.

4. **Differential diagnoses** include occult general medical conditions, normal health concerns, and delusional disorder, somatic type.

D. Clinical course

1. The onset is commonly during early adulthood but is variable.
2. Symptoms wax and wane, often in association with psychological stress.
3. Complete remission may occur, particularly in cases with a sudden onset.

E. Treatment includes psychotherapy directed at ameliorating psychological stress and resolving underlying psychological conflicts. Treatment of comorbid anxiety and depression is often necessary.

VIII. Body Dysmorphic Disorder. In this disorder, a normal-appearing individual has an excessive preoccupation with an imagined physical defect.

   A. Epidemiology. This disorder occurs at a **1:1 male to female ratio**. Cultural influences on the perception of physical characteristics may affect the presentation of symptoms.

   B. Diagnosis

   1. The preoccupation is not better explained by another mental disorder (e.g., avoidant personality disorder, anorexia nervosa).

   2. Associated features

   a. Patients may have minor physical anomalies.

   b. This disorder may be associated with additional diagnoses of delusional disorder, somatic type; major depressive disorder; social phobia, and obsessive-compulsive disorder.

   3. Differential diagnoses include normal concerns about appearance, anorexia nervosa, social phobia, avoidant personality disorder, and gender identity disorder.

   C. Clinical course

   1. The **onset** is usually during adolescence and may be gradual or sudden.

   2. The severity of the individual's preoccupation may fluctuate and is often kept secret.

   3. The exact nature of concern with appearance may vary over time.

   4. The individual may be preoccupied with checking his appearance and may engage in elaborate grooming or dressing behaviors to hide his perceived defect. Social avoidance may become severe and may cause interpersonal and occupational problems.

   5. Some individuals seek cosmetic surgery to correct their imagined defects; however, this does not usually resolve symptoms.

   D. Treatment. There is no definitive treatment for body dysmorphic disorder. Comorbid depression and obsession with physical anomalies may be ameliorated with use of serotonin reuptake inhibitors (e.g., fluoxetine).

Review Test

Directions: Each of the numbered items or incomplete statements in this section is followed by answers or by completions of the statement. Select the ONE lettered answer or completion that is BEST in each case.

Questions 1–3

A 37-year-old woman complains of persistent headaches, neck pain, intermittent lower abdominal cramps, "carpal tunnel" pain, nausea, food allergies, sexual aversion, and persistent tingling in her extremities upon awakening. According to her medical records, extensive physical and laboratory assessments have been unremarkable. The woman says that she has been in severe physical distress for more than 7 years and does not know how much longer she can bear these symptoms.

1. Which of the following is the most likely diagnosis?

(A) Body dysmorphic disorder
(B) Conversion disorder
(C) Hypochondriasis
(D) Pain disorder
(E) Somatization disorder

2. Which of the following associated conditions is this patient likely to have?

(A) Decreased serotonin levels
(B) Hallucinosis
(C) Substance abuse
(D) Schizoid personality disorder
(E) Somatic delusions

3. Which of the following steps is most appropriate for the management of this patient's case?

(A) Explain to the patient that her symptoms will gradually diminish and caution her not to overuse medical resources
(B) Explain to the patient that her symptoms will gradually diminish and prescribe a placebo
(C) Explain to the patient that she has no acute findings and schedule a follow-up appointment in 1 month
(D) Explain to the patient that her symptoms are caused by a psychological conflict and refer her to a psychiatrist
(E) Explain to the patient that she has no acute findings and refer her to a psychiatrist

4. A 17-year-old girl is brought to the emergency room by her parents because of sudden blindness. The patient is from an intensely religious background. She states that she cannot see anything, and she believes that her condition is divine punishment for her sinful behavior. She also states that she gracefully accepts "God's will." Physical examination shows intact visual reflexes. Which of the following is the most likely diagnosis?

(A) Conversion disorder
(B) Delusional disorder
(C) Factitious disorder
(D) Hypochondriasis
(E) Malingering

5. A 47-year-old man is hit by a forklift at the warehouse in which he works, injuring his knee. After successful surgical repair of his knee, the patient continues to complain of significant pain that prevents him from returning to work. Physical examination and imaging studies are unremarkable. He is unable to comfortably support his family with his disability income. The family has been forced to reduce their expenses, which has caused a strain on his marriage. The patient has stopped participating in weekend sports because of his pain, and he spends most of his time watching television, consuming analgesics, and drinking beer. Which of the following is the most likely diagnosis?

(A) Factitious disorder
(B) Hypochondriasis
(C) Malingering
(D) Pain disorder
(E) Somatization disorder

6. A 63-year-old man undergoes a left nephrectomy for a tumor that is subsequently determined to be benign. Following his operation and uneventful recovery, the man becomes preoccupied with the idea that he faces renal failure and worries when his urine is more or less yellow-colored than is typical. He insists on having weekly renal function tests. Although his physician reassures him that he will function well with one healthy kidney, the individual is convinced that he will have kidney failure. Which of the following is the most likely diagnosis?

(A) Body dysmorphic disorder
(B) Delusional disorder, somatic type
(C) Hypochondriasis
(D) Obsessive-compulsive disorder
(E) Somatization disorder

7. A 45-year-old man refuses to cut his shoulder-length hair for his new job and his employer threatens to dismiss him. The man hesitantly admits to his employer that he wears his hair long to cover what he considers are extremely prominent ears. The man believes that if his ears were visible, he would be ridiculed. The man actually has very mildly prominent ears that would not attract attention. Which of the following is the most likely diagnosis?

(A) Body dysmorphic disorder
(B) Delusional disorder, somatic type
(C) Hypochondriasis
(D) Malingering
(E) Somatization disorder

Answers and Explanations

1–E. This woman most likely has somatization disorder, which is characterized by multiple somatic complaints of pain and dysfunction in several organ systems. Body dysmorphic disorder involves misinterpretation of physical appearance. Conversion disorder involves a loss of sensory or motor function. Hypochondriasis is characterized by a belief that one has a serious disease; this belief is based on misinterpretation of physical symptoms. In pain disorder, an individual has a predominant focus on pain without other prominent physical complaints.

2–C. Substance abuse, including misusing medications, is a common associated finding in individuals with somatization disorder. Decreased serotonin levels are associated with violent suicide. Hallucinosis and somatic delusions are associated with psychotic disorders; however, there is no evidence of psychosis in this woman's case. Although histrionic, antisocial, and borderline personality disorders are associated with somatization disorder, schizoid personality disorder is not.

3–C. Management of a patient with somatization disorder includes careful documentation of symptoms and diagnosis in the patient's medical record and routine follow-up appointments in a general medical clinic. This course of treatment minimizes unnecessary diagnostic procedures, decreases the costs of emergency visits, and may improve the patient's sense of well being. Placebos, warnings, and psychological formulations have not proved effective for treatment of this disorder. Referring the patient to a psychiatrist may be helpful if the patient is extremely anxious or disturbed, or if there is uncertainty about the diagnosis of somatization disorder or other comorbid psychopathology.

4–A. The patient's symptoms include vision loss that does not appear to have a physiologic cause. It is likely that her condition is associated with a psychological conflict, which is characteristic of conversion disorder. Her emotional state is unusually bland ("la belle indifference"), which is an associated symptom of conversion disorder. Her symptoms are not volitional and do not appear to be produced for external gain or to assume the sick role; thus, factitious disorder and malingering are less likely diagnoses. Delusional disorder is likely if the patient presents with patently false beliefs. In this case, her beliefs are culturally appropriate religious convictions. Hypochondriasis is unlikely because she is not preoccupied with her deficits.

5–D. This patient most likely has pain disorder. His pain appears disproportionate to his physical lesions, which suggests that psychological factors may be contributing to his condition. However, chronic pain caused by only physical disease cannot be ruled out in this case. Other features of his presentation, including musculoskeletal disease, misuse of analgesics, marital problems, and alcohol abuse, are common in individuals with pain disorder. Treatment should include cessation of analgesic use. Also, the patient should return to work, even in a limited capacity, and begin counseling to reduce stress and resolve psychological conflicts.

6–C. Despite adequate assessment and reassurance, this man is not convinced that he can survive with one kidney and is worried. He most likely has hypochondriasis, which is characterized by a preoccupation with having a serious disease. The preoccupation is based on a misinterpretation of physical signs, and the individual is unresponsive to physician reassurance following a thorough evaluation. Although his worry may be considered an obsession, obsessive-compulsive disorder is not diagnosed if the nature of the obsession is purely somatic. Delusional disorder may be considered for a diagnosis if the patient's unrealistic belief has a delusional intensity. Body dysmorphic disorder involves a preoccupation with one's physical appearance. In somatization disorder, an individual has multiple physical complaints that involve many organ systems.

7–A. The man's symptoms suggest that he has body dysmorphic disorder, which is characterized by grossly misperceiving a minor physical anomaly. In this disorder, the individual's belief is not baseless and bizarre enough to be considered delusional. In hypochondriasis, the individual misinterprets the meaning of a physical symptom. Malingering is an unlikely diagnosis because the individual has no obvious external incentives for his behavior. Somatization disorder presents with multiple physical complaints.

17
Factitious Disorder and Malingering

I. **Overview**. Both factitious disorder and malingering involve the intentional production or feigning of medical symptoms.

   A. **Definitions**

      1. **Factitious disorder** is characterized by the intentional production or feigning of physical or psychological symptoms in **an attempt to assume the sick role**. This disorder was formerly called Munchausen syndrome.
      2. **Malingering** is the intentional production of false or grossly exaggerated physical or psychological symptoms and is **motivated by external incentives.**

   B. **Complications**

      1. Factitious disorder and malingering often provoke anger and exasperation in health care professionals, which may lead to suboptimal care and failure to diagnose general medical conditions.
      2. Some patients may harm themselves during attempts to produce symptoms, may inappropriately use medical and financial resources, and may suffer iatrogenic injury.

II. **Diagnostic Clues**

   A. **Presenting complaints** may include dramatic, peculiar, and changing medical complaints and medical complaints associated with potential environmental incentives for illness.
   B. **History** may include vague and complex medical problems, guardedness about revealing past complaints or medical assessments, multiple past medical workups with inconclusive findings, past or current treatment by many physicians, history of signing out of hospitals against medical advice, and noncompliance with diagnostic procedures.
   C. **Mental status examination** may show anxiety, peculiar indifference to significant medical complaints, and extreme familiarity with medical terminology and procedures.

D. **Physical examination and laboratory studies.** Findings may be inconsistent with medical complaints or with known physiologic mechanisms, and there may be signs of multiple surgical procedures.

III. Factitious Disorder

A. **Epidemiology.** This disorder is more common in men.

B. **Etiology.** Psychodynamic theories suggest that this behavior represents an expression of anger against authority figures or dependency needs.

C. **Diagnosis**

  1. **Subtypes** include:

     a. With predominantly psychological signs and symptoms
     b. With predominantly physical signs and symptoms
     c. With combined psychological and physical signs and symptoms

  2. **Associated features**

     a. The individual may have **iatrogenic conditions** caused by previous invasive diagnostic procedures or treatment of factitious symptoms.
     b. The individual may have **physical trauma** or **toxicosis** resulting from attempts to produce factitious symptoms.
     c. **Coexisting personality disorders**, particularly antisocial and dependent personality disorders, are common.
     d. The individual's familiarity with medical treatment and terminology may be remarkable because of a previous medical illness or an occupational association (e.g., the individual works in the health care field).
     e. **Munchausen syndrome by proxy.** This behavior, which is associated with factitious disorder, involves the production or feigning of symptoms in another individual. For example, a parent may deliberately induce symptoms in a child.

  3. **Differential diagnoses** include actual general medical conditions, somatoform disorders, other mental disorders, and malingering.

D. **Clinical course**

  1. The **onset** is usually during early adulthood. It often occurs following hospitalization for either a general medical condition or mental disorder.
  2. The **course** is usually chronic, and the individual may be hospitalized repeatedly on the basis of factitious symptoms. The individual may travel extensively, so that he can receive medical treatment where his previous history is unknown.
  3. Substance-induced mental disorders may occur because of the individual's attempts to produce psychological symptoms.

E. **Treatment**

  1. Individuals with this disorder are usually highly resistant to treatment for their primary condition. They often refuse to acknowledge that they intentionally produced their symptoms, despite being confronted with overwhelming evidence.

2. **Accurate diagnosis, careful documentation,** and **effective communication among health care providers** may decrease iatrogenic complications caused by unnecessary diagnostic procedures or treatment.

IV. Malingering

A. **Epidemiology.** Malingering occurs predominantly in men.
B. **Etiology.** By definition, the individual's motivation to malinger is an external incentive.
C. **Diagnosis**

1. **Associated features and diagnoses**

   a. There are external incentives (e.g., monetary reward, avoidance of unwanted duties, avoidance of blame or punishment, obtaining drugs or benefits) for the individual's medical conditions.

   b. **Antisocial personality disorder** is common.

2. **Differential diagnoses** include actual general medical conditions, factitious disorder, conversion disorders, other somatoform disorders, other mental disorders, and noncompliance with treatment for other reasons.

D. **Clinical course**

1. The **onset** of malingering is in response to environmental incentives. The behavior remits when external incentives are eliminated. Sometimes malingering may represent adaptive and nonpathologic behavior.

2. The individual is often uncooperative during diagnostic evaluation or treatment.

3. The individual's disability claims are often exaggerated relative to objective findings or subjective medical complaints.

E. **Treatment**

1. Malingering behavior is controlled by eliminating the external incentives that motivate the production of symptoms.

2. Appropriate diagnostic assessment and careful documentation are necessary to accurately diagnose malingering, prevent iatrogenic conditions that may be caused by unnecessary treatment, and rule out actual medical conditions.

Review Test

Directions: Each of the following items or incomplete statements in this section is followed by answers or by completions of the statement. Select the ONE lettered answer or completion that is BEST in each case.

1. A 23-year-old woman complains of severe neck pain following a minor traffic accident in which her car was hit from behind. She claims the pain prevents her from engaging in even light physical activity. After threatening litigation, her attorney secures a sizable settlement from the insurance company to compensate her for time lost from work. She is a waitress and an aspiring actress. While participating in an aerobics class, the woman tells her friend that she greatly exaggerated her pain to "get a paid vacation, courtesy of the insurance industry." Which of the following is the most likely diagnosis?

(A) Antisocial personality disorder
(B) Factitious disorder
(C) Malingering
(D) Pain disorder with physical and psychological factors
(E) Psychological factors contributing to physical illness

2. A 45-year-old man is brought to the emergency room by paramedics after he complains of dizziness and headache. Emergency room examination shows anisocoria, with a left pupillary diameter of 2 mm and a right pupillary diameter of 5 mm. The patient denies any precipitating events or general medical conditions. While awaiting further examination, he is observed surreptitiously placing eye drops in his right eye. When questioned about this action, he becomes angry, denies the behavior, and abruptly leaves the hospital. Which of the following is the most likely diagnosis?

(A) Conversion disorder
(B) Delusional disorder, somatic type
(C) Dependent personality disorder
(D) Factitious disorder
(E) Malingering

3. A 6-year-old child is brought to a physician by her mother. The mother states that the child has had intractable diarrhea for several hours. The mother denies any knowledge of the child ingesting unusual substances. Physical examination and laboratory studies show mild dehydration. After subsequent extensive questioning by the physician, the mother tearfully admits that she gave the child an over-the-counter laxative because she was concerned that the child was constipated and uncomfortable. The mother says that this is the first time she has given the child a laxative and that she was too frightened and embarrassed to initially admit it. She emphatically denies any intent to harm the child. Which of the following actions is the best initial intervention?

(A) Educate the mother about laxative use in children and schedule a follow-up appointment with a social service agency
(B) Hospitalize the mother in a psychiatric unit and summon relatives to assume temporary custody of the child
(C) Notify law enforcement authorities
(D) Refer the mother and child for outpatient counseling
(E) Separate the child from the mother and notify child protective services

4. A 25-year-old woman with epilepsy has a witnessed tonic-clonic seizure with urinary incontinence. She also has minor lacerations caused by biting her tongue and striking her head on the ground during the seizure. Laboratory studies show subtherapeutic blood levels of her prescribed anticonvulsant medication. In the hospital, a nurse sees the patient spit recently administered anticonvulsant medication into the toilet. When the patient is confronted, she demands to leave the hospital. Which of the following is the most likely diagnosis?

(A) Conversion disorder with seizures or convulsions
(B) Factitious disorder
(C) Malingering
(D) Pseudo seizures
(E) Psychotic disorder due to epilepsy

5. A 30-year-old man presents to the emergency room with tachycardia and diaphoresis. He tells the examining physician that he took poison and refuses to disclose what type of poison he ingested. He says, "If you're such a great doctor, why don't you figure out what I took. Otherwise, I don't mind dying." Which of the following is the best initial management of this case?

(A) Admit the patient voluntarily only if he divulges the substance he ingested
(B) Admit the patient voluntarily regardless of the information he does or does not provide
(C) Admit the patient involuntarily and obtain toxicologic studies
(D) Discharge the patient immediately
(E) Summon law enforcement authorities to detain the patient

Answers and Explanations

1–C. This woman is malingering because she has grossly exaggerated her symptoms to obtain financial compensation. Although she may have other antisocial traits, there is not enough information in this case to determine if she has antisocial personality disorder. In pain disorder, the individual actually experiences pain. Because the woman was able to participate in an aerobics class, it is unlikely that she was actually experiencing severe neck pain. Although malingering may play a role in psychological factors contributing to a physical illness, it does not assume a central role.

2–D. It is likely that this man placed mydriatic medication, such as atropine, into his right eye to induce anisocoria. Because this behavior is volitional and there is no known external incentive for his actions, factitious disorder is a more likely diagnosis than malingering. When he is confronted, he becomes angry, denies his actions, and leaves the situation, which is a typical response in factitious disorder. Because his symptoms are intentionally produced, he does not have conversion disorder. He shows no evidence of delusional beliefs. Although dependent and antisocial personality disorders are more common in individuals with factitious disorder, there is insufficient evidence in this case to make these diagnoses.

3–A. The child's symptoms were induced by the mother; however, it is likely that the mother did not intend to cause severe diarrhea. Therefore, parent education is the most appropriate intervention in this case. However, further investigation should be pursued to rule out neglect or child abuse. These types of child abuse cases are sometimes called Munchausen syndrome by proxy and are associated with factitious disorder.

4–B. This woman's signs and symptoms suggest that she intentionally produced a seizure by not taking her anticonvulsant medication, which is suggestive of factitious disorder. Factitious symptoms are commonly produced by individuals who have a general medical condition, which often complicates diagnosis of factitious disorder. Before concluding that this patient has factitious disorder, the clinician should explore other reasons for noncompliance with medication, such as ignorance or the presence of unpleasant adverse effects.

5–C. The patient has deliberately produced symptoms and is complicating the diagnostic assessment. Although this situation is distressing to health care personnel, appropriate treatment must be initiated. This patient's potentially self-destructive behavior and veiled suicidal rumination suggest that involuntary detention and treatment are necessary.

18

Dissociative Disorders

I. Overview

A. Definition. Dissociation is the fragmentation or separation of aspects of consciousness, including memory, identity, and perception.

B. Forgetfulness and dissociation. The pattern of forgetfulness is not random.

1. Typically, individuals remember things that are significant (e.g., work skills, their spouse's birthday), things that have many associated reminders (e.g., date for filing income tax returns, advertising slogans), and things that are pleasantly or unpleasantly emotionally charged.

2. Individuals tend to forget minor details, especially when the details have little association to other information (e.g., the names of the bones of the wrist). Mnemonics are used to lessen this effect.

3. **Dissociation.** Individuals may forget things that are particularly anxiety provoking, such as events that occurred during periods of threat or stress (e.g., how one managed to escape from a burning building).

C. Psychodynamic theory

1. In exploring the past memories of his patients, Freud noted that sometimes events that were highly significant and emotionally charged were forgotten, often to a striking degree. These events were often associated with emotional conflict and resultant anxiety.

2. **Defense mechanism of dissociation.** Psychodynamic theory suggests that the psyche protects itself from anxiety by banishing the memory of anxiety-provoking events or feelings from consciousness. This process represents a dissociation of some elements of consciousness from the whole consciousness.

D. Normal dissociative phenomena

1. Typically, consciousness seems relatively integrated throughout our lives, and individuals have some unified and enduring sense of self.

2. Individuals unknowingly partition off some elements of consciousness (e.g., memories, aspects of personality, perceptions) at any given time. For example, an individual may absently drive her car several miles past a planned stop and then wonder who was driving the car while she was lost in thought.

3. Because individuals tend to exclude anxiety-provoking thoughts, memories, or feelings and remember these unpleasant things less well, what may appear to be ordinary forgetfulness may actually have more significance. For example, forgetting a relative's birthday could involve emotionally conflicting feelings about that individual.

E. **Dissociative pathology**. Some degree of dissociation is always present; however, if an individual's consciousness becomes too fragmented, it may pathologically interfere with the sense of self and ability to adapt.

1. Dissociative pathology is more likely to occur during periods of great stress or fatigue.
2. Some individuals may be predisposed to developing pathologic dissociation because of early psychologically traumatic experiences.
3. Dissociative phenomena may be seen in a number of mental disorders, including:

a. **Dissociative disorders**, which includes **dissociative amnesia, dissociative fugue, dissociative identity disorder,** and **depersonalization disorder** (see III—VI)
b. **Conversion disorder**
c. **Somatization disorder**
d. **Acute stress disorder**
e. **Posttraumatic stress disorder (PTSD)**

II. Diagnostic Clues to Dissociative Disorders

A. **Presenting complaints** may include amnesia, personality change, erratic behavior, odd inner experiences (e.g., flashbacks, déjà vu), and confusion.
B. **History** may include peculiar forms of amnesia, particularly selective and generalized amnesia, recurrent episodes of amnesia, markedly different behavior at different times, unexplained absences for periods of time, and episodes of subjective perception of altered consciousness.
C. **Mental status examination** may show gaps in memory and suggestibility (e.g., susceptibility to hypnotic suggestions by the examiner).

III. Dissociative Amnesia

A. **Definition.** Dissociative amnesia is characterized by episodes in which the individual is unable to recall important and often emotionally charged memories. The memory disturbance is too significant to be attributed to ordinary forgetfulness.
B. **Epidemiology.** There is an increasing frequency of diagnosis of this disorder, which may represent either an increase in prevalence or an increase in diagnostic interest.
C. **Etiology** (see I C, E 2)
D. **Diagnosis.** The symptoms do not occur exclusively during the course of another dissociative disorders, stress disorders, or somatization disorder.

1. **Associated features**

a. Impulsiveness and interpersonal problems are often present.
b. Suggestibility is often high in these patients.
c. Mood disorders, conversion disorder, and personality disorders are commonly present.

2. **Differential diagnoses** include amnestic disorder due to a general medical condition, substance-induced amnestic disorder, delirium, dementia, dissociative fugue, dissociate identity disorder, PTSD, acute stress disorder, somatization disorder, factitious disorder, and malingering.

E. Clinical course

1. The **onset** is usually detected retrospectively by the discovery of memory gaps. The **duration** of memory gaps is extremely variable, ranging from minutes to years.

2. **Types.** The nature of the amnesia may vary.

   a. **Localized.** The individual has amnesia for events that occurred during a specific period of time.

   b. **Selective.** The individual has amnesia for only specific events that occurred in a circumscribed period of time.

   c. **Generalized.** The individual has amnesia for all events of his entire life.

   d. **Continuous.** The individual has amnesia for all events from a particular time to the present.

   e. **Systematized.** The individual has amnesia for only certain types of information (e.g., for a specific person).

3. The amnesia may suddenly or gradually remit, particularly when the traumatic circumstance resolves. Some amnesia may become chronic.

4. Future amnestic episodes are likely to occur.

F. Treatment includes:

1. Careful diagnostic evaluation for general medical conditions (e.g., head trauma, seizures, cerebrovascular disease) or substances (e.g., anxiolytic and hypnotic medications, alcohol) that may cause amnesia

2. Hypnosis, suggestion, and relaxation techniques

3. Removal of the patient from the stressful situation (e.g., a soldier with dissociative amnesia is moved from the field hospital to a distant location)

4. Psychotherapy directed at resolving underlying emotional stress

IV. Dissociative Fugue

A. Definition. The DSM-IV describes dissociative fugue as sudden, unexpected travel, accompanied by the inability to remember one's past and by confusion about personal identity, or by the assumption of a new identity.

B. Epidemiology. The **prevalence** of this disorder is 0.2%.

C. Etiology (see I C, E 2)

D. Diagnosis. The episodes do not occur exclusively during the course of dissociative identity disorder.

1. **Associated features**

   a. Mood disorders, PTSD, and substance-induced disorders are common comorbid conditions.

   b. A history of acute or chronic stressful events preceding the onset of symptoms may be present.

2. **Differential diagnoses** include dissociative symptoms due to general medical conditions (e.g., complex partial seizures), dissociative amnesia, dissociative identity disorder, psychotic disorders, factitious disorder, and malingering.

E. Clinical course

1. The onset, which is usually sudden, often follows a stressful life event.
2. Most episodes are isolated and last from hours to months.
3. **Resolution** is usually rapid, but amnesia may persist.

F. Treatment (see III F)

V. Dissociative Identity Disorder

A. Definition. Formerly termed multiple personality disorder, the DSM-IV describes dissociative identity disorder as the presence of multiple, distinct personalities that recurrently control the individual's behavior and is accompanied by the individual's failure to recall important personal information.

B. Epidemiology. This disorder has been reported more frequently in recent years, which may suggest an increased prevalence.

1. This disorder is more common in women.
2. Dissociative identity disorder is more common in relatives of individuals with this disorder.

C. Etiology

1. **Childhood sexual abuse** and its resultant dissociative defense mechanisms may be a cause of this disorder.
2. Some clinicians believe that a patient's susceptibility to suggestions of multiple personalities by the evaluator (i.e., suggestibility) plays a causative role.

D. Associated features and diagnoses

1. Borderline personality disorder and PTSD are often present.
2. Major depressive disorder and other mood disorders, substance-related disorders, sexual disorders, and eating disorders are sometimes present.
3. A history of childhood sexual abuse is often elicited, and suggestibility is common (see V C).
4. **Differential diagnoses** include borderline personality disorder and other personality disorders, bipolar disorder with rapid cycling, factitious disorder, and malingering.

E. Clinical course

1. The **onset** is usually occult, and the clinical presentation is noted several years later when disturbances in interpersonal functioning are present.
2. During the course of the disorder, individuals often have chaotic interpersonal relationships, demonstrate impulsivity and self-destructive behavior, make suicide attempts, and abuse substances.
3. The presence of distinct personalities is often subtle; in some cases, it is discovered only during treatment for associated symptoms.
4. **Symptoms** may fluctuate or be continuous.

F. Treatment. Psychotherapy may be directed at discovering psychologically traumatic memories from childhood and resolving the associated emotional conflict. Through psychotherapy, dissociated elements of consciousness are reintegrated.

VI. Depersonalization Disorder

A. Definition. The DSM-IV describes depersonalization disorder as the persistent or recurrent feeling of being detached from one's mental processes or body, accompanied by intact sense of reality.

B. Epidemiology

1. Although the prevalence of this disorder is unknown, individual episodes of depersonalization are common.
2. In many cultural rituals, symptoms of depersonalization are part of trance-like states.

C. Associated features and diagnoses

1. Symptoms of **anxiety** are often present during episodes.
2. **Derealization.** The individual's perception of the environment is often distorted or strange during episodes of depersonalization. For example, an individual with this disorder may be suddenly engulfed by an overwhelming sense of detachment while walking through a shopping mall and perceive the speech of those around him as unintelligible.

D. Differential diagnoses include substance-induced mental disorders with dissociative symptoms, including intoxication, withdrawal, and hallucinogen-induced persisting perceptual disorder; panic disorder; acute stress disorder; and PTSD.

E. Clinical course

1. The **onset** is usually in adolescence or early adulthood. In some cases, stressful events may precede the onset of the disorder or may exacerbate symptoms.
2. Presenting symptoms are usually accompanied by anxiety, panic, or depression.
3. The **course** is usually chronic, with exacerbations and remissions. The **duration** of episodes ranges from seconds to years.

F. Treatment. Psychotherapy and, occasionally, pharmacotherapy directed at decreasing anxiety are used to treat this disorder.

Review Test

Directions: Each of the numbered items or incomplete statements in this section is followed by answers or by completions of the statement. Select the ONE lettered answer or completion that is BEST in each case.

1. A 19-year-old man is brought to the emergency room by volunteers from a homeless shelter. The man claims that he cannot remember who he is. He says that he found himself in Los Angeles, but that he cannot remember where he comes from, the circumstances of his trip, or any other information about his life. He has neither identification nor money, but he has a bus ticket from New York. Which of the following is the most likely diagnosis?

(A) Depersonalization disorder
(B) Dissociative amnesia
(C) Dissociative fugue
(D) Dissociative identity disorder
(E) Substance-induced amnestic disorder

2. A 34-year-old woman survives the sinking of a ferryboat and claims no memory for the events surrounding the disaster. She cannot explain how she got ashore. Physical examination is unremarkable, and her cognitive ability is intact. She is distraught about the unknown fate of her husband, who was also aboard the ship, and is tormented by nightmares for the next several nights. Which of the following is the most likely diagnosis?

(A) Amnesia due to transient cerebral anoxia
(B) Dissociative amnesia
(C) Dissociative fugue
(D) Dissociative identity disorder
(E) Factitious disorder

3. A 39-year-old woman complains of impulsivity and moodiness. She says that her friends and coworkers often refer to personal incidents during which she was present, but for which she has no memory. She is hypnotized during a diagnostic evaluation and suddenly assumes a childlike voice, referring to herself in the third person. In subsequent hypnosis sessions, she describes episodes of sexual abuse by her now-deceased parents during her childhood. In an unhypnotized state, she is unable to recall these episodes of sexual abuse. Which of the following is the most likely diagnosis?

(A) Dissociative amnesia
(B) Dissociative fugue
(C) Dissociative identity disorder
(D) Malingering
(E) Posttraumatic stress disorder

4. A 41-year-old male business executive describes a highly disturbing episode of confusion during a tense business negotiating session. After 4 hours of heated discussion, he experienced a sense of physically floating far from the meeting and had difficulty understanding what the distant voices were saying. He said his body felt light and that he was acutely aware of his breathing. He has subsequently experienced several more similar episodes but with less intensity. Which of the following is the most likely diagnosis?

(A) Depersonalization disorder
(B) Dissociative amnesia
(C) Dissociative fugue
(D) Factitious disorder
(E) Brief psychotic disorder

Answers and Explanations

1–C. The symptoms of amnesia, unexplained travel, and identity confusion are most suggestive of dissociative fugue. Because of the generalized nature of his amnesia, substance-induced amnestic disorder an unlikely diagnosis. There is insufficient evidence of distinct alternative personalities to diagnose dissociative identity disorder.

2–B. Localized amnesia following a stressful event is most suggestive of dissociative amnesia. In this case, the woman also has accompanying anxiety and nightmares, both of which are commonly present with dissociative amnesia. Amnesia due to transient cerebral anoxia is a less likely diagnosis because the woman has no physical findings and her cognitive abilities are intact. Dissociative fugue and dissociative identity disorder are diagnosed only in the presence of identity disturbances. Factitious disorder is unlikely because there is neither evidence of intentional production of symptoms nor gratification from assuming the sick role.

3–C. The symptoms of distinct personalities accompanied by significant memory impairment is most suggestive of dissociative identity disorder. The identity disturbance that accompanies the amnesia is not fully explained by dissociative amnesia. The individual did not experience unusual travel, which would suggest dissociative fugue. Malingering is unlikely because there are no obvious external incentives for her symptoms. Posttraumatic stress disorder may be associated with dissociative identity disorder; however, in this case, there are no symptoms of intrusive recollections or anxiety.

4–A. The man's peculiar sense of detachment, particularly in association with a stressful circumstance, is most suggestive of depersonalization disorder. Symptoms of derealization (e.g., distorted sounds) are also present. Because the individual does not have memory disturbances, dissociative amnesia and dissociative fugue are less likely diagnoses. Factitious disorder is an unlikely diagnosis because there is no evidence of intentionally produced symptoms. Brief psychotic disorder is a less likely diagnosis because the individual's distorted perceptions are not accompanied by an inability to assess reality.

19
Sexual Disorders

I. Overview

A. Human sexuality. In addition to its reproductive function, human sexuality has important psychological and social implications.

    1. Sexual function involves many biologic systems, including the endocrine system, central nervous system (CNS), sensory systems, and the neuromuscular system.

    2. Sexuality is strongly influenced by the individual's previous learning. Adverse events during childhood are sometimes linked to sexual disorders during adulthood.

    3. Environmental factors also strongly influence sexuality.

B. Sexual disorders. There are three groups of sexual disorders described in the DSM-IV: **sexual dysfunctions, paraphilias,** and **gender identity disorders** (see II, III, and IV).

    1. Sexual dysfunction often leads to psychiatric disturbances, and psychiatric disturbances may lead to sexual dysfunction.

    2. The morbidity of sexual disorders may be associated with self-image problems, impaired reciprocal emotional relationships (e.g., romance), social ostracism, and legal problems.

    3. **Treatment** of sexual disorders requires the clinician to make judgments about cultural norms, age, physiology, and social issues.

II. Sexual Dysfunctions

A. Overview. Sexual dysfunctions are characterized by disturbances in sexual desire or in psychophysiologic changes during sexual response.

    1. Sexual dysfunction affects an individual's sexual satisfaction, self-image, and interpersonal relationships.

    2. Although sexual dysfunctions may be lifelong, they are usually acquired following a period of emotional stress or physiologic sexual compromise, such as that caused by alcohol intoxication or neurologic damage.

    3. Sexual dysfunction may be limited to certain situations or partners; however, it can become generalized.

    4. Some cases of sexual dysfunction may be caused exclusively by psychological factors, but others are caused by a combination of psychological factors and general medical conditions or substance use. Sexual dysfunction that is caused exclusively by physiologic factors is diagnosed as sexual dysfunction due to a general medical condition or substance-induced sexual dysfunction.

5. **Assessment** of sexual dysfunction must account for the individual's age, physical status, interpersonal milieu, and cultural background.

6. Because individuals are hesitant to report sexual dysfunction, estimates of the prevalence of these disorders are unreliable.

B. **Types.** The DSM-IV categorizes sexual dysfunctions according to the phase of the sexual response cycle in which they occur.

1. **Sexual desire disorders**

   a. The DSM-IV describes **hypoactive sexual desire disorder** as a deficiency in sexual fantasy and in the desire for sexual activity.

      (1) It is often associated with other sexual difficulties.

      (2) It usually develops following severe stress and may wax and wane in severity.

   b. The DSM-IV describes **sexual aversion disorder** as an aversion to sexual activity, ranging range from distaste to extreme revulsion. The aversion may be generalized or for a specific component of sexual activity.

      (1) When faced with potential sexual situations, individuals with this disorder may become very anxious.

      (2) Attempting to avoid sexual activity may in itself cause interpersonal problems.

2. **Sexual arousal disorders**

   a. The DSM-IV describes **female sexual arousal disorder** as the inability to attain or maintain the lubrication and swelling responses associated with sexual arousal. It is often associated with other sexual dysfunctions, including hypoactive sexual desire and orgasmic problems.

   b. The DSM-IV describes **male erectile disorder** as the inability to attain or maintain an erection.

      (1) Symptoms are often situational, and normal erectile function may be achieved in some circumstances (e.g., masturbation) but not in others (e.g., with a sexual partner who is perceived as making performance demands).

      (2) Failure to maintain erection often leads to anxiety in sexual situations, which further interferes with erectile ability.

3. **Orgasmic disorders**

   a. The DSM-IV describes **female orgasmic disorder** as a delay in, or absence of, orgasm following a normal sexual excitement phase.

      (1) Female capacity for orgasm appears highly variable and may increase with age.

      (2) It is unusual for a woman to acquire female orgasmic disorder once orgasmic capacity has been attained.

      (3) Although early literature inferred specific psychodynamic significance to anorgasmia, no clear associations have been demonstrated.

   b. The DSM-IV describes **male orgasmic disorder** as a delay in, or absence of, orgasm during sexual activity that follows a normal sexual excitement phase. This disorder is usually highly situational, frequently occurring only during coital activity.

   c. The DSM-IV describes **premature ejaculation** as achieving orgasm and ejaculation with minimal sexual stimulation before, on, or shortly following insertion and before the individual wants it to occur.

      (1) The disorder is usually highly situational; the clinician must account for age, sexual partner, and frequency of recent sexual activity when assessing an individual with this complaint.

      (2) The ability to delay ejaculation increases with age.

      (3) Premature ejaculation sometimes develops in association with male erectile disorder.

4. Sexual pain disorders

   a. The DSM-IV describes **dyspareunia** as genital pain associated with sexual intercourse. The pain is not caused exclusively by a general medical condition (e.g., endometriosis) or substance use.

      (1) The pain is not better accounted for as a component of somatization disorder or another Axis I disorder.

      (2) The disorder is seen in both sexes, and may be associated with any phase of the sexual response cycle.

   b. Vaginismus is involuntary contraction of the perineal muscles surrounding the vagina, which interferes with sexual intercourse. The disorder may occur exclusively during sexual activity or in other situations (e.g., during a gynecologic examination).

5. Sexual dysfunction due to general medical conditions. General medical conditions can interfere with sexual responses or cause painful sexual intercourse. Disorders that often cause sexual dysfunction include:

   a. Neurologic conditions, including neurodegenerative conditions, traumatic nerve injury, and focal CNS lesions

   b. Endocrine conditions, including disorders of the hypothalamic–pituitary axis, diabetes mellitus, thyroid and adrenal disorders, and hypogonadism

   c. Vascular conditions, including focal or general compromise of genital vascular supply

   d. Genitourinary conditions, including injury, infection, neoplasms, Peyronie disease, endometriosis, and atrophic vaginitis

6. Substance-induced sexual dysfunction is characterized by sexual dysfunction that is exclusively the result of a substance; the symptoms are in excess of those usually associated with intoxication.

   a. Substances can interfere with sexual response and can cause painful sexual intercourse.

   b. Abused substances that commonly produce sexual dysfunction include alcohol, amphetamines, cocaine, opioids, sedatives, hypnotics, and anxiolytics.

   c. Prescribed medications that commonly produce sexual dysfunction include antihypertensives, histamine H_2-receptor antagonists, antidepressants, neuroleptics, anxiolytics, anabolic steroids, and anticonvulsants.

d. **Specific psychopharmacologic medications** are commonly associated with sexual dysfunction.

(1) Trazodone is associated with priapism.

(2) Thioridazine is associated with retrograde ejaculation.

(3) Selective serotonin reuptake inhibitors, particularly fluoxetine, are associated with delayed orgasm.

C. **Treatment** of sexual dysfunctions often includes sexual education and psychotherapy directed toward resolving underlying emotional and interpersonal conflicts.

1. **Behavioral therapies** are used to decrease anxiety that may interfere with aspects of sexual function.

a. Behavioral therapies for sexual dysfunctions often require a cooperative sexual partner.

b. Specific behavioral techniques are often employed.

(1) The **squeeze technique** is used for treatment of premature ejaculation. The partner squeezes the glans of the penis before orgasm is reached.

(2) The **start-stop technique**, in which level of excitement is carefully modulated, is also used for treatment of premature ejaculation.

(3) **Masturbation** techniques are used for treatment of orgasmic disorders.

(4) The **sensate focus technique** is used for treatment of male erectile disorder. The focus of sexual interaction is initially on nongenital activity and progresses to genital activity as situational anxiety decreases.

2. **Pharmacotherapy.** Pharmacologic interventions for sexual dysfunctions are limited.

a. **Testosterone** is effective for treating male erectile disorder due to hypogonadism; otherwise, it is ineffective for treating sexual dysfunction.

b. **Selective serotonin reuptake inhibitors** may be effective for treating premature ejaculation.

c. Other **oral** and **topical medications** (e.g., yohimbine, topical anesthetics) have been used with varying success to treat both male erectile dysfunction and premature ejaculation.

d. Injection of **vasoactive substances** (e.g., papaverine, alprostadil, phentolamine) into the corpus cavernosum is often effective treatment of male erectile disorder; however, the pain and other adverse side effects limit its usefulness.

3. **Penile prostheses** can be surgically implanted to treat male erectile dysfunction.

III. Paraphilias

A. **Definition.** The DSM-IV describes paraphilias as recurrent intense sexually arousing fantasies, sexual urges, or behaviors that occur for at least 6 months and involve inanimate objects, the suffering or humiliation of oneself or one's partner, or children or other nonconsenting persons.

B. **Epidemiology.** The majority of cases of paraphilia are in males. The **prevalence** of paraphilia generally decreases after early adulthood; however, it is difficult to determine the specific prevalence of these disorders because the paraphilic behavior is often hidden.

C. Etiology

1. **Psychodynamic theory** postulates that adverse events during specific phases of psychosexual development can lead to paraphilias. Significant anecdotal evidence supporting this theory is derived from case histories.

2. Unknown inborn **biologic factors** have also been cited as possible causes of paraphilias; however, there is no clear evidence.

D. Diagnosis

1. **Diagnostic clues**

   a. **Presenting complaints** may include feelings of guilt or shame, spousal or societal disapproval of the paraphilia, interpersonal problems, and sexual dysfunction.

   b. **History** may include recurrent, unusual sexual fantasies or activities.

   c. **Mental status examination.** Dysphoria may be present.

   d. **Physical examination.** Signs of injury from practices associated with sexual masochism may be present.

   e. **Laboratory studies.** Penile plethysmography, which measures penile tumescence, may show arousal from unusual stimuli.

2. **Associated features**

   a. The fantasies or stimuli may be essential for the individual to become sexually aroused, or they may be employed only occasionally.

   b. Paraphilias may significantly interfere with interpersonal relationships, and they can lead to injury of others and to criminal prosecution.

   c. Individuals with paraphilias may present for clinical evaluation or treatment because of interpersonal difficulties or legal mandate.

   d. Individuals may feel a sense of shame, repugnance, or guilt; however, they sometimes believe that the only source of their problem is societal judgement.

   e. Individuals may become obsessed with activities or interests that put them near the paraphilic object, activity, or situation.

   f. Personality disorders and dysphoria are common.

3. **Other complications** of paraphilias include self-loathing, compromised interpersonal relationships, and sexually transmitted diseases acquired during high-risk sexual activity with prostitutes.

4. **Types.** The DSM-IV describes eight paraphilias.

   a. **Exhibitionism** is the exposure of one's genitals to a stranger.

   b. **Fetishism** is the use of inanimate objects for sexual arousal.

   c. **Frotteurism** is touching and rubbing against a nonconsenting person.

   d. **Pedophilia** is sexual activity with a child.

   e. **Sexual masochism** involves acts in which the individual derives sexual excitement from being humiliated, beaten, bound, or otherwise made to suffer.

   f. **Sexual sadism** involves acts in which the individual derives sexual excitement from the psychological or physical suffering, including humiliation, of the victim.

   g. **Transvestic fetishism** involves cross-dressing.

   h. Voyeurism is the act of observing unsuspecting individuals, typically strangers, who are naked, in the process of undressing, or engaging in sexual activity.

5. **Differential diagnoses** include nonpathologic sexual fantasy or activity and bizarre sexual activity occurring during the course of a cognitive or psychotic disorder.

E. **Clinical course.** The onset of paraphilic fantasies is usually during adolescence or earlier, and the course is often lifelong.

F. **Treatment.** The goals of treatment may include focusing sexual desire on more appropriate objects or situations, lessening intrapsychic conflict, and decreasing the frequency of paraphilic behavior.

1. Psychodynamic psychotherapy is effective in decreasing dysphoria and improving self-understanding.
2. Specific behavioral techniques, usually **aversive conditioning**, are sometimes used.
3. **Pharmacotherapy.** Antiandrogens, such as medroxyprogesterone, may be used to decrease sexual behavior.
4. Surgical castration is rarely used in this country.

IV. Gender Identity Disorder

A. **Overview.** The DSM-IV describes gender identity disorder as strong and persistent cross-gender identification that is accompanied by continual uneasiness with one's designated sex.

1. The individual's identification with the other gender is pervasive and usually lifelong, and it usually involves more than sexual orientation. This diagnosis is reserved for individuals without intersex abnormalities.
2. Children with this disorder have a desire to engage in play that is usually associated with the opposite sex. Often, the child has a conviction that he or she will grow into a member of the opposite sex.
3. As adults, individuals with this disorder usually make an effort to appear and live as members of the opposite sex. They may alter their physical appearance though hormonal treatment or surgery, including penectomy and castration.
4. Equal numbers of males with this disorder have a sexual preference for males or females; females with this disorder almost always have a sexual preference for other females.

B. **Epidemiology.** This disorder occurs at a **3 : 1 male to female ratio** in clinic populations.

C. **Etiology**

1. **Psychodynamic theory** postulates that abnormal events during early psychosexual development, particularly those concerning identification with male and female caregivers, can lead to gender identity disorder. There is significant anecdotal evidence supporting this theory.
2. Unknown inborn **biologic factors** have also been cited as possible causes of gender identity disorder; however, there is no clear evidence.

D. Diagnosis

1. **Diagnostic clues**

   a. **Presenting complaints** may include anxiety or dysphoria about one's gender identity.

   b. **History.** The individual may have a long history of dissatisfaction with his or her phenotypic sex and a long history of desire or attempts to live as a member of the opposite sex.

   c. **Mental status examination.** The individual is often depressed or anxious.

   d. **Physical examination** may show evidence of exogenous hormonal treatment (feminization or masculinization) or evidence of surgical alteration of primary or secondary sexual characteristics (e.g., electrolysis of hair, artificial genitals).

   e. **Laboratory studies** may show evidence of exogenous steroids.

2. **Subtypes** include:

   a. Sexual attraction for males
   b. Sexual attraction for females

3. **Associated features.** Individuals with this disorder are often socially isolated and rejected, and they are often anxious or depressed.

4. **Differential diagnoses** include nonconformity to stereotypical sex role behavior, transvestic fetishism, concurrent congenital intersex condition [e.g., Turner syndrome, Klinefelter syndrome, congenital virilizing adrenal hyperplasia, ambiguous genitalia (pseudohermaphroditism), androgen insensitivity syndrome], and schizophrenia with delusions.

E. Clinical course

1. **Onset** of recognizable symptoms usually occurs at 2 to 4 years of age, when sexual identity forms (IV A 2).

   a. Most individuals with symptoms do not develop gender identity disorder, and the behaviors usually gradually disappear.

   b. Those few children for whom cross-gender behaviors continue through childhood may have gender identity disorder.

2. By adulthood, 75% of males with a history of this behavior report a homosexual or bisexual orientation.

3. The disorder usually persists throughout the individual's life.

F. Treatment. The goal of treatment is rarely to change the individual's sexual identity, and these attempts are usually unsuccessful. Realistic goals include reduction of depression and anxiety and improvement of personal and social adjustment.

1. **Psychotherapy** is often employed to decrease depression and anxiety associated with the condition.

2. **Hormone treatment.** Testosterone or estrogen is often used to change the individual's physical characteristics and improve sense of well being; however, caution must be exercised in monitoring adverse effects.

3. **Gender reassignment** surgery may be, but is not always, successful in improving the individual's personal and social adjustment.

Review Test

Directions: Each of the following items or incomplete statements in this section is followed by answers or by completions of the statement. Select the ONE lettered answer or completion that is BEST in each case.

1. A 25-year-old woman presents with her spouse. The husband states that his wife has a "glandular problem" because she has no desire for sex. According to the husband, she agrees to intercourse reluctantly and infrequently. Assuming the accuracy of the husband's description which of the following statements about the patient is most likely accurate?

(A) If she has a sexual dysfunction, she is likely to have more than one
(B) She has a testosterone deficiency
(C) She is having an affair with another person
(D) She is taking antidepressant medication
(E) Unconscious conflicts about sexuality are responsible for her behavior

2. A 42-year-old man complains of inadequate erections. Since the initial episode a few months ago, he has been constantly worrying about maintaining an erection prior to insertion and can no longer enjoy sex. Which of the following is the most useful advice?

(A) Tell the patient that declining sexual function is a component of aging
(B) Advise the patient to find alternate ways to satisfy his partner
(C) Initiate administration of trazodone
(D) Ask the patient to bring in his partner for a frank discussion about relational problems
(E) Ask the patient to bring in his partner for a discussion of sensate focus techniques

3. A 31-year-old man complains that he often ejaculates within seconds after insertion during sexual intercourse. He says that he feels sexually inadequate and seeks treatment. Which of the following interventions is most likely useful to this patient?

(A) Begin administration of low doses of thioridazine
(B) Advise the patient to masturbate to orgasm several hours before having sexual intercourse
(C) Advise the patient to practice the squeeze technique with his partner
(D) Advise the patient to think about work problems during sex
(E) Advise the patient to use a topical anesthetic or a thick condom

4. A 55-year-old man states that he "can no longer stand" himself and seeks counseling. He says that he has been secretly dressing in women's underwear for years and has successfully concealed this from everyone, including his wife. He hides underwear in his car and changes in public restrooms. He finds this behavior "disgusting" and has tried to stop it, but ultimately he cannot resist the sexual arousal associated with it. Which of the following interventions is most likely useful?

(A) Discuss sexual reassignment surgery with the patient
(B) Have the patient explore the reasons that he finds the behavior disgusting
(C) Tell the patient that many men participate in this behavior
(D) Initiate treatment with medroxyprogesterone
(E) Suggest that the patient disclose his behavior to his wife and begin marital counseling

5. The parents of an 11-year-old boy are extremely disturbed about his teacher's comment that their son is teased at school about his effeminate behavior. The boy has not mentioned any problems to his parents. The parents are seeking advice. Which of the following interventions is most likely useful?

(A) Obtain chromosomal analysis of the boy
(B) Obtain psychiatric assessment of the boy
(C) Enroll the boy in a sports program
(D) Enroll the boy in a different school
(E) Withhold any specific intervention unless the boy has other evidence of emotional problems

Answers and Explanations

1–A. Based on the husband's statements, the woman most likely has hypoactive sexual desire disorder. This disorder is usually associated with other sexual disorders, such as dyspareunia or sexual arousal disorder, and may lead to sexual aversion disorder. It is likely that the couple has other problems in the marital relationship.

2–E The man's symptoms are most suggestive of male erectile dysfunction. Performance anxiety increased following his initial episode, as occurs in many cases. Initial treatment with sensate focus techniques involves decreasing the anxiety associated with sexual activity. Conjoint therapy, acceptance of aging, and exploring alternate types of sexual activity also address the man's presenting problem. Trazodone may cause priapism in rare instances.

3–C The man's symptoms suggest premature ejaculation. The squeeze technique, in which the partner squeezes the glans of the penis when the patient senses impending orgasm, is often an effective treatment. Use of a selective serotonin reuptake inhibitor may be a useful pharmacologic intervention. Thioridazine causes retrograde ejaculation. Decreasing penile sensation or thinking about nonsexual matters during intercourse often causes erectile problems.

4–B The man's symptoms are suggestive of transvestic fetishism. The morbidity associated with this case is self-loathing, a condition which may respond to psychotherapy. The prevalence of this disorder is unknown. Sexual reassignment is sometimes useful in treating gender identity disorder, not travestic fetishism. Medroxyprogesterone may decrease paraphilic urges; however, other sexual urges are likely to decrease as well. Disclosing this behavior to a spouse may or may not alter the condition or improve self-image; however, it may cause interpersonal conflict.

5–B The boy is most likely experiencing severe emotional difficulty because of the teasing. Psychiatric assessment is needed to determine the best way to ameliorate the stress and decrease the risk of future psychopathology. Chromosomal analysis will not be helpful. Altering the boy's environment by placing him in a sports program or sending him to a different school is unlikely to change his effeminate behavior quickly. Presuming that the boy has emotional difficulties because of this situation is well founded; therefore, only observing the boy before contemplating intervention is less effective.

20
Eating Disorders

I. **Overview.** Eating disorders involve problems with eating behaviors, weight maintenance, body image, and physiologic processes that are affected by an individual's diet.

 A. **Anorexia nervosa** and **bulimia nervosa** are described in the DSM-IV. They have two common features:

  1. Both disorders are characterized by abnormal eating behaviors.
  2. Both disorders are associated with a disturbance in perception of body shape and weight.

 B. **Abnormal eating behaviors** include:

  1. **Abnormal regulation of food intake.** The individual restricts food intake or binges (i.e., rapid, poorly controlled consumption of large amounts of food).
  2. **Abnormal diet.** The individual eats a restricted range of foods, low-calorie foods, unusual foods, or non-nutritive substances.
  3. **Purging.** The individual purges food through vomiting or taking laxatives, diuretics, or enemas.

 C. Some **symptoms** associated with eating disorders are secondary to the abnormal food behaviors and efforts to control weight. These symptoms include the complications of starvation, purging, and overexertion.

 D. **Mechanisms** that regulate food intake are complex and involve chemoreceptors, sensory stimuli, and psychological responses.

 E. **Psychological associations** with food are formed in early childhood. Food is associated with nurturing, control, and body image.

 F. **Other eating disorders** include pica, rumination disorder, and feeding disorder of infancy or early childhood (see Chapter 4 III B).

II. **Anorexia Nervosa**

 A. **Overview.** Individuals with anorexia nervosa fail to maintain a normal body weight, have a fear and preoccupation with gaining weight, unrealistically evaluate themselves as overweight, and have amenorrhea.

 B. **Epidemiology.** This disorder occurs at a **1:10 male to female ratio.**

  1. In young adult women, the prevalence of this disorder is 0.5%.

2. Anorexia nervosa and mood disorders are more common in relatives of individuals with this disorder.

C. Etiology

1. There is some evidence that **biologic factors** may have an etiologic role. Monozygotic twins have higher concordance for illness. Some abnormalities of the hypothalamic–pituitary axis, including amenorrhea, may precede abnormal eating behaviors.
2. Many clinicians believe that **psychological conflicts,** particularly those about family control and sexuality, may play a causative role.
3. The increasing frequency of anorexia nervosa in industrial societies suggests that **cultural factors** (e.g., emphasis on thinness) may contribute to the pathogenesis of the disorder.

D. Diagnosis

1. **Diagnostic clues**

    a. **Presenting complaints.** Family and friends may complain about the individual's weight loss and excessive food restriction. The individual usually has few subjective complaints, except about being overweight.

    b. **History** may include growing concern with body shape and diet and significant weight loss.

    c. **Mental status examination** may show a peculiarly energetic and unconcerned individual; however, obsessive rumination and depression may be present.

    d. **Physical examination**

    (1) **Signs of malnutrition** include emaciation, hypotension, bradycardia, lanugo (i.e., fine hair on the trunk), and peripheral edema.

    (2) **Signs of purging** include eroded dental enamel, which is caused by emesis; scarred or scratched hands, which occurs when teeth scratch the hand during self-gagging to induce emesis; parotid gland hypertrophy, and, rarely, esophageal or gastric tears caused by vomiting.

    e. **Laboratory studies**

    (1) **Signs of malnutrition** include normochromic, normocytic anemia; elevated liver enzymes; abnormal electrolytes; low estrogen and testosterone levels; abnormal neuroendocrine responses; sinus bradycardia; reduced brain mass; and abnormal electroencephalogram.

    (2) **Signs of purging** include metabolic alkalosis, hypochloremia, and hypokalemia caused by emesis; metabolic acidosis is caused by laxative abuse.

2. **Diagnostic features** include:

    a. **Refusal to maintain body weight** that is 85% or greater than a minimally normal weight for the individual's age and height. Individuals with this disorder lose weight by restricting their food intake and maintaining diets of low-calorie foods. Weight loss may also be achieved through purging (i.e., vomiting or taking laxatives, diuretics, or enemas) and exercise.

   b. **Intense fear of gaining weight** or becoming fat, despite being under-weight. Individual's with this disorder are greatly concerned with their appearance. They often spend a significant amount of time examining and denigrating themselves for self-perceived signs of excess weight.
   c. **A misperception of body shape or weight,** causing the individual to minimize or deny being underweight. Despite weight loss, individuals with this disorder regard themselves as overweight or "fat in some places," typically in the thighs, abdomen, or buttocks.
   d. **Amenorrhea in postmenarchal females.** Individuals with this disorder are amenorrheic; it is not entirely clear if amenorrhea is primary or secondary to weight restriction.

3. **Subtypes** include:
   a. **Restricting type,** in which the individual controls her weight by food restriction and exercise
   b. **Binge-eating/purging type,** in which the individual binge-eats and purges

4. **Associated features**
   a. **Obsessive-compulsive features** are often present.
      (1) An additional diagnosis of obsessive-compulsive disorder may be needed if the obsessions and compulsions are not related solely to food.
      (2) Obsessive-compulsive personality traits, such as inflexibility, limited spontaneity, and concern with control, are more common in individuals with anorexia nervosa.
   b. **Depressive symptoms** are common, and an additional diagnosis of major depressive disorder may be needed in some cases.
   c. **General medical conditions** caused by abnormal diets, starvation, and purging may be present (see II D 1 d, e).
   d. **Food interests.** Individuals with anorexia nervosa often have a paradoxical interest in recipes, cooking, or serving food.

5. **Differential diagnoses** include general medical conditions that cause weight loss, major depressive disorder, schizophrenia, obsessive-compulsive disorder, body dysmorphic disorder, and bulimia nervosa.

E. **Clinical course**
   1. **Onset**
      a. The average age of **onset** is 17 years of age, but a bimodal age of onset distribution has been described at 14 and 18 years of age.
      b. Late-onset (after age 30) anorexia nervosa has a poorer prognosis.
      c. Onset is often associated with emotional stressors, particularly conflicts with parents about independence, and sexual conflicts.
   2. The **course** is variable; some individuals recover following a single episode and others develop a waxing-and-waning course with gradual deterioration.
   3. **Mortality.** The long-term mortality rate of individuals hospitalized for anorexia nervosa is 10%, resulting from the effects of starvation and purging or suicide.

F. Treatment. The goals of treatment are to correct metabolic disturbances, restore a safe weight and normal food behaviors, and improve the accuracy of the individual's body image.

1. The primary objective always is to **correct significant physiologic consequences of starvation.** Hospitalization and forced feeding may be necessary.

2. **Behavioral treatment** is often employed, and contingencies (i.e., **rewards** or punishments) are always based on absolute weight, not on eating behaviors.

3. **Family therapy** is often employed to clarify conflicts about control issues.

4. Some evidence suggests that **antidepressants** may play a limited role in treatment of this disorder.

III. Bulimia Nervosa

A. Overview. Bulimia nervosa is characterized by frequent bingeing and purging and a self-image that is unduly influenced by weight.

B. Epidemiology. This disorder occurs at a **1:9 male to female ratio.**

1. In young adult females, the prevalence of this disorder is 2%.

2. Bulimia nervosa, mood disorders, and substance use disorders are more common in relatives of individuals with this disorder.

C. Etiology

1. **Psychological conflicts,** including issues about guilt, helplessness, and body image, are postulated as causative factors in bulimia nervosa.

2. **Biologic theories** about this disorder are usually based on its frequent association with mood disorders.

D. Diagnosis

1. **Diagnostic clues**

   a. **Presenting complaints** include inability to regulate food intake and feelings of guilt about purging.

   b. **History** may include frequent dieting, feelings of guilt about food and eating, mood symptoms, chaotic interpersonal relationships, impulsivity, and problems with self-image.

   c. **Mental status examination** may show borderline personality traits and depressive symptoms.

   d. **Physical examination.** The individual usually is a normal weight or is slightly obese. Complications of purging may be present (see II D 1 d).

   e. **Laboratory studies** may show complications of purging (see II D 1 e).

2. The DSM-IV describes the following **diagnostic features,** which occur at least twice weekly for 3 months.

   a. **Recurrent episodes of binge eating.** Individuals with this disorder are often obsessed with dieting but inevitably "lose control" and binge on high-calorie foods. Binges appear to be triggered by emotional stress and are followed by feelings of guilt, self-recrimination, and compensatory behaviors.

   b. **Recurrent, inappropriate compensatory behavior.** After a binge, individuals with this disorder attempt to prevent weight gain through self-induced vomiting; misuse of laxatives, diuretics, enemas, or other medications; fasting; or excessive exercise.

   c. Self-evaluation is unduly influenced by body shape and weight. Individuals with bulimia nervosa often castigate themselves for mild weight gain or lapses in control of their food intake.

   d. The disturbance does not occur exclusively during episodes of anorexia nervosa.

3. Subtypes include:

   a. Purging type

   b. Nonpurging type, in which the individual fasts or exercises but does not purge during bulimic episodes

4. Associated features

   a. Depressive symptoms are common, and dysthymic disorder or major depressive disorder may also be present.

   b. Substance abuse, usually of alcohol or stimulants, occurs in at least 33% of individuals with bulimia nervosa.

   c. Borderline personality disorder is present in about 50% of individuals with bulimia nervosa.

   d. Individuals with bulimia nervosa are often embarrassed by and secretive about their symptoms. They make significant efforts to conceal food and to isolate themselves during bingeing and purging. Also, they lie about these behaviors when confronted by family, friends, or roommates.

5. Differential diagnoses include anorexia nervosa, binge-eating/purging type; major depressive disorder with atypical features, and borderline personality disorder.

E. Clinical course

1. Onset is usually during late adolescence or early adulthood and often follows a period of dieting.

2. The **course** may be chronic or intermittent, with a total duration of several years.

F. Treatment. The goals of treatment are to restore normal eating behaviors, change the individual's self-image, and reduce the associated mood and personality symptoms.

1. Cognitive and **behavioral treatments** are often used to decrease bingeing and purging.

2. Antidepressant medications, particularly selective serotonin reuptake inhibitors, are frequently reported as efficacious.

3. Psychodynamic psychotherapies based on those used for borderline personality disorder are sometimes employed.

Review Test

Directions: Each of the numbered items or incomplete statements in this section is followed by answers or by completions of the statement. Select the ONE lettered answer or completion that is BEST in each case.

1. A 17-year-old girl is referred by a school counselor for progressive weight loss. She recognizes that other people have been concerned about her eating habits, but she says that she feels fine and does not think she is too thin. She emphatically states that she will not eat to please other people because she gets fat easily. Which of the following findings would be necessary to establish a diagnosis of anorexia nervosa?

(A) Amenorrhea
(B) Feelings of anger toward her controlling parents
(C) Bingeing or purging
(D) Complications of malnutrition
(E) Dental erosion

2. A 23-year-old woman with anorexia nervosa is involuntarily readmitted to the hospital after she fails to maintain her body weight at 80% of that considered ideal for her height. She insists that she has been eating regularly and wants to be discharged immediately. Which of the following conditions is the best for allowing this woman's release?

(A) The woman must agree to intranasal feeding
(B) The woman must agree to participate in outpatient psychotherapy regularly
(C) The woman must maintain an agreed-upon activity schedule
(D) The woman must maintain an agreed-upon weight
(E) The woman must maintain an agreed-upon diet

3. A 19-year-old woman is hospitalized for dehydration caused by severe, laxative-induced diarrhea. She is depressed about the recent breakup of a romantic relationship. She admits that she uses laxatives, because she has been bingeing frequently and is worried about gaining weight. Although the woman is very thin, she believes that she is overweight. She has never had a menses. Which of the following is the most likely diagnosis?

(A) Anorexia nervosa
(B) Brief psychotic disorder
(C) Bulimia nervosa
(D) Delusional disorder, somatic type
(E) Major depressive disorder

4. A 20-year-old woman seeks help for chronic bingeing and purging. She says that she is embarrassed by her behavior. She has been performing poorly academically in college, and she was recently caught shoplifting. The store did not file charges against the woman, and she is unable to explain her behavior. She also admits to using alcohol and marijuana frequently. She describes herself as easily distracted, restless, and impulsive. Which of the following medications would most likely be useful as part of a treatment plan for this patient?

(A) Disulfiram
(B) Fluoxetine
(C) Lithium
(D) Methylphenidate
(E) Valproate

190

5. A 24-year-old woman suffering from severe malnutrition is brought to the emergency room. She has been amenorrheic for six months, and she has been severely restricting her food intake. She states that because she quit her job, her former employers have been poisoning her food in an attempt to murder her. She says that she cannot risk eating food in a normal manner. Her thought processes are coherent, and she denies having hallucinations. Which of the following is the most likely diagnosis?

(A) Anorexia nervosa
(B) Bulimia nervosa
(C) Delusional disorder, persecutory type
(D) Obsessive-compulsive disorder
(E) Schizophrenia, paranoid type

Answers and Explanations

1—A. Amenorrhea is an essential feature of anorexia nervosa in women. A failure to maintain body weight, a distorted body image, and fear of obesity are other findings that must be present to diagnose anorexia nervosa. Although conflict about control is commonly found in the families of individuals with anorexia nervosa, it is not a finding required for diagnosis. Bingeing and purging may be present; however, food restriction is the sole cause of weight loss in anorexia nervosa. Complications of malnutrition (e.g., metabolic disturbances) may be noted but are not invariably present. Dental erosion may be caused by frequent vomiting.

2—D. Weight maintenance is the primary goal in the treatment of anorexia nervosa and supersedes all other issues. Intranasal feeding may be used as a final measure to help the individual achieve a safe weight.

3—A. The patient presents with low body weight, a distorted body image, a fear of obesity, and amenorrhea, all of which strongly suggest anorexia nervosa. Bingeing and purging behavior is commonly present with this disorder. Because this individual has the essential features of anorexia nervosa, the diagnosis of bulimia nervosa is not made. Because the woman shows no evidence of delusions, brief psychotic disorder or delusional disorder an unlikely diagnosis. Although depression commonly accompanies eating disorders, it does not appear to be the primary problem in this woman's case.

4—B. The woman's symptoms suggest that she has bulimia nervosa. Antidepressants, particularly selective serotonin reuptake inhibitors, are frequently efficacious in treating this disorder. Disulfiram is used to prevent relapse into alcohol dependence; however, alcohol dependence is not the primary problem in this woman's case. Lithium and valproate are indicated for the treatment of bipolar disorder; except for the woman's impulsivity, there is little indication of bipolar disorder. Methylphenidate is used to treat attention deficit hyperactivity disorder (ADHD). Although this woman may have ADHD, methylphenidate should not be initiated, because the potential for abuse is too significant.

5—C. This patient presents with plausible persecutory delusions, coherent thought processes, and an absence of hallucinations. These symptoms are most suggestive of delusional disorder. To diagnose anorexia nervosa, the patient must have a distorted body image, a fear of obesity, weight loss, and amenorrhea. To diagnose obsessive-compulsive disorder, the patient must have intrusive thoughts or commit senseless acts. To diagnose schizophrenia, the patient must have hallucinations, bizarre delusions, or disorganized speech or behavior.

21

Sleep Disorders

I. Normal Sleep

A. **Overview.** In typical circumstances, people sleep about 8 hours daily, usually at night.

1. **Sleep regulation** is a complex process that involves multiple brain structures, endogenous circadian rhythms, and the influence of experiencing night and day.

   a. The **dorsal raphe nucleus** influences sleep through serotonergic systems. Increases in serotonin levels promote sleep.

   b. The **locus ceruleus,** through norepinephrine-mediated systems, also influences sleep systems, and stimulation of this center disrupts sleep patterns by decreasing rapid eye movement (REM).

2. **Sleep periods** are often clinically described by **sleep architecture,** which is the profile of measurements recorded by polysomnography.

B. **Polysomnography** is the simultaneous recording of electrophysiologic parameters associated with sleep.

1. **Electrophysiologic recordings** usually measure electroencephalographic (EEG), electrooculographic (EOG), and electromyographic (EMG) activities.

   a. **Other parameters** measured include oral or nasal airflow, respiratory effort, chest and abdominal wall movement, oxyhemoglobin saturation, and exhaled carbon dioxide concentration.

   b. Although most polysomnography is conducted during normal sleeping hours, some measurements of daytime sleepiness may occur during normal waking hours.

2. **Polysomnographic terminology**

   a. **Sleep continuity** is the duration and number of sleep periods between wakeful periods during the sleep period.

   b. **Sleep latency** is the time needed to fall asleep.

   c. **REM latency** is the time between falling asleep and the first REM period.

   d. **Intermittent wakefulness** is the amount of time the individual is awake during the night after initially falling asleep.

  e. Sleep efficiency is the ratio of the time spent asleep to the time spent in bed.

C. Stages of sleep

 1. **Wakefulness.** An individual's EEG shows low voltage, fast waves.

 2. **Drowsiness.** An individual's EEG shows alpha waves [8–12 cycles per second (CPS)].

 3. **Non–rapid eye movement (NREM) sleep**

  a. Stage 1 represents the transition to sleep. The EEG shows theta waves (3–7 CPS). Stage 1 represents 5% of total sleep time.

  b. Stage 2 represents light sleep. The EEG shows sleep spindles (12–14 CPS) and triphasic complexes. Stage 2 represents 45% of total sleep time.

  c. Stage 3 represents slow-wave sleep. The EEG shows delta (i.e., high-amplitude, slow) waves (0.5–2.5 CPS). Stage 3 represents 12% of total sleep time.

  d. Stage 4 also represents slow-wave sleep. The EEG shows more than 50% delta waves. Stage 4 represents 13% of total sleep time.

 4. **REM sleep (stage 5)**

  a. During REM sleep, the EEG shows low-voltage, random, fast waves that have "sawtooth" (i.e., alpha-like) wave patterns.

  b. REM sleep represents 20%–50% of total sleep time, and dreaming occurs during these periods.

D. Sleep organization

 1. Sleep latency is usually 15–20 minutes.

 2. Sleep stages occur cyclically throughout the night; REM sleep alternates with NREM sleep about every 90 minutes.

 3. NREM stages 3 and 4 usually occur during the first one third to one half of the night and are absent during the last cycles of sleep.

 4. REM sleep periods increase in duration toward the morning.

E. Sleep deprivation

 1. The duration of NREM stages 3 and 4 in the sleep periods that follow sleep deprivation is increased.

 2. The amount of REM sleep in the sleep periods following REM sleep deprivation is increased.

F. Age and sleep patterns

 1. Children and adolescents have large amounts of slow-wave sleep.

 2. **Effects of aging**

  a. Sleep latency increases, and the endogenous sleep–wake cycle gradually shortens.

  b. Daytime napping occurs more frequently, sleep continuity decreases, and stage 1 sleep increases.

  c. Slow-wave and REM sleep decreases.

  d. Sleep satisfaction decreases, and more dyssomnias and parasomnias occur.

II. Sleep Disorders

A. Overview. Sleep complaints are common. One third of individuals feel that they have a sleep problem.

1. The most common **complaints** are having difficulty falling or staying asleep and feeling fatigue during the day.

   a. **Insomnia** and daytime fatigue are often the presenting complaints of many sleep disorders.

   b. Both insomnia and **hypersomnia** may cause daytime fatigue.

   c. Other less obvious sleep-related disturbances (e.g., sleep apnea) may lead to insomnia and daytime fatigue.

2. Sleep disorders may lead to depressive disorders and substance-related disorders because of distress or efforts to self-medicate.

B. Classification. Sleep disorders are classified by etiology.

1. **Primary sleep disorders**

   a. **Dyssomnias**

      (1) The DSM-IV describes dyssomnias as disorders characterized by difficulty falling asleep, staying asleep, or daytime fatigue.

      (2) These sleep disorders include primary insomnia, primary hypersomnia, narcolepsy, breathing-related sleep disorder, and circadian rhythm sleep disorder (see III–VII).

   b. **Parasomnias**

      (1) The DSM-IV describes parasomnias as disturbances that involve episodes of abnormal behavior or physiologic events that occur in association with sleep.

      (2) These disorders include nightmare disorder, sleep terror disorder, and sleepwalking disorder (see VIII–X).

2. **Sleep disorders related to another mental disorder** (see XI)
3. **Sleep disorders due to a general medical condition** (see XII)
4. **Substance-induced sleep disorders** (see XIII)

III. Primary Insomnia

A. Overview. Insomnia is commonly defined as difficulty initiating or maintaining sleep.

1. Insomnia is a common psychiatric complaint, and often has discernable causes, such as anxiety, depression, psychotic disorders, environmental disruption, substances, central nervous system (CNS) disease, pain, or respiratory problems. The term primary insomnia is used when there is no external cause for the disturbance.

2. Chronic insomnia often leads to frustration, daytime fatigue, and a preoccupation with restoring normal sleep.

B. Epidemiology

1. Women are more likely to complain of insomnia than men.
2. The **prevalence** of primary insomnia increases with age.

   a. The overall prevalence of complaints of insomnia is 35%.

b. It is estimated that about 20% of individuals with insomnia have primary insomnia.

3. Sleep problems are more common in relatives of individuals with this disorder.

C. Etiology

1. Presumptively, some patients have a constitutional predisposition to insomnia.

2. Because the typical onset of primary insomnia is associated with stressors, this disorder may originate from anxiety and distress about sleep, which then becomes self-perpetuating.

D. Diagnosis

1. Diagnostic clues

    a. Presenting complaints include difficulty falling asleep, frequent nighttime awakenings, early morning awakening, a sense of poor quality sleep, and daytime fatigue.

    b. Mental status examination may show fatigue.

    c. Physical examination is typically unremarkable.

    d. Laboratory studies may show abnormal polysomnographic findings (e.g., increased sleep latency, poor sleep continuity).

2. The major **diagnostic feature** is that for at least 1 month, the individual has difficulty falling or staying asleep; or, the individual has nonrestorative sleep.

    a. The disturbance does not occur exclusively during the course of another sleep disorder.

    b. The disturbance is not associated with another mental disorder, and it is not caused by substances or a general medical condition.

3. Associated features include:

    a. Anxious or depressed moods

    b. General preoccupation with health

    c. Substance abuse, which is often initiated in an effort to induce sleep or improve daytime alertness

4. Differential diagnoses include substance-induced insomnia, insomnia due to a general medical condition, and insomnia related to another mental disorder, other dyssomnias, parasomnias that disrupt sleep, other mental disorders with associated sleep disturbances, substance-induced sleep disturbances, and sleep disturbances due to general medical conditions.

E. Clinical course

1. Primary insomnia is often preceded by a long history of vague sleep complaints.

2. The **onset** is usually in adulthood and is often associated with a physical or psychological problem.

3. After the initial problems resolve, the insomnia continues and becomes a focus of complaint.

4. The course may consist of a relatively constant difficulty with sleep. The course also may be characterized by **exacerbations,** which may be associated with stressors, and **remissions**.

F. **Treatment.** The **goal** of treatment is to restore more satisfying sleep patterns, decrease subjective daytime fatigue, and decrease the individual's preoccupation with sleep.

1. **Modifying alcohol or drug use,** which may have developed in response to insomnia, is recommended.

2. **Improving sleep hygiene** may be useful. It involves:

   a. Setting a specific time to enter bed and a specific time to arise
   b. Using the bed only for sleep
   c. Avoiding daytime naps
   d. Exercising strenuously during the day and developing relaxing routines at night
   e. Abstaining from caffeine and alcohol, especially in the evening

3. Judicious administration of **benzodiazepine**s or other hypnotics is indicated in some cases. The clinician must monitor the development of tolerance and daytime cognitive impairment.

IV. Primary Hypersomnia

A. **Overview.** Hypersomnia is excessive somnolence and is a fairly common complaint. It is often caused by inadequate nighttime rest.

1. Inadequate nighttime rest may be caused by environmental disturbances, insomnias, dyssomnias, and parasomnias, which interfere with sleep duration and continuity.

2. Occasionally, excessive sleepiness occurs in the absence of other sleep problems and is manifested by extended sleep episodes (i.e., greater than 9 hours per night) or by frequent and extended daytime napping.

3. Some mental disorders, particularly mood disorders, and some general medical conditions (e.g., CNS tumors) can cause general hypersomnia.

4. Primary hypersomnia is diagnosed in the absence of other conditions that lead to this problem.

B. **Epidemiology**

1. Five percent of the population complains of daytime sleepiness.

2. Kleine-Levin syndrome is three times more common in males (see IV D 3).

3. Sleep disorders are more common in relatives of individuals with primary hypersomnia.

C. **Etiology.** Presumptively, there is an abnormality in the mechanisms that regulate the sleep–wake cycle.

D. **Diagnosis**

1. **Diagnostic clues**

   a. **Presenting complaints** include excessive duration of nighttime sleep with difficulty awakening, excessive daytime sleepiness, and nonrestorative daytime naps.
   b. **Mental status examination** may show fatigue.

c. **Physical examination** is usually unremarkable. Obesity is present in individuals with Kleine-Levin syndrome.

d. **Laboratory studies.** Nocturnal polysomnography is typically normal, and daytime recordings demonstrate increased drowsiness and sleep episodes.

2. **Diagnostic features.** The DSM-IV characterizes primary hypersomnia as at least 1 month of excessive nighttime sleep episodes or extreme daytime somnolence.

a. The sleepiness is not caused by insomnia or another sleep disorder.

b. The problem is not caused by another mental disorder, substances, or a general medical condition.

3. A **subtype** of recurrent primary hypersomnia is **Kleine-Levin syndrome.** It is characterized by prolonged somnolence that is accompanied by impulsivity, hypersexuality, obesity, and disorganized thinking.

4. **Associated features**

a. **"Sleep drunkenness,"** which is a state of confusion after awakening, is common in individuals with primary hypersomnia.

b. Individuals with this disorder have a higher incidence of major depressive disorder and stimulant abuse.

c. Individuals with primary hypersomnia have difficulty meeting social and occupational obligations, have impaired daytime performance caused by their sleepiness, and are embarrassed when sleep episodes occur at inopportune times.

d. Individuals with this disorder have a higher incidence of major depressive disorder and stimulant abuse.

5. **Differential diagnoses** include lack of sufficient nocturnal sleep, primary insomnia, other sleep disorders that interrupt nocturnal sleep, sleep disturbances related to major depressive episodes and other mental disorders, substance-induced sleep disorders, and sleep disorders due to general medical conditions.

E. **Clinical course**

1. **Onset** occurs during adolescence and early adulthood. The initial symptoms may last for weeks to months and then remain chronic.

2. Kleine-Levin syndrome may remit in middle age.

F. **Treatment.** The goals of treatment are to improve daytime alertness and shorten sleep periods. **Psychostimulants** are used in some cases.

V. Narcolepsy

A. **Overview.** Narcolepsy is a relatively rare disorder characterized by irresistible attacks of sleep, cataplexy, and recurrent intrusions of REM sleep during stage 1 sleep. Episodes of sudden loss of muscle tone when awake and episodes of paralysis when falling asleep or awakening also occur.

B. **Epidemiology**

1. Narcolepsy occurs at a **1:1 male to female ratio.** The prevalence of this disorder is 0.05% of the population.

2. Narcolepsy and other sleep disorders are more common in relatives of individuals with this disorder.

C. Etiology. Presumptively, narcolepsy is caused by a disturbance in CNS mechanisms underlying the regulation of REM sleep.

D. Diagnosis

1. Diagnostic clues

a. Presenting complaints almost always include daytime sleepiness.

(1) **Cataplexy.** Individuals also complain of loss of muscle tone, although respiration is always preserved. The loss of muscle tone varies in degree from minimal to complete flaccidity and is always bilateral.

(2) Individuals may also complain of brief episodes of **sleep paralysis**, which is an inability to move immediately before falling asleep or immediately upon awakening.

(3) **Hypnogogic and hypnopompic hallucinations.** Individuals may complain of peculiar episodes of vivid hallucinations when falling asleep (hypnogogic) or awakening (hypnopompic).

b. History. The individual may have a long history of involuntary daytime sleep episodes and episodes of muscle tone loss during emotionally charged situations.

c. Mental status and **physical examinations** are typically unremarkable.

d. Laboratory studies. Polysomnographic recordings indicate short sleep latency, sleep-onset REM, and an increase in the duration and intensity of REM sleep.

2. The DSM-IV describes the following **diagnostic features:**

a. Overpowering, daily attacks of refreshing sleep that occur for at least 3 months

b. The presence of one or both of the following:

(1) Cataplexy

(2) Elements of REM sleep that intrude during the transition period between sleep and wakefulness that is manifested by either hypnopompic or hypnagogic hallucinations or sleep paralysis

c. The disturbance is not caused by a substance or a general medical condition.

3. Associated features and diagnoses

a. Multiple other sleep complaints, including interrupted nocturnal sleep, vivid dreaming, and daytime functional impairment due to sleepiness are common.

b. Cataplexy can lead to accidents or attempts to control the onset of attacks by restricting emotionality.

c. Depressive episodes and anxiety are common.

4. Differential diagnoses include sleep deprivation, hypersomnias, other sleep disorders, other mental disorders with associated sleep disturbances, substance-induced sleep disturbances, and sleep disturbances due to general medical conditions.

E. Clinical course

1. The **onset** is usually during adolescence or early adulthood and is associated with emotional stressors in some cases.
2. The individual often has a long history of daytime somnolence that precedes the onset of narcolepsy.
3. Cataplexy usually develops after sleep attacks are present for months or years.
4. Sleep attacks and cataplexy usually remain constant; however, hallucinations and sleep paralysis may wax and wane in frequency or may never occur.

F. **Treatment** goals are to ameliorate daytime sleepiness and associated symptoms.

1. Scheduling daytime naps is occasionally effective.
2. **Pharmacotherapy**
   a. Psychostimulants are often effective in decreasing daytime somnolence.
   b. Antidepressants combined with psychostimulants may decrease episodes of cataplexy.

VI. Breathing-Related Sleep Disorder

A. Overview. Nocturnal breathing problems often lead to sleep disturbances.

1. **Breathing problems** during sleep include:
   a. **Apnea** (i.e., the cessation of breathing) of variable duration
   b. **Hypopnea**, which is slow or shallow respiration
   c. **Hypoventilation**, which is characterized by reduced blood oxygen saturation and increased carbon dioxide levels
2. The DSM-IV describes three major categories of breathing problems that lead to breathing-related sleep disorder:
   a. **Obstructive sleep apnea syndrome**
   b. **Central sleep apnea syndrome**
   c. **Central alveolar hypoventilation syndrome**
3. Although individuals with these conditions may be unaware of respiratory difficulties during sleep, they almost always complain of the daytime somnolence that is caused by interrupted sleep.
4. **Obesity** is a major risk factor for breathing-related sleep disorder caused by obstructive sleep apnea (pickwickian syndrome).
5. Breathing-related sleep disorder may be responsible for some cases of "crib-death" in infants.

B. Epidemiology. The prevalence of this disorder is about 5% of the population, depending on diagnostic threshold.

1. Obstructive sleep apnea occurs at an **8:1 male to female ratio.**
2. Sleep apnea is more common in relatives of individuals with this disorder.

C. Etiology

1. **Obstructive sleep apnea syndrome** may be caused by congenital upper airway obstruction, obesity, or space-occupying lesions that compromise the airway.
2. **Central sleep apnea syndrome** may be caused by lesions in the brain stem.
3. **Central alveolar hypoventilation syndrome** may be caused by chronic obstructive pulmonary disease and other general medical conditions.

D. Diagnosis

1. **Diagnostic clues**

   a. **Presenting complaints** may include daytime drowsiness, complaints from spouse about snoring or nocturnal restlessness, and frequent awakenings during the night.

   b. **History** usually includes increasing problems with daytime fatigue and disrupted sleep.

   c. **Mental status examination** is essentially unremarkable, although the individual may be sleepy.

   d. **Physical examination.** The individual is often obese.

   e. **Laboratory studies.** Nocturnal polysomnography may show short sleep duration, increased time in stage 1 sleep, decreased time in REM and slow-wave sleep, and frequent awakenings.

      (1) In **obstructive sleep apnea syndrome,** the individual may have apneic episodes of varying duration, reduced arterial oxygen saturation, and evidence of airway obstruction in imaging studies.

      (2) In **central sleep apnea syndrome,** the individual may have irregular breathing (e.g., Cheyne-Stokes), apneic episodes, and reduced arterial oxygen saturation.

      (3) In **central alveolar hypoventilation syndrome,** the individual may have reduced airflow, reduced arterial oxygen saturation, and increased carbon dioxide levels.

2. The DSM-IV describes the major **diagnostic feature** as a sleep disruption, which causes insomnia or daytime somnolence, that is caused by a sleep-related breathing condition. The disturbance is not caused by another mental disorder, substances, or a general medical condition (other than a breathing-related disorder).

3. **Subtypes.** The specific breathing problem is classified as a general medical condition on Axis III in the DSM-IV.

4. **Associated features**

   a. **General medical conditions** associated with breathing-related sleep disorder include:

      (1) Obesity (in obstructive sleep apnea)
      (2) Mild hypertension
      (3) Pulmonary hypertension and signs of right-sided cardiac failure
      (4) Neurologic conditions affecting respiratory control
      (5) Space-occupying lesions causing airway obstruction

     b. Signs of respiratory distress during sleep include loud snoring, apneic episodes, thrashing in bed, peculiar sleeping positions, frequent awakenings, and nocturia or enuresis.

     c. Children with obstructive sleep apnea may have disturbed sleep; however, they have fewer complaints about daytime sleepiness. They also may breathe through their mouths during the day, have difficulty with phonation, and have learning disabilities.

    5. Differential diagnoses include asymptomatic snoring, other sleep disorders, general medical conditions that affect sleep by mechanisms other than breathing disturbance, and substance-induced sleep disorders.

E. Clinical course

    1. Onset may occur at any age; however, most men with obstructive sleep apnea present in middle age. It is usually gradual, with progressive severity.

    2. In obstructive sleep apnea, weight loss may improve symptoms.

    3. Cardiovascular complications, including cardiac arrhythmias, may develop.

    4. Apneic episodes may increase with age.

F. Treatment. The goal of treatment is to improve nocturnal ventilation.

    1. Obstructive sleep apnea. Weight reduction, removal of space-occupying lesions, and nasal continuous positive airway pressure are helpful.

    2. Central sleep apnea. Treatment of the underlying neurologic condition when possible and mechanical ventilation are used.

    3. Central alveolar hypoventilation. Mechanical ventilation is used.

    4. Contraindications. Use of benzodiazepines and other sedative hypnotics to treat disrupted sleep in this disorder is contraindicated, because it may further compromise ventilation.

VII. Circadian Rhythm Sleep Disorder

A. Overview

    1. An individual's internal sleep–wake cycle may not always match desired sleeping and waking times.

     a. Delayed sleep phase. Internal and desired circadian rhythms may not be in accord; the individual never falls asleep until late in the night and never feels fully awake until late in the morning.

     b. Jet lag. An individual who travels may have difficulty adjusting to a different time zone.

     c. Shift work. An individual is forced by work requirements to have a sleep–wake cycle that does not coincide with the typical nocturnal sleep period; or, the individual may continually shift from one schedule to another.

    2. Although many individuals experience transient sleep difficulties under certain conditions, circadian rhythm sleep disorder is diagnosed if the problems persist and cause significant impairment.

B. Epidemiology

1. Symptoms are more common with aging, and adolescents commonly have delayed sleep phase.
2. The **prevalence** of delayed sleep phase disturbances in adolescents is 7%, and the prevalence of shift work disturbances in night-shift workers is 60%.

C. Etiology

1. Depending on the individual, this disorder is caused by a combination of social or biologic inabilities to reset the endogenous sleep–wake cycle to a more desired one.
2. The endogenous sleep–wake cycle may be influenced by light exposure. The biologic mechanisms that accomplish this may be impaired in individuals with this disorder.

D. Diagnosis

1. **Diagnostic clues**

    a. **Presenting complaints** include persistent morning drowsiness, severe jet lag, inability to maintain full wakefulness during shift work, and inability to sleep during desired sleep time.
    b. **History.** The individual may be a "night owl." Also, the individual may have traveled recently or frequently by jet to different time zones, particularly west to east. The individual may perform shift work, particularly with changing schedules.
    c. **Mental status** and **physical examinations** are typically unremarkable.
    d. **Laboratory studies.** Polysomnographic findings are usually normal during periods when the individual feels sleepy. During the desired externally imposed sleep periods, sleep latency is increased and sleep continuity is decreased.

2. **Diagnostic features**

    a. There is a significant disaccord between the sleep–wake cycle required by an individual's environment and the individual's circadian sleep–wake pattern.
    b. The disturbance is not exclusively a manifestation of another sleep disorder, another mental disorder, substance use, or a general medical condition.

3. **Subtypes** include:

    a. Delayed sleep phase type (see VII A 1 a)
    b. Jet lag type (see VII A 1 b)
    c. Shift work type (see VII A 1 c)
    d. Unspecified type

4. **Associated features**

    a. Occupational, social, and family problems may be more common in affected individuals.
    b. Schizoid, schizotypal, and avoidant personality features may be present in delayed sleep phase type.
    c. The disorder may exacerbate other psychiatric conditions.

5. **Differential diagnoses** include typical variations in sleep patterns, other sleep disorders, other mental disorders with associated sleep disturbances, substance-induced sleep disturbances, and sleep disturbances due to general medical conditions.

E. **Clinical course**

1. Delayed sleep phase type starts in adolescence and may attenuate with aging.
2. Phase shift types may persist unless the work schedule changes.
3. Jet lag type usually resolves over several days in new time zones.
4. A susceptibility to future episodes of circadian rhythm sleep disorder may persist after the current episode remits.

F. **Treatment.** The goal of treatment is to shift the sleep–wake cycle to a more desirable one.

1. The individual **gradually changes bed times** toward the desired time, paying careful attention to **sleep hygiene.**
2. Occasionally, **short-term use of benzodiazepines** or other hypnotics may be helpful.

VIII. Nightmare Disorder

A. **Overview.** Disturbing dreams have disrupted the sleep of the fictional and nonfictional, and they have been ascribed to everything from a profoundly guilty conscience to indigestion.

1. As described in the DSM-IV criteria for nightmare disorder, the content of these dreams usually involves threats to an individual's survival, security, or self-esteem.
2. The individual often remembers the nightmares in great detail on awakening, making it difficult to return to sleep.

B. **Epidemiology.** Although nightmares are common, the prevalence of nightmare disorder is unknown. Children often have nightmares, and women report nightmares more often than men.

C. **Etiology.** Although most clinicians believe that intrapsychic emotional conflict is associated with nightmares, biologic predisposition to this condition has been proposed.

D. **Diagnosis**

1. **Diagnostic Clues**

   a. **Presenting complaints** include nightmares and disrupted sleep.
   b. **History.** The individual often recalls nightmares in some detail.
   c. **Mental status** and **physical examinations** are essentially unremarkable.
   d. **Laboratory studies.** Polysomnographic recordings show sudden awakenings from REM sleep at the time the individual reports nightmares.

2. **Diagnostic features**

   a. The DSM-IV describes the major diagnostic feature as repeated, clinically significant awakenings from sleep with a detailed recall of disturbing dreams. The individual rapidly becomes alert and oriented after awakening from the nightmares.

b. The nightmares are not caused by another mental disorders (e.g., posttraumatic stress disorder), substances, or general medical conditions.

3. **Associated features.** Anxiety and depressive symptoms are common in individuals with this disorder.

4. **Differential diagnoses** include sleep terror disorder; substance-induced sleep disorder, parasomnia type; sleep disorder due to a general medical condition, parasomnia type; and nightmares caused by other mental disorders.

E. Clinical course

1. Frequent nightmares often begin in childhood, and usually resolve quickly.

2. In some individuals, the symptoms may persist for years without resolving.

F. Treatment

1. **Reassurance** may be useful for managing the anxiety caused by nightmare disorder.

2. Discussing the emotional significance of the dream content and resolving the associated intrapsychic conflict may help decrease anxiety and improve sleep.

3. **Benzodiazepines** and other hypnotics are sometimes used to improve sleep continuity.

IX. Sleep Terror Disorder

A. Overview

1. **Episodes.** Individuals, especially children, sometimes have isolated episodes of sudden arousal from sleep in a condition of terror and confusion. These episodes are distinguished from nightmares by the absence of any storylike recall of disturbing dream events and by subsequent amnesia for the episodes.

2. Sleep terror disorder is diagnosed when these episodes are frequent and cause clinically significant distress.

B. Epidemiology. The prevalence of this disorder is about 1% of the population.

1. The disorder is more common in children, and it is more common in boys than in girls.

2. In adults, this disorder occurs at a **1:1 male to female ratio.**

3. Sleep terror and sleepwalking are more common in relatives of individuals with this disorder.

C. The **etiology** is unknown, although a biologic predisposition is suggested.

D. Diagnosis

1. **Diagnostic clues**

   a. Presenting complaints are often from spouses or parents about the individual's sudden screams and confusion upon awakening.

   b. Mental status examination is essentially unremarkable, except during episodes.

      c. Physical examination is typically unremarkable.

      d. Laboratory studies. Polysomnographic recordings show sudden partial awakenings from slow-wave sleep (with theta and alpha waves), accompanied by autonomic arousal. The awakenings frequently occur early in the sleep period and not during REM sleep.

  2. The major **diagnostic feature** is abrupt, recurrent, and clinically significant awakenings from sleep, accompanied by panic and autonomic arousal, with relative unresponsiveness to the environment and subsequent amnesia for the episode.

  3. Associated features

      a. Some semi-purposeful motor activity, including sleepwalking, may occur during episodes.

      b. Environmental sleep disruptions, emotional stress, and use of depressant drugs increase the likelihood of episodes.

      c. More depressive and anxiety symptoms and more psychopathology are diagnosed in individuals with this disorder.

  4. Differential diagnoses include nightmare disorder, sleepwalking disorder, other parasomnias, hypnogogic hallucinations in narcolepsy, nocturnal seizures, and substance-induced sleep disorders, parasomnia type.

E. Clinical course

  1. The **onset** is usually in middle childhood, and the disorder usually resolves during adolescence.

  2. If the onset is during adulthood, the course may be more chronic.

F. Treatment. The goal of treatment is to decrease the frequency of sleep terror episodes.

  1. Treatment is directed at ameliorating environmental sleeping disturbances and emotional stress through education about sleep hygiene and reassurance. Psychotherapy is also helpful to resolve emotional conflicts.

  2. Diazepam is often effective, perhaps by decreasing the amount of slow-wave sleep.

X. Sleepwalking Disorder

A. Overview. Sleepwalking describes a spectrum of motor behavior that occurs during sleep that ranges from confused arousal to getting up out of bed. The individual may walk about and engage in activities, such as eating or responding to other people.

  1. Usually, the individual has reduced responsiveness during the episode and amnesia for the sleepwalking events.

  2. Episodes terminate when the individual awakes in a confused state or returns to bed and resumes normal sleep.

  3. Isolated sleepwalking episodes are fairly common, especially in childhood.

B. Epidemiology

  1. This disorder occurs at a **1:1 male to female ratio.** The prevalence of this disorder is 2% of the population.

2. Sleepwalking and sleep terrors are more common in relatives of individuals with this disorder.

C. **Etiology.** Because of the strong familial aggregation of this disorder, heritable factors may cause this disorder. Presumptively, these factors involve dysregulation of sleep events.

D. **Diagnosis**

1. **Diagnostic Clues**

   a. **Presenting complaints** include sleepwalking, which is reported by the individual or others, and awakening in different locations (e.g., in the kitchen or front yard) with amnesia for events that transpired.

   b. **History** includes recurrent episodes of sleepwalking.

   c. **Mental status examination** is unremarkable, except during sleepwalking episodes.

   d. **Physical examination** is unremarkable.

   e. **Laboratory studies.** Polysomnography, when not obscured by movement artifact (e.g., disruptions in tracing electrical events because of attempts to walk while electrodes are attached), shows episodes of arousal, which start during slow-wave NREM sleep.

2. **Diagnostic features.** Sleepwalking disorder is diagnosed when an individual has repeated and clinically significant episodes of complex motor behavior that begins during sleep, reduced environmental responsiveness during the episodes, and amnesia for the events the following morning.

   a. Shortly after awakening from the episodes, mental status returns to normal.

   b. The episodes are not substance-induced and are not caused by a general medical condition.

3. **Associated features**

   a. Other parasomnias are common in individuals with sleepwalking disorder.

   b. Stress and alcohol and other sedatives may increase the frequency of sleepwalking episodes.

4. **Differential diagnoses** include nonclinical sleepwalking episodes, sleep terror disorder, breathing-related sleep disorder, sleep-related epilepsy, and substance-induced sleep disorder, parasomnia type.

E. **Clinical course**

1. Sleepwalking usually remits spontaneously in adolescence.

2. The course of sleepwalking disorder in adults is usually characterized by waxing and waning of symptoms for many years.

F. **Treatment.** The goals of treatment are to decrease the intensity, frequency, and potential danger of sleepwalking events.

1. Often, discontinuation of alcohol or other substance use markedly improves the clinical picture.

2. Stress reduction may also be helpful.

3. Administration of **diazepam** may be useful; it decreases the amount of NREM sleep.

XI. Sleep Disorders Related to Another Mental Disorder. These sleep disturbances are diagnosed if the sleep disturbance requires a separate clinical focus.

    A. Overview. Many mental disorders cause insomnia or hypersomnia, and separate diagnoses are usually not needed.

        1. Disorders that most commonly cause sleep disturbances include deliriums, dementias, schizophrenia and other psychotic disorders, mood disorders, and anxiety disorders.

        2. When a sleep disturbance is clinically significant and warrants independent attention, insomnia or hypersomnia related to another mental disorder is diagnosed.

    B. The **course** and **treatment** of these disorders are usually determined by the related mental disorder.

XII. Sleep Disorder Due to a General Medical Condition. This disorder is characterized by sleep disturbances that are caused by the physiologic effects of general medical conditions.

    A. Overview. Sleep disturbances commonly occur during the course of a general medical condition; however, a sleep disorder is diagnosed when the disturbance becomes a separate focus of clinical attention.

    B. Subtypes include:

        1. Insomnia type
        2. Hypersomnia type
        3. Parasomnia type
        4. Mixed type

    C. General medical conditions that often cause sleep disturbances include degenerative neurologic diseases, cerebrovascular disease, endocrine disease, CNS infections, and pain.

    D. Treatment. In addition to treating the related general medical condition, sleep hygiene and the judicious use of hypnotic agents may be effective in treating the sleep disturbance.

XIII. Substance-Induced Sleep Disorder. This disorder involves significant complaints of sleep disturbance that result from the concurrent use, or recent cessation of use, of a substance, including medication.

    A. Diagnosis. This disorder is diagnosed when sleep disturbances occur exclusively during the course of intoxication or withdrawal from substances.

    B. Subtypes include:

        1. Insomnia type
        2. Hypersomnia type
        3. Parasomnia type
        4. Mixed type

    C. Substances that induce sleep disturbances during intoxication and withdrawal include alcohol, amphetamines, caffeine, cocaine, opioids, sedatives, hypnotics, and anxiolytics.

Review Test

Directions: Each of the numbered items or incomplete statements in this section is followed by answers or by completions of the statement. Select the ONE lettered answer or completion that is BEST in each case.

1. A 45-year-old man states that he has experienced severe, recurrent insomnia since a stressful business failure two years ago. At the time that his business failed, he worked extremely long and irregular hours, and he often was unable to fall asleep. Although his business problems have been resolved and are no longer a source of worry for him, he says that he still has trouble falling asleep and staying asleep. He denies having other medical problems or abusing alcohol. Which of the following is the most likely diagnosis?

(A) Adjustment disorder with anxious mood
(B) Circadian rhythm sleep disorder, shift work type
(C) Generalized anxiety disorder
(D) Insomnia due to another mental disorder
(E) Primary insomnia

2. A 52-year-old man complains of falling asleep too easily. He drifts off to sleep when he is working at his desk, after lunch, and during work conferences or dinner with a friend. He is embarrassed by his behavior. He states that he fights the urge to sleep, but the urge is irresistible. Which of the following polysomnographic findings would he most likely have?

(A) Apneic episodes
(B) Decreased sleep latency
(C) Increased sleep efficiency
(D) Intrusive rapid eye movement (REM) activity
(E) Poor sleep continuity

3. A 27-year-old woman complains of irresistable daytime sleep episodes from which she awakes refreshed. She says that she sleeps well at night. A polysomnographic study shows rapid eye movement (REM) periods that begin during stage 1 sleep. Which of the following is the best initial treatment plan?

(A) Initiate flurazepam
(B) Instruct the woman about sleep hygiene
(C) Initiate methylphenidate
(D) Initiate trazodone
(E) Initiate valproate

4. A 64-year-old man complains of daytime fatigue and nocturnal sleep that is not refreshing. His wife confirms that he sleeps restlessly during the night and frequently awakens. She also states she knows when he is awake, because that is the only time his loud snoring ceases. Which of the following treatment plans is most likely to be effective?

(A) Initiate diazepam
(B) Initiate methylphenidate
(C) Nasal continuous positive airway pressure
(D) Nasal decongestant spray

5. A 10-year-old boy is brought in by his parents who state that he has frequent nightmares. They describe numerous episodes in which he suddenly cries out in his sleep and awakens. During these episodes, he appears frightened and confused. After being soothed, he drifts back into sleep. The boy says that he is unable to remember these episodes. Which of the following is the most likely diagnosis?

(A) Circadian rhythm sleep disorder
(B) Insomnia due to another mental disorder
(C) Nightmare disorder
(D) Sleep apnea, central type
(E) Sleep terror disorder

Answers and Explanations

1—E. The man has difficulty initiating and maintaining sleep, suggesting a diagnosis of primary insomnia. Primary insomnia often begins during a period of stress and persists after the stressor has resolved. Because the initial stressor has resolved in this case, adjustment disorder or insomnia due to another mental disorder is an unlikely diagnosis. Circadian rhythm sleep disorder is associated with ongoing disruptions of an individual's sleep–wake cycle. Generalized anxiety disorder is characterized by excessive anxiety that is difficult to control.

2—B. The patient's presenting complaint is rapid sleep onset, which is also called decreased sleep latency. Irresistable daytime sleepiness may suggest either hypersomnia or disturbed sleep periods characterized by decreased sleep efficiency, poor sleep continuity, or both. Apneic episodes cause disturbed sleep. Intrusive rapid eye movement (REM) activity is characterized clinically by hypnogogic hallucinations or cataplexy.

3—C. Narcolepsy is characterized by attacks of refreshing daytime sleep and intrusive rapid eye movement (REM) episodes. Methylphenidate is the treatment of choice for narcolepsy. Used alone, flurazepam, trazodone, or valproate has no clear efficacy for this disorder. Sleep hygiene does not improve the symptoms of narcolepsy.

4—C. Restless sleep, frequent awakenings during sleep, and daytime sleepiness are symptoms of a breathing-related sleep disorder. The patient's snoring suggests an obstructive etiology. Nasal continuous positive airway pressure, in addition to weight loss and removing any space-occupying lesion, are the treatments of choice. Benzodiazepines and other hypnotics are contraindicated in sleep apnea.

5—E. Sleep terror disorder is characterized by sudden awakening accompanied by autonomic arousal, with subsequent amnesia for the episode. The episodes occur during non–rapid eye movement (NREM) sleep. Nightmare disorder is characterized by disturbing dreams and occurs during rapid eye movement (REM) sleep. There is limited data in this case to suggest the diagnosis of circadian rhythm sleep disorder, insomnia due to another mental disorder, or sleep apnea, central type.

22

Impulse-Control Disorders

I. Overview

A. **Impulses.** Individuals are continuously barraged by impulses that arise from psychological drives.

1. Psychosocial development involves learning to control and channel these impulses.

2. Numerous **mental disorders** are characterized by problems with impulse control, including substance dependence, paraphilias, and antisocial and borderline personality disorders.

B. **Impulse-control disorders.** The primary pathology in these disorders is an inability to resist impulses that are harmful to the individual or others. The impulse control disorders are intermittent explosive disorder, kleptomania, pyromania, pathological gambling, and trichotillomania (see II–VI).

1. In each impulse-control disorder, the nature of the impulse is different, but the sequence of psychological events surrounding the impulse and act is similar.

    a. The individual experiences tension, excitement, or arousal before committing the act or while attempting to resist the impulse.

    b. The individual feels enjoyment, satisfaction, or relief while committing the act or witnessing the results of the act.

    c. The individual may feel a sense of remorse or guilt following the act.

2. **Characteristics.** The pathological impulses in these disorders do not stem from understandable motives, such as monetary gain, vengeance, or ideologic beliefs.

    a. The impulses are not responses to hallucinations or delusions.

    b. The impulses are not better accounted for by other disorders, such as conduct disorder, antisocial personality disorder, or manic episodes.

C. The **etiology** of impulse-control disorders is poorly understood; however, it may involve both neurobiologic and psychological factors.

D. **Treatment.** The goals of treatment are to reduce the frequency and severity of pathological impulses.

1. Although various **behavioral** and **cognitive approaches** have been used to treat these disorders, there is limited data about their effectiveness.

2. Pathological gambling may be ameliorated through **self-help groups** that are modeled after Alcoholics Anonymous.

II. Intermittent Explosive Disorder

A. Definition. Intermittent explosive disorder is characterized by at least several instances of impulsive assaults or destruction of property.

B. Prevalence. Intermittent explosive disorder is rare, and it predominantly occurs in men.

C. Associated features

1. Although the individual may describe these episodes as peculiar events of loss of control, the individuals are often aggressive between episodes.
2. Narcissistic, obsessive, paranoid, and schizoid personality traits are associated with this disorder.

D. Clinical course. Symptoms of this disorder are more common during late adolescence and early adulthood.

1. **Physical injuries** may be sustained because of fighting.
2. Symptoms may lessen in severity in later years.

III. Kleptomania

A. Definition. Kleptomania is characterized by an inability to resist impulses to steal objects. The impulses are not motivated by a perceived usefulness or worth of the objects.

B. Prevalence. The disorder is rare and is significantly more common in women.

C. Associated features

1. Individuals with this disorder are often subjectively aware of the senselessness of the theft and feel regretful.
2. Individuals with this disorder often have social and legal difficulties when they are caught stealing.
3. This disorder is sometimes associated with bulimia nervosa.

D. The **clinical course** may be characterized by chronic or sporadic stealing.

IV. Pyromania

A. Definition. Pyromania is characterized by episodes of intentional fire setting.

B. Associated features

1. Individuals with this disorder are often fascinated by fires and firefighting.
2. They may experience pleasure because of the destruction they caused.

C. Course and prevalence. Pyromania is rare and little is known about its course. Fire setting is much more common in adolescents but is usually secondary to other behavioral disorders.

V. Pathological Gambling

A. Definition. Pathological gambling is characterized by chronic, progressive, and maladaptive gambling behavior.

1. Individuals with this disorder develop a preoccupation with gambling, losing control over the frequency of gambling and amounts wagered.

2. They may attempt to conceal their behavior and losses from others, and they often jeopardize both social relationships and financial situations.

B. Prevalence. This disorder may be relatively common (i.e., approximately 2% of the population) and occurs at a **2:1 male to female ratio.**

C. Associated features

1. Associated **personality traits** include competitiveness, restlessness, mood lability, and erratic work habits.
2. Individuals with this disorder have a higher incidence of substance abuse, mood disorders, and personality disorders.

D. Clinical course. The disorder usually has an insidious onset, with exacerbations during stress and a gradually increasing overall severity.

VI. Trichotillomania

A. Definition. Trichotillomania is characterized by chronic hair pulling that causes obvious hair loss.

1. Individuals most commonly pull hair from their scalp, eyebrows, and eyelashes; however, any body hair may be involved.
2. The behavior increases during stress and sometimes during times of relaxation.
3. Individuals may attempt to conceal resulting alopecia.

B. Epidemiology

1. The **prevalence** is approximately 1% of the population.
2. It appears to be equally common in males and females during childhood. During adulthood, it occurs more often, or is more noticeable, in females.

C. Associated features. Trichophagia, nail biting, and scratching may also be present.

D. Clinical course. The **onset** is usually during childhood. The disorder may last for decades and vary in severity.

Review Test

Directions: Each of the numbered items or incomplete statements in this section is followed by answers or by completions of the statement. Select the ONE lettered answer or completion that is BEST in each case.

1. A 7-year-old girl has excoriated areas on her hands caused by scratching, and her fingernails are bitten to the quick. Physical examination shows several alopecic patches on her head. The girl says that she likes to pull her hair and chew it when she is upset. Which of the following is the most likely diagnosis?

(A) Attention deficit hyperactivity disorder
(B) Autistic disorder
(C) Generalized anxiety disorder
(D) Pica
(E) Trichotillomania

2. A 15-year-old boy is accused of setting his neighbor's car on fire to destroy evidence that he had broken into the car and stolen a wallet. The boy has been linked to several suspicious fires that followed burglaries. He has a recent history of truancy and fighting. Which of the following is the most likely diagnosis?

(A) Antisocial personality disorder
(B) Attention deficit hyperactivity disorder
(C) Conduct disorder
(D) Kleptomania
(E) Pyromania

3. A 20-year-old woman complains of being unable to maintain the body weight she desires. She says that she often has irresistible urges to consume large quantities of junk food and feels guilty after acting on these urges. She also says that she steals small items from stores, although she can easily afford to pay for them. She says that stealing gives her "a thrill" when she leaves the store undetected. In addition to bulimia nervosa, which of the following is the most likely diagnosis?

(A) Antisocial personality disorder
(B) Borderline personality disorder
(C) Intermittent explosive disorder
(D) Kleptomania
(E) Schizophrenia, disorganized type

4. A 24-year-old man is repeatedly brought to the emergency room of a local hospital for injuries he sustains fighting with strangers at a bar. He says that he becomes belligerent and aggressive, even before he begins to drink. He notes that he usually regrets his actions immediately afterward and often drinks heavily to decrease his agitation and physical pain. Which of the following is the most likely diagnosis to account for his fighting?

(A) Alcohol intoxication
(B) Antisocial personality disorder
(C) Delirium
(D) Intermittent explosive disorder
(E) Oppositional defiant disorder

5. A 67-year-old man complains of being unable to stop spending his retirement fund gambling in Las Vegas. He says that he has gambled for most of his life and has occasionally won large sums of money. He says that he now feels like he is "losing control." He says that he is depressed about living on a fixed income and the thought of aging. Which of the following is the most likely diagnosis?

(A) Bipolar II disorder
(B) Dementia
(C) Major depressive disorder
(D) Obsessive-compulsive disorder
(E) Pathological gambling

Answers and Explanations

1—E. The alopecic patches are evidence of hair pulling, which the girl engages in to decrease anxiety. This behavior is most suggestive of trichotillomania. Hair chewing, nail biting, and scratching are behaviors that commonly accompany this disorder. There is little evidence of attention deficit hyperactivity disorder or autistic disorder in this case. Generalized anxiety disorder would be a more likely diagnosis if the girl's anxiety was excessive and difficult to control. Pica is characterized by ingesting, not simply chewing, nonnutritive substances.

2—C. The boy's behaviors represent a violation of major age-appropriate norms in several areas, which is most consistent with a diagnosis of conduct disorder. Antisocial personality disorder is not diagnosed before adulthood, and there is little evidence of attention deficit disorder in this case. Kleptomania would be a more likely diagnosis if the objects stolen had no value to the boy. Pyromania would also be a more likely diagnosis if the fire was set for pleasure or gratification; instead, the boy set the fire to conceal a burglary.

3—D. Impulsive and pleasure-inducing stealing of objects that an individuals does not need is most suggestive of kleptomania. This disorder is commonly associated with individuals who have bulimia nervosa. There is little evidence of a larger pattern of violations that would suggest a diagnosis of antisocial personality disorder. Although borderline personality disorder is also commonly associated with bulimia nervosa, there is little evidence for the diagnosis in this case. There is no evidence of uncontrolled aggressiveness to suggest intermittent explosive disorder or psychosis to suggest schizophrenia.

4—D. Irresistible episodes of aggressiveness are most suggestive of intermittent explosive disorder. If the episodes only occurred following alcohol ingestion, his behavior would more likely be caused by intoxication. Antisocial personality disorder is often associated with intermittent explosive disorder; however, there is little evidence in this case to suggest a pattern of rule violations. There is no evidence of delirium. Oppositional defiant disorder would be a more likely diagnosis if his aggressiveness was directed toward authority figures.

5—E. An irresistible urge to gamble, despite the serious problems it is causing, is most suggestive of pathological gambling. Bipolar II disorder would be a more likely diagnosis if the individual had other signs of hypomania (e.g., grandiosity). Although dementia is associated with decreased impulse control, the man has no signs of cognitive impairment. The man is unhappy, but there are no additional symptoms that strongly suggest he has major depressive disorder. Obsessive-compulsive disorder may be characterized by irresistible impulses, but the impulses are irrational.

23

Adjustment Disorders

I. Overview

A. Environmental stressors. Many individuals encounter difficult environmental stressors during certain periods of their lives. Stressors include interpersonal problems (e.g., divorce), occupational problems (e.g., job loss), and medical problems (e.g., onset of a serious illness).

1. During these periods, individuals may experience anxiety, depression, or behavioral symptoms (e.g., erratic actions) that interfere with functioning.
2. As the stressors resolve or new coping skills develop, the symptoms remit.

B. Adjustment disorders are diagnosed when environmental stressors have a clinically significant effect on the individual's functioning. The risk that a stressor will cause an adjustment disorder depends on the individual's emotional strength and coping skills.

II. Epidemiology. These disorders are very common.

III. Diagnosis

A. Diagnostic Clues

1. **Presenting complaints** include a "nervous breakdown," inability to manage problems of life, and overwhelming anxiety or depression associated with specific life stressors.
2. **History.** The individual experiences essentially normal functioning before the onset of the stressor.
3. **Mental status examination** shows symptoms of anxiety, depression, or disturbed conduct.

B. Diagnostic features. The DSM-IV describes these disorders as maladaptive reactions to an identifiable psychosocial stressor. The reactions occur within 3 months of the initial presence of the stressor and last 6 months or less after the stressor ends or is resolved. The individual's reactions are not merely a pattern of overreaction to stress and do not meet the criteria for other psychiatric disorders.

1. **Subtypes** include:

   a. With depressed mood
   b. With anxiety

      c. With disturbance of conduct
      d. With mixed disturbances of emotions and conduct

  2. Acute and chronic adjustment disorders. Adjustment disorders are acute if the symptoms last less than 6 months and chronic if the symptoms last longer than 6 months.

C. Associated features. Social and occupational performance may be compromised. The individual may become unpredictable, less conscientious, or socially withdrawn.

D. Differential diagnosis. These disorders may be difficult to distinguish from a normal reaction to stress or from other psychiatric disorders that occur following stress (e.g., generalized anxiety disorder, acute or posttraumatic stress disorders, major depressive disorder).

IV. Clinical course

A. The **onset** of an adjustment disorder begins shortly following a significant environmental stressor.

B. If the stressor ceases, the individual's symptoms usually remit quickly.

C. If the stressor persists, the individual's symptoms may also continue unless he develops new ways of coping with the stressor and adapts to the new situation.

V. Treatment

A. Etiologic stressors should be removed or ameliorated when possible.

B. Brief **cognitive** or **psychodynamic psychotherapy** is usually the treatment of choice. The focus of psychotherapy is on improving coping skills, strengthening defense mechanisms, or changing the way the individual evaluates a stressful situation.

C. Adjunctive **anxiolytic** or **antidepressant medication** may be used to decrease intolerable anxiety, improve secondary insomnia, or alleviate severe depression.

Review Test

Directions: Each of the numbered items or incomplete statements in this section is followed by answers or by completions of the statement. Select the ONE lettered answer or completion that is BEST in each case.

1. A 28-year-old woman without previous behavioral problems becomes angry and bitter after her husband of 5 years leaves her to live with his female business partner. One week later, the woman quits her job without giving notice and begins drinking heavily. For the next several weeks, the woman telephones friends and tearfully expresses suicidal rumination. She also makes several threatening calls to her husband's new girlfriend. Which of the following is the most likely diagnosis?

(A) Adjustment disorder
(B) Alcohol-induced mood disorder
(C) Bipolar I disorder
(D) Bipolar II disorder
(E) Borderline personality disorder

2. A 53-year-old man who was laid off 3 months ago from his job as a graphics designer complains of paralyzing anxiety. He says that he is unable to concentrate on reading help wanted advertisements or arranging job interviews. He has difficulty making even simple decisions (e.g., about what to wear) and has trouble falling asleep. Which of the following is the most likely diagnosis?

(A) Adjustment disorder with anxiety
(B) Adjustment disorder with depressed mood
(C) Adjustment disorder with disturbance of conduct
(D) Generalized anxiety disorder
(E) Social phobia

3. A 77-year-old man is demoralized following sudden, unilateral hearing loss. He describes difficulty driving his car because of his decreased ability to hear local sound. He no longer enjoys music as much as he used to, and he is embarrassed when conversing with others because he has difficulty hearing from his left side. He has started to avoid social events and ruminates about the problems of aging. Which of the following is the best initial treatment regimen?

(A) Antidepressant medication
(B) Biofeedback training
(C) Brief psychotherapy
(D) Group psychotherapy
(E) Systematic desensitization

4. Four months after witnessing the murder of her parents and younger brother during a burglary of her home, a 19-year-old woman begins behaving in an increasingly irresponsible manner. She visits bars and dance clubs alone, accepts rides home from strangers, and engages in high-risk sexual activity. Which of the following is the most likely diagnosis?

(A) Acute stress disorder
(B) Adjustment disorder with disturbance of conduct
(C) Alcohol intoxication
(D) Bipolar I disorder, single manic episode
(E) Posttraumatic stress disorder

Answers and Explanations

1–A. Depression and erratic behavior following an interpersonal stressor are most suggestive of adjustment disorder with mixed disturbance of emotions and conduct. The cause of the symptoms is most likely the stressor and not the physiologic result of alcohol. Bipolar disorders I and II are unlikely diagnoses for an individual who has no history of mood episodes. Borderline personality disorder is a less likely diagnosis for an individual who has no history of past behavioral and interpersonal difficulties.

2–A. The man's symptoms of anxiety following a serious stressor (i.e., job loss) are most suggestive of adjustment disorder with anxiety. He has no symptoms of erratic behavior, which would suggest a conduct disturbance, and significant depressive symptoms are not elicited. Generalized anxiety disorder is characterized by excessive anxiety about multiple matters and persists for at least 6 months. Social phobia is characterized by anxiety that is caused by a fear of embarrassment in social situations and, similar to generalized anxiety disorder, persists for at least 6 months.

3–C. The man's symptoms suggest that he has adjustment disorder with anxious mood. In this case, his symptoms of anxiety are serious and significantly interfere with daily functioning. Adjustment disorders often respond to brief courses of psychotherapy that focus on better methods of coping with current stressors. Antidepressant medication may be used if the symptoms persist or intensify. Biofeedback training and systematic desensitization are behavioral techniques that are useful for treating anxiety symptoms, but are not commonly used to treat depression. Group psychotherapy would be difficult, at least initially, for a withdrawn and embarrassed individual.

4–B. Erratic behavior following a severe stressor is most suggestive of adjustment disorder with disturbance of conduct. Posttraumatic stress disorder would be a more likely diagnosis if the woman had intrusive recollections of her family's murder, emotional numbness, and persistent hyperarousal. Acute stress disorder is diagnosed only within 1 month following a severe stressor. Bipolar I disorder, single manic episode, would be a more likely diagnosis if other symptoms of mania (e.g., sleeplessness, grandiosity, expansiveness) were present. Alcohol intoxication is unlikely to cause this woman's marked change of behavior.

24

Personality Disorders

I. Overview

A. Personality is composed of an individual's different personality traits.

    1. Personality traits are described by the DSM-IV as enduring modes of comprehending and relating to the environment and oneself. These modes are present in many settings.

    2. A **personality disorder** is described by the DSM-IV as a long-term, stable pattern of unusual and inflexible personality traits that lead to functional impairment or distress.

B. Axis II. Personality disorders are described by the DSM-IV as qualitatively different from other psychiatric disorders and are placed on a separate diagnostic axis—Axis II.

II. Diagnosis

A. Diagnostic features. Individuals with a personality disorder exhibit markedly deviant, inflexible, and maladaptive patterns of inner perception and behavior.

    1. These patterns have been present since adolescence or early adulthood.

    2. These patterns are not exclusively a manifestation of another mental disorder, and they are neither substance-induced nor caused by a general medical condition.

    3. The patterns occur in several of the following areas:

        a. Cognition, which is the way individuals perceive and interpret themselves and others

        b. Affect, which is the quality of emotional responsiveness

        c. Interpersonal functioning, which is how an individual interacts with others

        d. Impulse control, which is the ability to restrain actions

B. Diagnostic clues

    1. Presenting complaints include impaired interpersonal relationships, chronic unhappiness, and low self-esteem.

2. **History.** The individual may have a long pattern of impaired interpersonal relationships, problems with adapting to environmental stress, and failure to achieve social or occupational goals.

3. **Mental status examination** may reveal characteristic abnormalities.

   a. In **Cluster A** disorders, the individual may have peculiar thought processes or content and inappropriate affect.

   b. In **Cluster B** disorders, the individual may have mood and affect lability, dissociative symptoms, and a preoccupation with rejection.

   c. In **Cluster C** disorders, the individual may have anxiety and may be preoccupied with criticism or rigidity.

4. **Physical examination** is usually unremarkable. However, there may be evidence of violence (e.g., bruises and knife and gunshot wounds) in those with antisocial personality disorder and evidence of self-destructive behavior (e.g., wrist cuts and scars, burns) in those with borderline personality disorder.

5. **Laboratory studies** are usually unremarkable, although evidence of substance abuse is more likely in those with antisocial and borderline personality disorders.

C. **Types.** The DSM-IV classifies three **clusters** of personality disorders that share trait patterns.

   1. **Cluster A: Odd or eccentric**

      a. **Paranoid personality disorder** is characterized by distrust and suspiciousness (see VII A).

      b. **Schizoid personality disorder** is characterized by detachment and restricted emotionality (see VII B).

      c. **Schizotypal personality disorder** is characterized by a discomfort with social relationships, thought distortion, and eccentricity (see VII C).

   2. **Cluster B: Dramatic, emotional, or erratic**

      a. **Antisocial personality disorder** is characterized by a disregard and violation of the basic rights of others (see VII D).

      b. **Borderline personality disorder** is characterized by social and emotional instability (see VII E).

      c. **Histrionic personality disorder** is characterized by emotionality and attention-seeking behavior (see VII F).

      d. **Narcissistic personality disorder** is characterized by an inflated self-esteem, demands for admiration, and a lack of concern for others (see VII G).

   3. **Cluster C: Anxious or fearful**

      a. **Avoidant personality disorder** is characterized by social inhibition, feelings of inadequacy, and hypersensitivity to criticism (see VII H).

      b. **Dependent personality disorder** is characterized by submissive and clinging behavior associated with a need to be taken care of (see VII I).

      c. **Obsessive-compulsive personality disorder** is characterized by a preoccupation with orderliness, perfection, and control (see VII J).

4. Other personality disorders

a. Some clinicians believe that several additional personality disorders exist, including passive-aggressive (negativistic) and depressive personality disorder. Other clinicians believe that attempts to classify personality disorders are reductionistic, and that there are an infinite number of possible personality disorders.

b. Personality disorder not otherwise specified is described in the DSM-IV for personality disorders that have a pattern of pathologic traits that are not clearly accounted for by any of the specific personality disorders.

D. Distinguishing features. Personality disorders may be distinguished by the associated interpersonal interactions or self-perceptions.

1. For example, individuals with schizoid and avoidant personality disorders have similar interpersonal behavior (i.e., both types avoid interaction with other individuals) but different self-perceptions (i.e., schizoid individuals feel indifferent to isolation; avoidant individuals perceive themselves as lonely).

2. Individuals with avoidant and dependent personality disorders have different interpersonal behavior (i.e., avoidant individuals isolate themselves; dependent individuals seek closeness) but similar self-perceptions (i.e., both types have low self-esteem).

III. Etiology of Personality Disorders

A. Early theories. Before the twentieth century, aberrant personality was believed to be a manifestation of faulty parental stock, "low breeding," or moral decay.

1. In the early nineteenth century, Pinel described **"manie sans delire"** as irrationality with intact intellect.

2. Pritchard described **"moral insanity,"** which was an early description of antisocial personality disorder.

3. **"Constitutional psychopathic inferiority"** was a late nineteenth century diagnosis similar to the description of an antisocial personality.

B. Freudian psychodynamic theory reshaped the way Western civilization conceptualized personality and pathology with several central tenets.

1. Adult personality is a product of the interaction between inborn factors and childhood experience. The way a person learns to solve emotional problems during various stages of childhood development determines adult personality traits.

2. Emotional problems of childhood are resolved by creating **defense mechanisms**, which are intrapsychic methods of decreasing anxiety. Specific types of childhood emotional conflict yield specific kinds of defense mechanisms, and these defense mechanisms underlie personality traits in adulthood.

3. Faulty resolution of childhood emotional conflict leads to adult psychopathology, and emotional traumas during specific stages of child development lead to specific adult personality disorders.

C. **Later psychodynamic theory**. Psychodynamic personality theory was further developed by Anna Freud, Heinz Hartmann, and others. According to these theorists, some personality traits (e.g., curiosity, creativity) are not based solely on emotional conflict, but may be realistic attempts at problem solving or exist because they are intrinsically pleasurable.

1. **Alloplastic versus autoplastic defenses (Franz Alexander)**. Alloplastic defense mechanisms distort the individual's perception of the environment and cause personality pathology; autoplastic defenses distort the individual's self-perceptions and cause "neurosis."

2. **"Character armor" (Wilhelm Reich)**. Aberrant personality traits are an individual's "armor" against the suffering generated by intrapsychic conflicts.

3. **Object relations theory (Masterson) and self-psychology (Kohut).** These similar theories emphasize the role of interpersonal relationships in forging adult personality. A faulty sense of self, caused by pathologic childhood interactions with caregivers, creates personality pathology.

4. **Temperament theory** (Chess and Thomas and others). Some researchers have examined the relationship between innate temperament and adult personality. **"Goodness of fit"** describes the quality of interaction between a child's temperament and his interpersonal environment; it is a determinant of future psychopathology.

D. **Biologic theories**. Some familial studies indicate genetic relationships between personality disorders and other psychiatric disorders, and patients with personality disorders are at higher risk for developing other psychiatric disorders.

1. There is a relationship between Cluster A personality disorders and psychotic disorders.

2. There is a relationship between Cluster B personality disorders and substance use disorders, somatoform disorders, and mood disorders.

3. There is a relationship between Cluster C personality disorders and anxiety disorders.

IV. Clinical Course of Personality Disorders

A. **Personality traits.** Inflexible and maladaptive personality traits may be apparent during childhood, but are usually evident only in some environmental contexts during this period.

1. The stability of personality traits increases with adolescence and adulthood.

2. By definition, a personality disorder is present if pathologic personality traits persist into early adulthood.

B. **Lifestyle.** Personality disorders may strongly influence an individual's choice of lifestyle, often encouraging those that minimize apparent disability.

1. For example, individuals with personality disorders that cause them to isolate themselves (e.g., schizoid or avoidant personality disorders) may choose occupations that minimize contact with others.

2. Personality disorders limit an individual's flexibility and life choices.

C. **Symptoms.** During the course of a lifetime, symptoms of specific personality disorders can exacerbate or remit.

1. **Remittance.** Symptoms of borderline, antisocial, and avoidant personality disorders often lessen with age.
2. **Exacerbations.** Symptoms of paranoid and schizoid personality disorders often exacerbate with age.

V. Differential Diagnosis of Personality Disorders

A. **Distinguishing personality disorders from normal behavior.** The inflexible and maladaptive traits in personality disorders are often present in more flexible and adaptive forms in a nonpathologic personality.

1. **"State versus trait."** Clinicians may have difficulty distinguishing innate personality traits from behavior that is induced by specific environments.
2. Some clinicians believe that dimensional approaches to describing personality—i.e., viewing personality traits as spectra between normality and pathology—are more useful than the distinct diagnostic categories in the DSM-IV.

B. **Distinguishing personality disorders from Axis I disorders**

1. The **distinction between Axis I and II disorders** is not clear-cut, and there are strong associations between disorders on different axes.
   a. Individuals with psychotic disorders often present with schizoid, schizotypal or paranoid traits.
   b. Individuals with social phobia often present with avoidant traits.
   c. Individuals with somatoform disorders often present with histrionic traits.

2. **Personality pathology** that occurs only during periods of another psychiatric disorder is not considered a separate personality disorder. If a personality disorder predates the onset of an Axis I diagnosis that contains similar traits, the personality disorder may be noted as a premorbid condition.

C. **Personality changes due to a general medical condition** are usually distinguished by an onset that coincides with the onset of the general medical condition.

D. **Postconcussional disorder.** This cognitive disorder may be associated with personality changes, as well as with cognitive problems, fatigue, sleep difficulties, headaches, and emotional lability.

E. **Comorbid conditions.** Individuals with personality disorders frequently have mood, anxiety, and substance-related disorders.

VI. Treatment

A. **Overview**

1. Treatment for personality disorders is generally directed at improving the individual's adaptation and sense of well-being by making traits more flexible and adaptive.
2. Often, individuals with a personality disorder are unaware of their personality pathology and seek treatment because of associated unhappiness, anxiety, or interpersonal problems.

B. **Psychodynamic** and **cognitive therapies** are the treatments of choice for most personality disorders.

1. The focus of psychotherapeutic exploration and recommended psychotherapeutic techniques may differ for specific personality disorders.
2. Lengthy treatment is often required for successful outcome.

C. **Psychiatric medication** may ameliorate some symptoms of certain personality disorders.

1. **Antipsychotic medication** may be useful for treatment of thought disturbances in borderline, paranoid, and schizotypal personality disorders.
2. **Antidepressant medications**, particularly selective serotonin reuptake inhibitors and monoamine oxidase inhibitors, may be useful for treatment of depressed mood and impulsivity in borderline personality disorder.
3. **Mood stabilizers** are occasionally useful in treating impulsivity in borderline and antisocial personality disorders.
4. **Anxiolytic medications** may be useful for treating anxiety associated with avoidant personality disorder.

VII. Specific Personality Disorders

A. **Paranoid personality disorder.** Individuals with this disorder tend to be mistrustful and suspicious of the motivations and actions of others. They are often secretive and isolated, and they tend to be emotionally cold and odd.

1. **Epidemiology**
   a. This disorder is more common in males and is sometimes associated with social separation imposed by culture or economics.
   b. The prevalence of this disorder is 1% of population.
   c. Schizophrenia and delusional disorder are more common in relatives of individuals with paranoid personality disorder.
2. **Associated features.** Individuals with this disorder may be socially isolated, have brief episodes of psychosis with persecutory delusions, and have preexisting sensory impairment.
3. **Differential diagnoses** include psychotic disorders with persecutory delusions, personality changes due to general medical conditions, substance-induced personality changes, and other personality disorders.
4. **Clinical course.** Symptoms may intensify in later life in association with social or sensory isolation, and delusional disorder may supervene.
5. **Treatment.** The goal of treatment is to decrease the individual's suspiciousness and isolation.

   a. Initially, supportive **psychotherapy** may be the treatment of choice. The psychotherapist should avoid ambiguous comments and not create demands for warmth and intimacy, because these may be threatening to individuals with this disorder.
   b. Individuals with severe paranoid ideation may be responsive to low doses of **antipsychotic medications**.

B. **Schizoid personality disorder.** Individuals with this disorder are usually emotionally distant and seemingly derive little joy from living. They appear uninterested in interacting with others and indifferent to praise or criticism.

1. **Epidemiology**
   a. This disorder is more common in males, but its prevalence is unknown because few individuals come to clinical attention.

b. Schizophrenia is more common in relatives of individuals with this disorder.

2. Associated features include social drifting and dysphoria.

3. Differential diagnoses include residual symptoms in schizophrenia, autistic disorder, Asperger disorder, and other personality disorders.

4. Clinical course. Symptoms are often obvious in childhood, and schizophrenia occasionally supervenes in adolescence or early adulthood. Social isolation often persists or worsens as the individual ages.

5. Treatment. The goal of treatment is to facilitate greater pleasure in life through more meaningful relationships with others.

  a. Individual psychotherapy is the initial treatment of choice, and the patient may often tolerate and even enjoy extended psychodynamic exploration.

  b. Antidepressant medication may be beneficial for individuals with marked anhedonia (i.e., inability to experience pleasure).

C. Schizotypal personality disorder. Similar to individuals with schizoid personality disorder, individuals with schizotypal personality disorder are socially isolated and uncomfortable interacting with others. In contrast to individuals with schizoid personality disorder, individuals with schizotypal personality disorder have peculiar patterns of thinking, including ideas of reference and persecution; preoccupation with metaphysical, occult, or religious phenomena; and odd manners of speech and affect.

1. Epidemiology

  a. This disorder is more common in males.

  b. The prevalence of this disorder is 3% of the population.

  c. Schizotypal personality disorders and schizophrenia are more common in relatives of individuals with this disorder.

2. Associated features include anxiety, dysphoria, other personality disorders, and occasional brief psychotic episodes.

3. Differential diagnosis (see VII B 3)

4. Clinical course. The onset of symptoms is often during childhood, and schizophrenia may supervene.

5. Treatment. The goals of treatment are to reduce idiosyncratic thinking and improve social functioning.

  a. Psychotherapy is useful for both goals. However, the therapist must be careful not to demonstrate unqualified acceptance of eccentric behavior.

  b. Antipsychotic medication may be useful to decrease the individual's bizarre ideas.

D. Antisocial personality disorder. Individuals with this disorder behave poorly toward others; repeatedly violate the law; lie; behave impulsively, irresponsibly, and aggressively; disregard the safety of themselves and others; and show a lack of remorse for their actions. These individuals may use manipulative means, such as charm or guilt, to induce others into serving their ends.

1. Epidemiology

  a. This disorder occurs at a 3:1 male to female ratio and is more common in lower socioeconomic environments.

b. The prevalence of this disorder in the male population is 3%.

c. Familial pattern. Antisocial personality disorder, somatization disorder (in female relatives), and substance-related disorders are more common in both biologic and adoptive relatives of individuals with this disorder.

2. **Diagnosis.** To diagnose this disorder, the individual must be at least 18 years of age and must have the onset of conduct disorder before 15 years of age.

3. **Associated features**

   a. Individuals with this disorder are often immersed in social strife. They may participate in criminal activity and have a history of incarcerations, failed relationships, and abandoned responsibilities. They may experience injuries or death because of violent behavior.

   b. Attention deficit hyperactivity disorder, substance-related disorders, and other personality disorders are common premorbid or comorbid conditions.

4. **Differential diagnoses** include substance-related disorders, manic episodes in bipolar or schizoaffective disorder, and other personality disorders.

5. **Clinical course**. The onset of symptoms is often during childhood, and the course of early adulthood is often complicated by drug abuse, poor academic and occupational performance, and criminal behavior. Symptoms often remit in middle age.

6. **Treatment.** The goals of treatment are to decrease impulsivity and increase the individual's conformity with societal values regarding interpersonal relationships.

   a. Individual psychotherapies have not been overwhelmingly efficacious.

   b. Group and **milieu therapies**, particularly those that strongly promote group identity and cohesion, are sometimes effective.

   c. Limit-setting for antisocial behaviors (e.g., refusal of relatives to tolerate abuse, incarceration) is often necessary during treatment.

   d. Mood stabilizers may be used to control impulsivity; however, this intervention has not demonstrated clear efficacy.

E. **Borderline personality disorder.** Individuals with this disorder have unstable interpersonal relationships, emotions, and self-image. They are also notably impulsive and often self-destructive.

1. **Epidemiology**

   a. This disorder occurs at a 1:3 male to female ratio.

   b. The prevalence of this disorder is 2% of the population.

   c. Borderline personality disorder, antisocial personality disorder, substance-related disorders, and mood disorders are more common in relatives of individuals with this disorder.

2. **Additional diagnostic features**

   a. Individuals with borderline personality disorder may be demanding and capricious in relationships, prone to irresponsibility, and emotionally labile.

    b. Suicide threats and attempts as well as other forms of self- destructive behavior are common.

    c. Their intrapsychic life may be characterized by fears of abandonment and chronic feelings of identity confusion or emotional emptiness.

    d. During times of stress, they may have paranoid ideation or severe dissociative symptoms that resemble brief psychotic episodes.

3. Associated features

    a. The interpersonal histories of individuals with borderline personality disorder are characterized by crises.

    b. A history of childhood abuse, particularly sexual abuse, is common.

    c. Mood disorders, substance-related disorders, eating disorders, posttraumatic stress disorder, and other personality disorders are frequent comorbid conditions.

4. Differential diagnoses include mood disorders, other personality disorders, and adolescent angst.

5. Clinical course. Symptoms are most severe in young adults but often decrease with age.

6. Treatment. The goals of treatment are to improve emotional stability, sense of identity, and interpersonal relationships and to decrease self-destructive behavior.

    a. Psychotherapy

        (1) Specialized, intensive individual psychotherapy, sometimes in hospital environments, is considered the treatment of choice by many clinicians.

        (2) The course of therapy is often complicated by self-destructive threats and acts, abrupt termination precipitated by the patient's anger, or intervening financial or interpersonal chaos.

        (3) Therapist countertransference is common and may adversely affect the course of treatment.

    b. Pharmacotherapy. Many classes of psychoactive medications are advocated for treatment of associated emotional instability and impulsiveness, but outcome studies have not uniformly supported their efficacy.

F. Histrionic personality disorder. Individuals with this disorder have extreme emotional lability and constantly attempt to attract attention to themselves through dramatic behavior or dress. They often appear inappropriately seductive, emotionally shallow, obsessed with their physical appearance, over-dramatic, and are unduly influenced by others.

1. Epidemiology

    a. This disorder is more commonly diagnosed in females.

    b. The prevalence of this disorder is 2% of the population.

2. Associated features include difficult interpersonal relationships, social ostracism, somatization disorder, conversion disorder, major depressive disorder, and other personality disorders.

3. Differential diagnosis is other personality disorders, particularly borderline and narcissistic personality disorders.

4. **Clinical course.** Symptoms are often most severe in early adulthood and decrease with age.

5. **Treatment.** The goals of treatment are to decrease behaviors used to inappropriately seek attention and to improve interpersonal relationships. Individual psychodynamic therapy, with a focus on exploring underlying motivations for behavior, is the treatment of choice.

G. **Narcissistic personality disorder.** Individuals with this disorder have an overriding sense of entitlement and self-importance that is coupled with a lack of understanding and concern for the feelings of others. They may be preoccupied with their own self-described accomplishments and demand attention from others, and they also may envy, dismiss, or exploit others individuals.

1. **Epidemiology**
   a. This disorder occurs at a 3:2 male to female ratio.
   b. The prevalence of this disorder is less than 1% of the population.

2. **Associated features** include hypersensitivity to real or imagined slights from others, difficult interpersonal relationships, extreme ambitiousness, periods of anger and self-pity, psychostimulant abuse, and other personality disorders.

3. **Differential diagnoses** include other personality disorders, particularly antisocial, borderline, and narcissistic personality disorders, and manic or hypomanic episodes.

4. **Clinical course.** Symptoms may increase as aging-related problems (e.g., debilitating general medical conditions, decreasing social and occupational status) accumulate.

5. **Treatment.** The goal of definitive treatment is a far-reaching reorganization of the individual's relationship to self and others. Psychotherapy is complicated by the breadth of the goal and by the individual's limited motivation for change.

H. **Avoidant personality disorder.** Individuals with this disorder shy away from or avoid almost all occupational or social relationships because of fears of rejection that are based on feelings of inadequacy.

1. **Epidemiology**
   a. This disorder occurs at a 1:1 male to female ratio.
   b. The prevalence of this disorder is 1% of the population. The prevalence may vary in cultures, depending on the acceptability of diffident behavior.

2. **Additional diagnostic features.** Individuals with this disorder perceive themselves as substandard and are preoccupied with rejection, often avoiding activities because of fear of failure. Unlike individuals with schizoid personality disorder who avoid relationships because of indifference, individuals with avoidant personality disorder are lonely and seek human contact, albeit only in circumstances in which acceptance is certain.

3. **Associated features** include social phobia, panic disorder with agoraphobia, and other personality disorders.

4. **Differential diagnoses** include panic disorder with agoraphobia and other personality disorders.

5. Clinical course

  a. The disorder is rarely diagnosed in young children, because fear of separation and shyness with strangers may be normal.

  b. Symptoms of this disorder are apparent when childhood shyness increases rather than attenuating during adolescence and disrupts further psychosocial development.

  c. Social phobia often supervenes.

  d. Symptoms may remit with aging.

6. Treatment. The goals of treatment are to improve social assertiveness, decrease sensitivity to criticism, and improve self-confidence.

  a. Psychotherapy

   (1) Several forms of individual and group psychotherapies, most notably assertiveness training, have proved efficacious.

   (2) The difficult first task of therapy is to establish trust, because the patient may be hypersensitive to perceived rejection by the therapist or group members.

  b. Pharmacotherapy. Anxiolytic medications may be useful to control severe anxiety in social situations.

I. Dependent personality disorder. Individuals with this disorder are consumed by the need to be taken care of. They exhibit clinging behavior, allow others to assume responsibilities for important decisions, avoid initiating activities independently, worry unrealistically about abandonment, and feel inadequate and helpless.

1. Epidemiology

  a. This disorder occurs at a 1:1 male to female ratio.

  b. The prevalence of this disorder is common; however, the prevalence in different cultures may be influenced by the acceptability of dependent behaviors.

2. Additional diagnostic features

  a. Individuals with this disorder may avoid disagreements with others because of a fear of losing their support.

  b. They lack the confidence to make even unimportant decisions independently, and they constantly seek support from others.

  c. Often, these individuals focus their dependency on a family member or spouse and desperately seek a substitute when this person is unavailable.

3. Associated features include self-doubt, excessive humility, poor independent functioning, mood disorders, anxiety disorders, adjustment disorder, and other personality disorders.

4. Differential diagnoses include dependency caused by unrealistic environmental concerns or by disability resulting from another psychiatric disorder, and other personality disorders.

5. The **clinical course** often depends on the characteristics of the person on whom the individual depends.

6. Treatment. The goals of treatment are to decrease inappropriate dependency on others and to improve self-reliance and self-esteem.

a. Cognitive, behavioral, and psychodynamic psychotherapies have all been highly efficacious.

b. The therapist must be careful not to foster undue dependency in the therapeutic relationship.

J. Obsessive-compulsive personality disorder. Individuals with this disorder are preoccupied with details and lose a sense of overall goals. They are strict, perfectionistic, overconscientious, and inflexible. They are also obsessed with work and productivity and are hesitant to delegate tasks to others.

1. **Epidemiology**

   a. This disorder occurs at a 2:1 male to female ratio.

   b. The prevalence of this disorder is 1% of the population.

2. **Additional diagnostic features**

   a. Individuals with this disorder may be miserly and unable to give up even useless possessions.

   b. This disorder should not be confused with obsessive-compulsive disorder, which has distinct diagnostic features.

3. **Associated features** include indecisiveness, dysphoria, anger, social inhibition, and difficulty with interpersonal relationships.

4. The **differential diagnoses** are other personality disorders, particularly paranoid and narcissistic personality disorders.

5. **Clinical course.** The severity of symptoms may wax and wane in association with environmental stressors. Depressive mood disorders or schizophrenia may supervene.

6. **Treatment**. The goals of treatment are to decrease behavioral rigidity and increase enjoyment of life.

   a. **Psychotherapy** is the treatment of choice, although it is not uniformly efficacious. Patients in psychotherapy may become engrossed in the minutiae of self-examination and must be redirected toward therapeutic goals.

   b. **Serotonergic antidepressants** may be useful for some patients, especially those with an additional diagnosis of obsessive-compulsive disorder.

Review Test

Directions: Each group of items in this section consists of lettered options followed by a set of numbered items. For each item, select the **one** lettered option that is **most** closely associated with it. Each lettered option may be selected once, more than once, or not at all.

Questions 1–10

Match each of the following clinical cases with its corresponding personality disorder.

(A) Antisocial personality disorder
(B) Avoidant personality disorder
(C) Borderline personality disorder
(D) Dependent personality disorder
(E) Histrionic personality disorder
(F) Narcissistic personality disorder
(G) Obsessive-compulsive personality disorder
(H) Paranoid personality disorder
(I) Schizoid personality disorder
(J) Schizotypal personality disorder

1. A 57-year-old man living in a condominium complex constantly accuses his neighbors of plotting to avoid paying their share of maintenance. He writes angry letters to other owners and has initiated several lawsuits. He lives alone and does not socialize.

2. A 24-year-old man lives alone and works at night as a security guard. He ignores social invitations from coworkers, and he has no outside interests.

3. A 30-year-old man is completely preoccupied with studying and brewing herbal teas. He associates many peculiar powers with consumption of these teas, and he says that plants sometimes whisper to him. He spends all of his time alone, often taking walks in the wilderness for days to collect plants for teas. He has no history of disorganized behavior.

4. A 21-year-old man is arrested for beating a motorist during a car jacking. The man has a history of repeated incarcerations for robbery, driving while under the influence of alcohol, and credit card fraud. When he was 16 years of age, he was expelled from high school for fighting.

5. A 27-year-old woman is taken to the emergency room after she calls paramedics and tells them that she has taken an overdose of fluoxetine. She has a history of multiple previous suicide gestures, which usually follow the breakup of a stormy relationship. She also has a history of substance abuse.

6. A 30-year-old woman becomes highly agitated and vocal during an argument with another person while waiting in line for a theater performance. Security is called, and the woman screams loudly and falls limp when guards attempt to detain her. She shouts, "They are killing me for speaking out!"

7. A 50-year-old man who is a partner in a law firm refuses to comply with the otherwise unanimous wishes of his partners. He states that he is only interested in getting his share of the firm's profits and that he has no interest in the well-being of the other employees. He states that he is the firm's "rainmaker" (i.e., the partner who obtains new clients) and therefore is not required to compromise with anyone else.

8. A 43-year-old man dreads the upcoming office Christmas party, because he believes that he is incapable of making social conversations or dancing. He thinks that he will become an object of pity or ridicule if he tries. He anticipates another lonely holiday season as a result.

9. A 26-year-old man is brought to the emergency room after sustaining severe lacerations during a sadistic episode with his partner. The patient is extremely concerned that the police will be called. The patient does not want the police to be informed because he does not want to upset his partner and cause him to leave.

10. A 37-year-old woman seeks psychotherapy because of her impending divorce. She says that she has driven her spouse away with her demands that the house is kept spotless, that extremely detailed and fixed work and recreational schedules are maintained, and that rigid dietary habits are maintained.

Answers and Explanations

1–H. The man's symptoms suggest paranoid personality disorder, which is characterized by distrust and suspiciousness. These individuals are often isolated and litigious.

2–I. The man's symptoms suggest schizoid personality disorder, which is characterized by detachment and restricted emotionality. These individuals commonly have a narrow range of interests and are aloof from other individuals.

3–J. The man's symptoms suggest schizotypal personality disorder, which is characterized by a discomfort with social relationships, thought distortion, and eccentricity. These individuals are commonly preoccupied with peculiar ideas and are often isolated socially.

4–A. The man's symptoms suggest antisocial personality disorder, which is characterized by a disregard and violation of the basic rights of others. These individuals commonly commit violence against others, lie, and are incarcerated for criminal activity.

5–C. The woman's symptoms suggest borderline personality disorder, which is characterized by social and emotional instability. Suicide gestures, emotional crises following termination of stormy relationships, and substance abuse are all common features of this disorder.

6–E. The woman's symptoms suggest histrionic personality disorder, which is characterized by excessive emotionality and attention-seeking behavior. These individuals commonly engage in dramatic behavior that attracts inappropriate public attention, and they commonly exaggerate their feelings.

7–F. The man's symptoms suggest narcissistic personality disorder, which is characterized by inflated self-esteem, demands for admiration, and a lack of concern for others. These individuals are commonly selfish and lack empathy for others.

8–B. The man's symptoms suggest avoidant personality disorder, which is characterized by social inhibition, feelings of inadequacy, and hypersensitivity to criticism. These individuals often avoid others, which often results in loneliness.

9–D. The man's symptoms suggest dependent personality disorder, which is characterized by submissive and clinging behavior associated with a need to be taken care of. These individuals often tolerate abuse from others to avoid the loss of a relationship.

10–G. The woman's symptoms suggest obsessive-compulsive personality disorder, which is characterized by a preoccupation with orderliness, perfectionism, and control. These individuals are often obsessed with rules and schedules and are rigid in their demands.

25
Other Treatment Problems

I. Overview

    A. Although possibly severe, some problems that come to clinical attention do not represent symptoms of a mental disorder, or they may warrant attention separate from a coexisting mental disorder.

    B. DSM-IV. These problems are described in the DSM-IV in the section titled Other Conditions That May Be a Focus of Clinical Attention.

II. Psychological Factor Affecting Medical Condition

    A. Although psychological factors influence the presentation of most general medical conditions, they sometimes play a distinct adverse role and may become a separate focus of treatment.

    B. These factors may include mental disorders, isolated psychological symptoms, personality traits, responses to stress, or maladaptive health behaviors (e.g., smoking, excessive alcohol use, overeating, not exercising regularly).

    C. These factors may influence the course of the general medical condition or interfere with treatment.

III. Medication-Induced Movement Disorders

    A. Overview. Medication-induced movement disorders are often caused by antipsychotic medication (i.e., neuroleptics). Additionally, tremor may be caused by lithium, antidepressants, and valproate.

    B. Types. Movement disorders include:

        1. Neuroleptic-induced parkinsonism
        2. Neuroleptic malignant syndrome
        3. Neuroleptic-induced acute dystonia
        4. Neuroleptic-induced acute akathisia
        5. Neuroleptic-induced tardive dyskinesia
        6. Medication-induced postural tremor

C. The signs of these disorders are described in Chapters 26 through 29.

IV. Other Medication-Induced Disorders. This category describes other adverse effects of medications, including severe hypotension, cardiac arrhythmias, and priapism.

V. Relational Problems

   A. Problems relating to other individuals may be caused by mental disorders or general medical conditions, or they may be independent problems.

   B. Examples. These problems, including parent–child relational problems, partner relational problems, sibling relational problems, or relational problems with other people (e.g., coworkers, employees, service personnel), may become separate foci of clinical attention.

VI. Problems Related to Abuse or Neglect

   A. Mistreatment of one or more individuals by another individual may become a focus of clinical attention.

   B. Examples. These situations include physical abuse of child, sexual abuse of child, neglect of child, physical abuse of adult, and sexual abuse of adult.

VII. Additional Conditions That May Be a Focus of Clinical Attention (Table 25-1)

Table 25-1.   Other Conditions That May Be a Focus of Clinical Attention (DSM-IV)

Noncompliance with treatment
Malingering
Adult, child, or adolescent antisocial behavior
Borderline intellectual functioning
Age-related cognitive decline
Bereavement
Academic problems
Occupational problems
Identity problems
Religious or spiritual problems
Acculturation problems
Phase of life or other life circumstance problem

Review Test

Directions: Each of the numbered items or incomplete statements in this section is followed by answers or by completions of the statement. Select the ONE lettered answer or completion that is BEST in each case.

1. Several months after suffering a myocardial infarction, a 53-year-old man complains of recurrent angina. He remains significantly overweight, continues to smoke, and dismisses his physician's advice to exercise regularly and decrease the amount of fat in his diet. He states with intended irony, "Every year doctors have some new diet fad. Next year it will probably be to eat more food." Which of the following psychological factors has the most significant effects on the course of his medical condition?

(A) Bulimia nervosa
(B) Maladaptive health behaviors
(C) Major depressive disorder
(D) Personality traits
(E) Stress-related physiologic response

2. A 4-year-old girl is sent home from preschool after biting several children in the classroom. The mother consoles the child and tells her that the other children must have "done something bad" to deserve being bitten. The mother then angrily calls the teacher and threatens legal action against the school. The following day, the girl says to the teacher, "I can bite anyone I want," and then shortly afterward bites another child. Which of the following conditions is the most likely cause of the child's behavior?

(A) Antisocial personality disorder
(B) Attention deficit hyperactivity disorder
(C) Autistic disorder
(D) Parent–child relational problem
(E) Separation anxiety disorder

3. A 13-year-old girl with Down syndrome is brought to the emergency room by her parents with a dislocated shoulder. Physical examination reveals bruises on her back and buttocks. The parents report that she becomes agitated and unmanageable at home and can be controlled only with corporal punishment. Which of the following conditions should be the immediate focus of clinical attention?

(A) Conduct disorder
(B) Mental retardation
(C) Neglect of a child
(D) Oppositional defiant disorder
(E) Physical abuse of a child

4. A 32-year-old man complains of a lack of purpose to his life. He left a close-knit religious community 1 year ago because of philosophical differences and has since drifted from one menial job to another and moved several times. He feels isolated and estranged from others and says, "I no longer know what I stand for." Which of the following conditions is the most appropriate focus of clinical attention?

(A) Avoidant personality disorder
(B) Identity problem
(C) Occupational problem
(D) Schizoid personality disorder
(E) Social phobia

5. A 40-year-old woman is grief-stricken 2 weeks after the death of her mother. She says that she thinks of her mother often, cries frequently, and has difficulty sleeping. She denies suicidal ideation, psychomotor retardation, or feelings of guilt or worthlessness. Which of the following conditions is most likely present?

(A) Adjustment disorder with depressed mood
(B) Bereavement
(C) Bipolar II disorder
(D) Dysthymic disorder
(E) Major depressive disorder

Answers and Explanations

1–B. The man's physical symptoms suggest continued coronary artery disease. The course of his condition will be most affected by his maladaptive health behaviors, including lifestyle and diet. Although some of his behaviors may reflect personality traits or a problematic coping style, there is insufficient evidence to ascribe the course of his medical condition to these factors. Noncompliance with treatment may become an additional factor affecting this case.

2–D. The child's symptoms suggest a relational problem between the child and her mother that involves inadequate discipline. The child is at risk for developing oppositional defiant or conduct disorder; however, the most appropriate focus of treatment in this case is the mother–child relationship.

3–E. The girl's presentation suggests that her parents are physically abusing her, and this problem must be addressed immediately. Children with mental disorders are at higher risk for abuse than other children. The girl is likely to have mental retardation and may also have oppositional defiant or conduct disorder; however, these conditions are a secondary concern in this case.

4–B. The man's complaints most suggest an identity problem, which is characterized by difficulty in defining one's goals, values, and social status. Individuals who voluntarily or involuntarily separate from close-knit groups commonly have problems defining a new identity. Occupational problems and spiritual concerns may also be present, but they are most likely secondary to the identity problem in this case. Although the individual may be exhibiting avoidant or schizoid traits or symptoms of social phobia, there is little evidence to suggest that these are pervasive and enduring patterns of behavior.

5–B. The woman's symptoms suggest that she is in bereavement, which is characterized by symptoms of sadness and grief following the death of a loved one. It is less likely that she has major depressive disorder, because the duration of symptoms is short and there are few other symptoms suggestive of a depressive episode. Adjustment disorder is also a less likely diagnosis, because there is little evidence of a significant impairment in social or occupational functioning.

Part Three

Clinical Psychopharmacology

26
Antipsychotic Medication

I. Overview

   A. General considerations. Antipsychotic medications block postsynaptic receptors, particularly dopamine receptors, and are used to treat manifestations of psychosis and other psychiatric disorders.

      1. History. The first antipsychotic medications were developed in the 1950s, beginning with **chlorpromazine**.

      2. Chemical classes. Antipsychotic medications are derived from several different chemical classes, including phenothiazines, thioxanthenes, and butyrophenones.

   B. Mechanism of action

      1. The precise mechanism of antipsychotic action is unknown; however, antipsychotic medication blocks several populations of dopamine receptors in the brain.

      2. Some newer antipsychotic medications (e.g., clozapine, risperidone, olanzepine, sertindole) also block some serotonin receptors, a property that may be associated with increased efficacy.

      3. Antipsychotic medication also variably blocks central and peripheral cholinergic, histaminic, and α-adrenergic receptors.

   C. Treatment guidelines. Informed consent and involuntary treatment are difficult issues associated with the use of antipsychotic medication.

II. Indications

   A. Psychomotor agitation (see V A). Antipsychotics are among the most efficacious pharmacologic agents for the medical treatment of psychomotor agitation.

   B. Schizophrenia and other psychotic disorders

      1. Schizophrenia (see V B). Antipsychotic medication is the treatment of choice for acute psychotic episodes and for prophylaxis against further episodes. However, it has less effect on residual symptomatology.

2. **Psychoses and cognitive disorders due to a general medical condition** (see V D, F). Antipsychotic medication is useful for treating agitation and psychosis that may accompany delirium, dementia, and other general medical conditions.

3. **Substance-induced psychosis** (see V E). Antipsychotic medication is useful in the treatment of agitation and psychosis induced by various substances. Clinicians must be careful to avoid adverse interactions between the antipsychotic medication and the offending substance.

4. **Other psychotic disorders.** Antipsychotic medication may be effective in treating delusional disorder, brief psychotic disorder, schizophreniform disorder, and other rarer psychotic disorders.

C. **Mood disorders.** Antipsychotic medication is useful for the treatment of agitation and psychosis during mood episodes.

D. **Sedation.** Antipsychotic medication may be useful when benzodiazepines are contraindicated or as an adjunct during anesthesia.

E. **Movement disorders** (see V I). Antipsychotic medication is the treatment of choice for Huntington disease and Tourette disorder.

III. Adverse Effects

A. **Sedative effects** may occur secondary to antihistaminic activity.

B. **Hypotension** is caused by α-adrenergic blockade and most commonly occurs with use of low-potency antipsychotic medication.

C. **Anticholinergic symptoms.** Dry mouth, blurred vision, urinary hesitancy, constipation, bradycardia, confusion, and delirium may occur.

D. **Movement syndromes.** There is a high incidence of extrapyramidal syndromes (EPS), and they affect patient compliance.

1. **Pathophysiology.** EPS may be caused by blockade of subpopulations of dopamine receptors in the basal ganglia.

2. **Types.** There are several more-or-less discrete types of acute EPS (e.g., pseudoparkinsonism, acute dystonia, akathisia) and at least one long-term EPS, tardive dyskinesia (see III D 4).

3. **Acute syndromes**

a. **Dystonia** is spasms of various muscle groups. Depending on the muscle groups involved, it may be called oculogyric crisis, buccolingual spasm, or opisthotonos.

(1) **Presentation** can be dramatic and frightening to patients, and it can be a major contributing factor to subsequent noncompliance with treatment.

(2) Young men may be at higher risk for developing these dystonias.

b. **Bradykinesia (pseudoparkinsonism).** This syndrome is characterized by slowed volitional movement, increased muscle tone, and resting tremor.

(1) **Signs** include decreased facial expression, small steps and a festinating gait, cogwheel rigidity, and pill-rolling.

(2) The **elderly** may be more predisposed to developing these symptoms.

(3) Antipsychotic-induced bradykinesia may be mistaken for catatonic rigidity or apathy and withdrawal.

c. **Akathisia.** Antipsychotic-induced akathisia is characterized by motor restlessness. It is often mistaken for anxiety and agitation.

d. **Treatment of acute syndromes.** Acute EPS may be treated by decreasing the patient's dosage of antipsychotic medication, administering antiparkinsonian medication, or switching the patient to an antipsychotic medication with fewer EPS effects.

(1) Antiparkinsonian medication is used for acute treatment and for prophylaxis against future EPS episodes.

(a) Anticholinergic drugs, such as benztropine and trihexyphenidyl, are the most commonly used treatment for acute EPS. Benztropine can be administered intravenously or intramuscularly to treat acute dystonia.

(b) Amantadine can be used to treat EPS when anticholinergic agents are contraindicated, but it may exacerbate psychosis.

(c) Propranolol may be effective for treating akathisia.

(d) Other drugs used to treat acute movement syndromes include benzodiazepines and antihistamines (e.g., diphenhydramine).

(2) Low-potency antipsychotic medication (e.g., chlorpromazine, thioridazine) causes less EPS but has more sedative effects. Clozapine and risperidone cause minimal or no EPS.

4. **Tardive movement disorders**, most commonly tardive dyskinesia, are a complication of long-term use of antipsychotic medication.

a. **Tardive dyskinesia** is characterized by choreoathetosis and other involuntary movements. These movements often first occur in the tongue or fingers and later involve the trunk. Variants of tardive dyskinesia include **tardive dystonia** and **tardive akathisia.**

b. The **etiology** is presumptively a form of "chemical denervation hypersensitivity," which is caused by chronic dopamine blockade in the basal ganglia.

c. **Risk.** Patients who take high doses of antipsychotic medication for long periods of time are at highest risk for developing this disorder. Many patients taking these medications ultimately develop some symptoms, which may gradually worsen with continued use.

d. **Treatment of tardive movement disorders** is difficult, because discontinuing the offending antipsychotic medication exacerbates psychotic symptoms in many patients.

(1) Prophylaxis involves the use of the lowest possible dose of antipsychotic medication, administering it for the shortest possible period of time. If tardive dyskinesia supervenes, the agent should be gradually discontinued if possible.

(2) Increasing dosage. Symptoms of tardive dyskinesia can be briefly eliminated by increasing the dosage of antipsychotic medications; however, this intervention should be reserved for emergency situations, because choreoathetosis will reemerge at the higher dosage.

(3) **Changing medication.** Switching the patient to clozapine may be indicated, because the incidence of tardive dyskinesia with this agent is low.

(4) Tardive dyskinesia may not be as irreversible as formerly believed, and choreoathetosis may gradually decrease when the antipsychotic medication is discontinued.

E. **Neuroleptic malignant syndrome** is a fairly rare and potentially life-threatening condition characterized by muscular rigidity, hyperthermia, autonomic instability, and delirium. It is usually associated with high dosages of high-potency antipsychotic medication. Treatment involves immediate discontinuation of the medication and physiologic supportive measures, and dantrolene or bromocriptine may be used.

F. **Dermal** and **ocular syndromes** include photosensitivity, abnormal pigmentation, and lenticular opacities. At high dosages, thioridazine may cause pigmentary retinopathy.

G. **Endocrine effects** include gynecomastia, galactorrhea, and amenorrhea.

H. **Other adverse effects** include cardiac conduction abnormalities, particularly with the use of thioridazine, leukopenia, and thrombocytopenia. Agranulocytosis occasionally occurs, usually with the use of clozapine. Seizures may occur and are more common with the use of clozapine.

IV. Differences Among Antipsychotic Medications (Table 26-1)

A. **Efficacy.** The overall efficacy among antipsychotic medications for the treatment of schizophrenia appears to be the same, except for clozapine, risperidone, and other newer antipsychotic medications such as sertindole and olanzapine.

1. **Clozapine** may be effective in treating some cases of schizophrenia that are resistant to other antipsychotic medications. It may also be particularly effective for the treatment of negative symptoms.

2. **Risperidone** and other newer antipsychotic medications may also be effective when other antipsychotic medications are ineffective.

B. **Potency.** Antipsychotic medication varies widely in potency.

1. Potency is sometimes expressed in relation to 100 mg of chlorpromazine. The higher the potency, the less medication is required to equal the antipsychotic efficacy of 100 mg of chlorpromazine. For example, fluphenazine is a high-potency antipsychotic medication, because only 5 mg are required to equal the antipsychotic efficacy of 100 mg of chlorpromazine.

2. In order of decreasing potency, haloperidol is rated at 5 mg, thiothixene is rated at 10 mg, trifluoperazine is rated at 20 mg, and thioridazine is rated at 100 mg.

C. **Adverse effects profile**

1. Although **high-potency agents** have less sedative and anticholinergic effects, they are more likely to cause acute EPS.

2. **Low-potency agents** have more sedative and anticholinergic effects, and cause more hypotension; however, they are associated with a lower incidence of EPS.

3. **Newer medications** such as clozapine, risperidone, sertindole, and olanzapine produce few extrapyramidal symptoms.

Table 26-1. Differences Among Antipsychotic Medications

Classification	Examples	Therapeutic Dosage Range	Adverse Effects	Indications
High-potency agents	Fluphenazine, haloperidol, pimozide, thiothixine, trifluoperazine	2–30 mg/day	Minimal sedative, hypotensive, and anticholinergic effects; high incidence of EPS	Acute treatment of psychomotor agitation; treatment of schizophrenia, particularly for patients who have general medical conditions or take other medications that make additional hypotensive or anticholinergic effects dangerous; treatment of movement disorders (e.g., Tourette disorder, Huntington disease)
Medium-potency agents	Loxapine, molindone, perphenazine	10–200 mg/day	Moderate sedative, hypotensive, and anticholinergic effects; moderate incidence of EPS	Treatment of schizophrenia; used particularly for patients in whom moderate sedative effects are tolerable or desirable
Low-potency agents	Chlorpromazine, thioridazine	100–800+ mg/day	Marked sedative, hypotensive, and anticholinergic effects; low incidence of EPS	Treatment of schizophrenia and other psychotic disorders; used particularly for patients who have general medical conditions (e.g., Parkinson disease) that may be exacerbated by EPS, and for patients in whom sedative effects are desirable and moderate hypotensive and anticholinergic effects are not dangerous
Newer agents	Clozapine, olanzepine, risperidone, sertindole	Clozapine: 200–900 mg/day Risperidone: 4–12 mg/day	Clozapine: Resembles low-potency agents; EPS and tardive dyskinesia almost absent; high incidence of seizures	Clozapine: Treatment of schizophrenia in patients who do not respond well to other antipsychotic agents, but who can tolerate increased risk for seizures and granulocytopenia; also used for patients who cannot tolerate acute EPS or exacerbation of tardive dyskinesia
			Others: Low incidence of acute EPS; some are sedating	Others: Especially useful for patients with schizophrenia who do not respond well to other antipsychotic agents or those who have EPS that is difficult to manage

EPS = extrapyramidal syndromes

V. Treatment guidelines. A clinician should select an antipsychotic medication based on the patient's diagnosis, symptoms, previous record of response, adverse effect profile, and the route of administration.

A. Psychomotor agitation

1. **High-potency antipsychotic medication** is generally preferred for decreasing psychomotor agitation, because the desired effect is different from merely sedating the individual.

   a. A **standard regimen** may be **5 mg of haloperidol** administered intramuscularly hourly until the patient is calm, which usually occurs after one to three doses. Intramuscular administration is preferable, because absorption is quick and reliable, and patient compliance issues are lessened.

   b. The **target symptom** is psychomotor agitation, not psychosis, and response occurs within 1 hour following an effective dose.

2. **Adverse effects** (e.g., EPS and hypotension) must be closely monitored and treated if necessary.

3. Some clinicians also administer a benzodiazepine (e.g., 2 mg of lorazepam) to a high-potency antipsychotic medication when treating agitation.

B. Schizophrenia

1. **Acute psychotic episodes**

   a. **Target symptoms** are hallucinations, delusions, disorganized speech and behavior, and catatonia.

   b. **Dose.** The lag time for response to an effective dose is often several days.

      (1) **Moderate doses** of antipsychotic medication (i.e., equivalent to 10–20 mg/day of haloperidol) are usually as effective as higher doses for this indication and cause fewer side effects.

      (2) **Higher doses** of antipsychotic medication should be used only when lower doses are ineffective or when psychomotor agitation is an additional target symptom.

      (3) When psychotic symptoms remit, antipsychotic medication should be gradually tapered to the lowest effective dose.

2. **Residual schizophrenia.** Most antipsychotic medications are not effective in ameliorating residual symptoms (e.g., social withdrawal, amotivation, and poor social functioning). However, they are effective in low dosages (e.g., 5 mg/day of haloperidol) for prophylaxis against recurrent psychosis.

   a. **Depot antipsychotic medication** (e.g., fluphenazine decanoate, haloperidol decanoate) has a role in treatment of residual schizophrenia. These agents are administered intramuscularly by a clinician on a bimonthly or monthly schedule and are gradually absorbed from the injection site into the general circulation, decreasing problems with patient compliance.

   b. **Clozapine** and other newer antipsychotic medications may have greater efficacy in treating residual symptoms, but clozapine requires a weekly white cell count to monitor for agranulocytosis.

c. **Dosage**

    (1) Attempts to taper the dosage of antipsychotic medication should be made at least once yearly to minimize the risk of tardive dyskinesia.

    (2) Some patients can discontinue antipsychotic medication for extended periods, restarting it only when signs of impending psychosis recur.

d. Clinicians should carefully attempt to distinguish the decreased psychomotor activity caused by an antipsychotic medication from the negative symptoms (i.e., amotivation, alogia, and affectual flattening) of schizophrenia.

C. **Schizoaffective disorders**. Antipsychotic medication is often needed during the treatment of schizoaffective disorders. It is often used in combination with mood stabilizers (e.g., lithium, anticonvulsants) and antidepressants.

D. **Psychosis due to a general medical condition.** Antipsychotic medication is useful in managing the symptoms of these disorders, but the patient's underlying condition must be also be treated.

E. **Substance-induced psychosis.** Antipsychotic medications are useful to treat this type of psychosis, but interactions between the offending substance and the antipsychotic medication must be avoided.

F. **Cognitive disorders**

1. **Delirium.** The benefits of controlling psychomotor agitation and psychotic symptoms in delirium with antipsychotic medication must be weighed against the risk of obscuring other acute changes in the individual's level of mentation or further compromising the patient's metabolic functioning.

2. **Dementia.** Antipsychotic medications play a major role in treating the psychomotor agitation and psychotic symptoms in dementia; however, they must be used with caution, often sparingly, in elderly patients.

G. **Bipolar disorders**

1. **Manic episodes.** Antipsychotic medication may be used to treat psychomotor agitation and psychosis during manic and possibly hypomanic episodes in bipolar disorders.

    a. After mood-stabilizing medication is initiated, antipsychotic medication should be tapered if possible.

    b. Concurrent use of mood-stabilizing and antipsychotic medications on a continuous basis in bipolar mood disorders should be initiated only when mood-stabilizing medication alone has been ineffective.

2. **Depressive episodes.** Antipsychotic medication may be used adjunctively with antidepressants, mood stabilizers, or electroconvulsive therapy to treat psychosis during depressive episodes in bipolar disorders.

H. **Major depressive disorder with psychotic features**. Antipsychotic medication is used in conjunction with antidepressants to treat depressive episodes with psychosis in major depressive disorder. The clinician should be careful to avoid additive anticholinergic effects from antipsychotic medications and antidepressants.

I. **Movement disorders**

1. **Huntington disease.** Antipsychotic medication is effective in controlling both choreoathetosis and psychotic symptoms associated with dementia in this disease.

2. **Tourette disorder.** Very low doses of high-potency antipsychotic medication (e.g., haloperidol or pimozide) may be useful for treating the tics and vocalizations that occur in this disorder. However, patients often experience slowed mentation.

Review Test

Directions: Each of the numbered items or incomplete statements in this section is followed by answers or by completions of the statement. Select the ONE lettered answer or completion that is best in each case.

Questions 1–2

A 23-year-old man with an exacerbation of schizophrenia has the onset of dysarthria and a twisted neck (opisthotonos) shortly after starting a course of haloperidol.

1. Which of the following is the most likely etiology for these findings?

(A) Akathisia
(B) Catatonic posturing
(C) Dystonia
(D) Pseudoparkinsonism
(E) Tardive dyskinesia

2. Which of the following is the most appropriate initial treatment for the patient's motor symptoms?

(A) Administer 2 mg of benztropine intramuscularly
(B) Administer 2 mg of trihexyphenidyl orally
(C) Discontinue all antipsychotic medication and observe the patient
(D) Switch antipsychotic medication to clozapine
(E) Switch antipsychotic medication to thiothixene

3. A 69-year-old man with dementia of the Alzheimer type and prostatic hypertrophy becomes increasingly belligerent toward his wife, accusing her of stealing his financial papers from his desk. Which of the following is the most appropriate initial treatment?

(A) Administer 25 mg of chlorpromazine orally twice daily
(B) Administer 100 mg of chlorpromazine orally twice daily
(C) Administer 2 mg of haloperidol orally twice daily
(D) Administer 5 mg of haloperidol orally three times daily
(E) Do not initiate antipsychotic medication and initiate marital therapy

4. A 44-year-old woman who has no previous psychiatric problems has the gradual onset of writhing movements of her tongue and hands, slowed mentation, and persecutory delusions. Which of the following is the most appropriate initial treatment?

(A) Initiate benztropine
(B) Initiate chlorpromazine
(C) Initiate clozapine
(D) Initiate pimozide
(E) Observe patient without medication for several weeks

5. A 35-year-old woman with a long history of bipolar disorder has a manic episode characterized by increased psychomotor activity, insomnia, and grandiose delusions. She is started on haloperidol and lithium. Her manic and psychotic symptoms resolve after 1 week, but she complains of sedation. Which of the following is the most reasonable next step in treatment?

(A) Continue both medications at current dosage and monitor the patient closely
(B) Gradually discontinue both medications over the next 2 weeks
(C) Gradually discontinue the haloperidol but continue lithium
(D) Gradually discontinue the lithium but continue the haloperidol
(E) Immediately discontinue both medications and initiate a different mood-stabilizing medication

Answers and Explanations

1–C. The onset of muscle spasms shortly after beginning antipsychotic medication, particularly high-potency antipsychotic medication, most suggests neuroleptic-induced dystonia. This dystonia is more common in younger men.

2–A. Acute dystonia is often an extremely uncomfortable condition and is most rapidly treated with intramuscular or intravenous administration of an anticholinergic medication, such as benztropine. Oral administration of trihexyphenidyl may be difficult because of the patient's buccolingual dystonia, and would take longer to work because of the need for gastrointestinal absorption. Discontinuing antipsychotic medication is likely to cause an exacerbation of the patient's psychosis. Clozapine has no associated extrapyramidal symptoms; however, it would not quickly alleviate this patient's dystonia and the drug has other serious risks (e.g., seizures, agranulocytosis). Thiothixene is another high-potency antipsychotic medication and is therefore also associated with dystonia. A low-potency antipsychotic is recommended if switching the patient's medication.

3–C. The agitation associated with dementia is often effectively lessened with use of an antipsychotic medication such as haloperidole. Elderly patients usually need smaller doses of antipsychotic medication than younger patients. Chlorpromazine, a low-potency antipsychotic medication, has marked anticholinergic effects, which may exacerbate the patient's urinary difficulties. Marital therapy is unlikely to be effective if the patient's belligerence is caused by dementia.

4–B. The woman's symptoms suggest choreoathetosis, dementia, and psychosis that is associated with Huntington disease. Antipsychotic medication, such as chlorpromazine, is effective in treating both the abnormal movements and delusions. Clozapine is an atypical antipsychotic medication and is not a first-choice drug in the treatment of Huntington disease. Clozapine is often used to treat patients who have developed tardive dyskinesia, which also presents as choreoathetosis. Pimozide is a high-potency antipsychotic medication that is used to treat Tourette disorder when haloperidol is ineffective; a higher incidence of seizures is associated with its use. Benztropine is ineffective for treating Huntington disease or tardive dyskinesia.

5–C. After successfully stabilizing a patient with a manic episode, during which both mood-stabilizing and antipsychotic medications were used, patients are usually continued on the mood stabilizer whereas the antipsychotic medication is tapered. It is less common to continue these patients on both classes of medications.

27
Anxiolytic Medication

I. **Overview**. Anxiolytic medication is used primarily to control anxiety.

   A. **Recognizing anxiety**

   1. **Anxiety is common** and represents a variety of conditions, ranging from daily stress to paralyzing psychiatric illness.
   2. **Etiologic theory** (see Chapter 15)

      a. **Freud** and others described unconscious conflicts as a cause of anxiety.
      b. **Wolpe** and others described behavioral conditioning as a cause of anxiety.
      c. **Klein** and others described physiologic problems as a cause of primary anxiety.

   B. **Treatment of anxiety**

   1. Effective **psychotherapies**, including support and reassurance, psychodynamic and cognitive psychotherapies, relaxation training, and biofeedback, are available to treat anxious people.
   2. **Pharmacotherapy.** Some types of anxiety respond to **anxiolytic medication**. The clinician must determine the type of anxiety that may respond to medication, which drugs to try, how to use them, and how to gauge responses.

II. **Types of Anxiolytic Medication** (Table 27-1)

   A. **Benzodiazepines** are the first-choice anxiolytic medication for most indications, because they have relatively few adverse effects when used appropriately (see V B).

   1. **Mechanism of action.** Benzodiazepines bind to specific receptors in the central nervous system (CNS) that are involved in the modulation of γ-aminobutyric acid (GABA) transmission.
   2. **Elderly individuals** require relatively lower doses of benzodiazepines and are more susceptible to adverse effects, particularly cognitive impairment.

Table 27-1. Commonly Used Anxiolytic Medications

Agent	Potency (High=1)	Dosage Range	Speed of Onset	Duration of Action	Comments
Alprazolam	0.5	0.75–6 mg/day	Rapid	Brief	Benzodiazepine of choice for treatment of panic disorder; three or four times daily dosage schedule is often necessary; high risk of withdrawal and dependence
Buspirone	***	15–30 mg/day	Lengthy delay	***	Used for treatment of generalized anxiety disorder; causes minimal sedation and cognitive and motor impairment; onset of therapeutic effect may take several weeks
Chlordiazepoxide	15	10–100 mg/day	Rapid	Long	Often used to treat alcohol withdrawal; less potential for dependency than diazepam
Clonazepam	1	1–6 mg/day	Rapid	Long	Effective in treatment of panic disorder, and less frequent dosing than alprazolam is needed; may be useful for treating the agitation associated with manic episodes
Diazepam	5	2–30 mg/day	Rapid	Long	Often used to treat generalized anxiety disorder; significant dependency; once or twice daily dosage is feasible
Flurazepam	15	15–30 mg/day	Rapid	Long	Used almost exclusively for treating insomnia; duration of action is associated with daytime "hangover"
Lorazepam	1	1–6 mg/day	Intermediate	Brief	Often used to treat anxiety associated with adjustment disorders and other acute states; often combined with antipsychotic medication to treat anxiety associated with acute psychosis; two or three times daily dosage schedule is often necessary
Temazepam	15	15–30 mg/day	Intermediate	Intermediate	Used almost exclusively for treating insomnia; duration of action is associated with minimal daytime "hangover"

B. Buspirone has a different clinical profile than benzodiazepines. There is a delayed onset of therapeutic effect and minimal motor or cognitive impairment.

C. Other drugs with some utility in treating various anxiety disorders and syndromes include some antidepressants (e.g., imipramine, paroxetine), antipsychotic medication, and antihistamines.

III. Indications

A. Anxiety disorders

1. **Adjustment disorder with anxious mood** (see V D 2). Anxiolytic medication is used in conjunction with brief psychotherapy to decrease anxiety surrounding specific stressors.
2. **Panic disorder** (see V D 3). Anxiolytic medication is used to decrease frequency and intensity of panic attacks.
3. **Generalized anxiety disorder** (see V D 1). Anxiolytic medication is used to decrease overall anxiety.
4. **Agoraphobia.** Anxiolytic medication is used to decrease fear associated with leaving sheltered surroundings.
5. **Obsessive-compulsive disorder.** Anxiolytic medication is used to decrease obsessional worries.

B. Other conditions

1. **Psychosis and mania.** Anxiolytic medication is used adjunctively with antipsychotic medication to decrease agitation.
2. **Sleep disorders** (see V D 6). Anxiolytic medication is used to decrease insomnia and to treat some parasomnias.
3. **Substance withdrawal** (see V D 7). Anxiolytic medication is used to decrease agitation during withdrawal from some substances, including alcohol, anxiolytics, sedatives and hypnotics, cocaine, and amphetamines.
4. **Epilepsy.** Anxiolytic medication is used to treat certain forms of epilepsy (e.g., myoclonic).
5. **Orthopedic problems.** Anxiolytic medication is used to treat some painful musculoskeletal conditions (e.g., muscle spasms surrounding injury sites).
6. **Uncomfortable diagnostic or treatment procedures.** Anxiolytic medication (e.g., diazepam, midazolam) is used to decrease anxiety and induce amnesia for individuals undergoing various invasive procedures, such as endoscopy or cardiac catheterization.

C. Inappropriate use of anxiolytic medication

1. **Avoiding useful anxiety.** Some anxiety is necessary for optimum functioning, and avoiding it with medication can quickly lead to a lower level of overall functioning and drug dependency.
2. **Avoiding withdrawal.** Continued use of anxiolytics for the sole purpose of avoiding the anxiety related to withdrawal from these medications is a sign of drug dependency.

IV. General Guidelines for Using Anxiolytic Medications

A. Clarify the purpose of treatment. The clinician must identify a patient's specific diagnosis, target symptoms, and treatment goals.

1. **Target symptoms** include:
   a. **Excessive anxiety** that is difficult for the individual to control
   b. **Hyperalertness** and sleep disturbances
   c. **Autonomic arousal**, including rapid heart rate and breathing, tremulousness, sweating, dry mouth, and gastrointestinal distress
   d. **Motor tension**, including increased muscle tone and restlessness
   e. **Anxiety attacks**
   f. **Agoraphobia**
   g. **Obsessions and compulsions**

2. **Treatment goals** are to lessen destructive anxiety symptoms, improve the individual's social and occupational functioning, and improve quality of life.

B. Select an appropriate anxiolytic. The clinician must select an anxiolytic that is indicated for a given diagnosis, weighing both risks and benefits.

C. Discontinuing treatment. The clinician should discontinue the medication if it is ineffective at treating the identified symptoms, if it is being used inappropriately, or if the patient's condition has improved and the medication is no longer needed.

D. Dosage

1. The clinician should avoid abruptly changing a patient's benzodiazepine dosage and should always gradually taper the dosage when ending treatment.
2. Clinicians should generally use **lower dosages for the elderly**.

E. Drug interactions. The clinician should avoid prescribing combinations of anxiolytics and other sedative–hypnotic medications. The clinician should also warn the patient not to mix the anxiolytic medication with alcohol.

V. Benzodiazepines

A. Indications for treatment with benzodiazepines include:

1. Generalized anxiety disorder
2. Adjustment disorder with anxious mood
3. Panic disorders
4. Acute and posttraumatic stress disorders
5. Other anxiety states
6. Some sleep disorders
7. Substance withdrawal

B. Adverse effects of benzodiazepines include sedation, impaired cognitive and motor performance, disinhibition, tolerance and withdrawal, abuse potential, and potential teratogenicity.

1. Adverse cognitive effects include difficulty with focusing attention, memory impairment, and confusion.
2. Benzodiazepine withdrawal is characterized by anxiety, insomnia, and tremulousness. Severe withdrawal, which usually occurs following prolonged use of high doses, may be complicated by delirium and seizures.

C. Differences among benzodiazepines (see Table 27-1)

1. **Pharmacokinetic profiles** of benzodiazepines differ regarding speed of tissue uptake, half-life, and mode of excretion.

2. **Efficacy**

   a. **Alprazolam** may be particularly useful in treating panic disorders.

   b. **Long-acting benzodiazepines** (e.g., diazepam) may be particularly useful in treating generalized anxiety disorder.

   c. **Clonazepam** may be particularly useful in controlling agitation during manic episodes.

3. **Abuse potential.** Benzodiazepines with a rapid onset (e.g., alprazolam) may have higher abuse potential.

D. Treatment guidelines

1. **Generalized anxiety disorder.** Long-acting benzodiazepines are generally used to facilitate a single daily dose without plasma level peaks and troughs.

   a. Relatively high doses, sometimes equivalent to 20 mg/day of diazepam, are often required.

   b. The patient should be instructed in other methods of anxiety management, and the clinician should attempt to gradually reduce the dose of benzodiazepine at regular intervals.

   c. The clinician should avoid abruptly ending use of a benzodiazepine, because the resulting withdrawal syndrome may resemble the symptoms of the original disorder.

2. **Adjustment disorder with anxious mood**. Short-term psychodynamic or cognitive psychotherapy is the treatment of first choice for this disorder, but benzodiazepines may be useful adjuncts to manage severe anxiety and insomnia.

   a. **Short-acting benzodiazepines** are often used to allow closer modulation of dosage.

   b. The patient should be on a time-limited course, and frequent attempts should be made to reduce the dose.

   c. Clinicians may want to avoid using alprazolam for treatment of this disorder because of the associated severe withdrawal problems.

3. **Panic disorder.** Benzodiazepines are the treatment of first choice for this disorder; however, these medications may have less overall efficacy for this indication than for other disorders.

   a. **Alprazolam** and **clonazepam** may have more efficacy than other benzodiazepines for treating this disorder. Currently, clonazepam is often substituted for alprazolam, because it has a lower incidence of dependency and longer duration of action.

   b. **Doses** are often relatively high (e.g., 2–10 mg/day of alprazolam).

   c. **Psychotherapy.** Although benzodiazepines as well as some antidepressants are useful in decreasing the frequency of panic attacks, psychotherapy is often necessary for decreasing anticipatory anxiety.

4. **Acute and posttraumatic stress disorders.** Benzodiazepines are used to treat the anxiety and insomnia that often accompany these disorders.

    a. The clinician should carefully avoid exacerbating the dissociative symptoms (e.g., emotional detachment, numbing) of these disorders.

    b. Medication use must be closely monitored to prevent benzodiazepine abuse and dependence in patients with posttraumatic stress disorder, because this diagnosis is associated with substance abuse and dependence.

  5. Other anxiety states. Benzodiazepines are often used adjunctively to treat severe anxiety that occurs during the course of other psychopathology (e.g., acute psychosis, mania).

    a. A **short-acting benzodiazepine** (e.g., lorazepam, clonazepam) is usually used for this indication.

    b. Advantages of using benzodiazepines instead of antipsychotic medications for this indication include a lower incidence of hypotension, anticholinergic effects, extrapyramidal syndromes, and dysphoria.

    c. Disadvantages of using benzodiazepines for this indication include sedative effects, an increased risk of exacerbating confusion, disinhibitory phenomena, and potential withdrawal symptoms when the medication is discontinued.

  6. Sleep disorders. Benzodiazepines are the treatment of first choice for many insomnias; however, they should not be substituted for an adequate diagnostic evaluation, possible psychotherapy, and environmental changes.

    a. Type. Choosing a benzodiazepine is a controversial issue. The data regarding the clinical consequences of differences in pharmacokinetic factors, including speed of tissue uptake and half-life, are unclear.

    b. The individual should be given a time-limited course at the lowest effective dose.

    c. Adverse effects include daytime drowsiness ("hangover"), cognitive and motor impairment, additive effects when used with alcohol, rebound insomnia, withdrawal symptoms, and psychological dependence.

    d. Diazepam may be particularly useful in treating sleep terror disorder and sleepwalking disorder.

  7. Alcohol, cocaine, and opioid withdrawal

    a. Benzodiazepines are the treatment of choice in alcohol withdrawal and alcohol delirium with onset during withdrawal ("delirium tremens").

    b. Clinicians often initially administer relatively high doses at frequent intervals, with a fairly rapid taper over several days.

    c. Benzodiazepines are a useful adjunct in treating anxiety and insomnia during psychostimulant and opioid withdrawal.

VI. Buspirone

A. Indications. Buspirone is effective in the treatment of **generalized anxiety disorder** and may be particularly useful if the patient has contraindications to benzodiazepines. It may also be useful during treatment of **social phobia**.

B. The **mechanism of action** is unclear but may involve alterations in dopaminergic or serotonergic activity in the CNS.

C. Generally, there is about a **1-week lag time** before clinical response.

D. Adverse effects

1. Buspirone does not appear to cause additive effects when taken with sedative–hypnotics. It also does not cause a clear withdrawal syndrome, significant sedation, or cognitive impairment.
2. Some patients complain of nausea or headaches while taking the drug.

Review Test

Directions: Each of the numbered items or incomplete statements in this section is followed by answers or by completions of the statement. Select the ONE lettered answer or completion that is BEST in each case.

1. A 47-year-old man with generalized anxiety disorder who is being treated with 10 mg/day of diazepam complains of daytime drowsiness and difficulty focusing his thoughts. He notes some decrease in his anxiety but still has significant worry and hyperarousal. Which of the following is the most appropriate next step in management?

(A) Increase diazepam to 20 mg/day
(B) Switch to buspirone
(C) Switch to fluoxetine
(D) Switch to lorazepam
(E) Taper the diazepam to 5 mg/day

2. A 25-year-old woman complains of frequent anxiety attacks that occur without warning. She has been hesitant to leave her house, because she fears that she will have an attack in public. Which of the following is the most appropriate medication for initial treatment?

(A) Alprazolam
(B) Buspirone
(C) Chlorpromazine
(D) Diazepam
(E) Lorazepam

3. A 30-year-old woman suddenly stops taking the 6 mg/day of lorazepam that she has been using for several weeks to treat the insomnia and anxiety that followed a difficult breakup with her husband. The following day, she has severe anxiety attacks and is restless and tremulous. Which of the following is the most appropriate management?

(A) Initiate alprazolam
(B) Initiate buspirone
(C) Restart lorazepam at the original dose
(D) Restart lorazepam at half of the original dose
(E) Withhold all medications and follow the woman closely

4. A 26-year-old man with schizophrenia describes severe anxiety and insomnia associated with the onset 2 weeks ago of auditory hallucinations, in which voices tell him he is about to die. He was started yesterday on 5 mg of haloperidol given orally twice daily; however, his anxiety and insomnia remain severe today. Which of the following interventions is the most appropriate next step in management?

(A) Continue the haloperidol and initiate chlorpromazine
(B) Continue the haloperidol at current dosage and initiate clonazepam
(C) Discontinue haloperidol and initiate clonazepam
(D) Increase the dose of haloperidol
(E) Increase the dose of haloperidol and initiate clonazepam

5. A 21-year-old medical student seeks treatment for her severe anxiety associated with studying for final examinations that she will take in 3 weeks. Which of the following is the most appropriate initial pharmacologic intervention?

(A) Buspirone
(B) Diazepam
(C) 0.5 mg of lorazepam given twice daily
(D) 2 mg of lorazepam given twice daily
(E) No pharmacologic intervention

Answers and Explanations

1–B. The drowsiness and cognitive impairment are most likely caused by the diazepam. Switching the patient's medication to buspirone may minimize these symptoms and successfully treat his anxiety. Increasing the dose of diazepam may control his anxiety symptoms but would further exacerbate his drowsiness and cognitive impairment. Fluoxetine is not used to treat generalized anxiety disorder. Lorazepam would have the same adverse effects as diazepam. Tapering the diazepam dose may decrease the adverse effects, but would likely exacerbate his anxiety symptoms, which are still not completely controlled.

2–A. The woman's symptoms suggest that she has panic disorder, which is most appropriately initially treated with alprazolam. Clonazepam may be another good initial choice. Buspirone and chlorpromazine are not used for treating panic disorder. Diazepam and lorazepam are usually less effective than alprazolam for controlling panic symptoms.

3–C. The woman's symptoms suggest she is experiencing benzodiazepine withdrawal. Because of the potential for seizures and delirium, rapid treatment is essential. Lorazepam at the original dose is most likely effective; her dose can then be gradually tapered if it is no longer necessary to control her original symptoms. Alprazolam may effectively stop her withdrawal symptoms, but it is difficult to taper this benzodiazepine subsequently. Buspirone has no effect on benzodiazepine withdrawal symptoms.

4–B. Benzodiazepines are often useful adjuncts for managing the anxiety associated with psychotic symptoms. Use of benzodiazepines may allow the clinician to avoid increasing the dosage of antipsychotic medication. The clinician may instead switch the patient to a lower potency antipsychotic medication (e.g., chlorpromazine) with more sedation. Concurrent use of more than one antipsychotic medication is rarely indicated. Benzodiazepines alone are not effective for treating psychosis.

5–E. The information available in this case suggests that the individual's anxiety is probably normal and may help create motivation to study. Counseling and instruction in anxiety management (e.g., relaxation exercises, biofeedback) may be useful. Benzodiazepines should not be used for these situations unless nonpharmacologic interventions fail. If nonpharmacologic intervention fails, the benefits of benzodiazepines must be weighed against the potential adverse cognitive effects.

28

Antidepressant Medication and Electroconvulsive Therapy

I. Antidepressant Medication

A. General considerations

1. Antidepressants are derived from a variety of chemical classes and are used to alleviate depressive symptoms in mood, adjustment, and psychotic disorders. They are also used to treat various anxiety disorders, bulimia nervosa, enuresis, and chronic pain.

2. Some antidepressants are extremely dangerous when an overdose is ingested. When used to treat individuals with depressive symptoms, clinicians should generally prescribe in small doses and only after determining the absence of suicidal intent.

B. Mechanism of action

1. The mechanism of therapeutic action of these drugs is unknown, and it is unclear whether all antidepressants share a single mode of action.

2. Many antidepressants affect **monoamine neurotransmission** in the central nervous system (CNS), through reuptake inhibition and modulation of receptor function.

   a. Many antidepressants inhibit reuptake of serotonin, norepinephrine, or both.

   b. Some antidepressants block acetylcholine (muscarinic), α-adrenergic, and histamine (types 1 and 2) receptors.

C. Efficacy in depressive disorders. There is no single antidepressant that has proved to have more overall efficacy than others; however, some individuals clearly respond to certain antidepressants but not others.

1. **Overall efficacy** of antidepressants in the treatment of major depressive disorder is approximately 70%.

2. A patient may undergo trials of several antidepressants before finding an effective one.

3. Currently, there is no clinically accepted method of predicting which patient will respond to which antidepressant.

4. **Nonpharmacologic somatic therapies for mood disorders. Electroconvulsive therapy (ECT)** is used to treat major depressive episodes, especially when individuals do not respond to antidepressants or are extremely suicidal (see VI). Other modalities for treating depressive disorders include light therapy for seasonal depression, sleep deprivation, and, rarely, psychosurgery.

II. Classes of Antidepressants

A. Overview

1. In addition to mood elevation, each antidepressant medication has a characteristic profile of adverse effects, including changes in arousal (e.g., from marked sedation to mild activation), orthostatic hypotension, anticholinergic effects, decrease in seizure threshold, and changes in cardiac conduction.

2. Classes of antidepressants also differ according to their pharmacologic properties, efficacy in specific non-mood disorders, and margin of safety.

B. Tertiary amine tricyclic antidepressants (TCAs), which were some of the earliest antidepressants to be widely used, are converted to secondary amines in the body.

1. **Specific medications** include imipramine, amitriptyline, doxepin, clomipramine, and trimipramine.

2. **Efficacy.** In addition to the use of tertiary amine TCAs for treatment of mood disorders, imipramine is often used to treat panic disorder; clomipramine is used to treat obsessive-compulsive disorder; and amitriptyline is used to treat chronic pain.

3. **Adverse effects.** Tertiary amine TCAs tend to cause significant sedation, orthostatic hypotension, and anticholinergic effects. They are the most dangerous antidepressants in overdose.

C. Secondary amine TCAs

1. **Specific medications** include desipramine, nortriptyline, and protriptyline.

2. **Adverse effects.** Secondary amines are generally less sedating and cause less hypotension and anticholinergic effects. However, they may be more likely to exacerbate psychosis.

D. Heterocylic antidepressants

1. **Specific medications** include maprotiline and amoxapine.

2. **Specific efficacy.** Amoxapine is unique because it blocks dopamine receptors and may have antipsychotic efficacy.

3. **Adverse effects.** Maprotiline is more likely to cause seizures than many other antidepressants, and amoxapine may cause acute movement disorders.

E. Selective serotonin reuptake inhibitors (SSRIs)

1. **Specific medications** include fluoxetine, fluvoxamine, paroxetine, and sertraline.

2. **Efficacy.** In addition to treating depressive disorders, SSRIs are particularly efficacious in the treatment of obsessive-compulsive disorder and bu-

limia nervosa. Because they have relatively mild adverse effects, they are safer to use by potentially self-destructive patients and patients with certain general medical conditions.

3. **Adverse effects** include appetite loss, nausea, vomiting, diarrhea, and anorgasmia. SSRIs cause minimal or no cardiac, anticholinergic, or hypotensive effects.

F. **Other non-monoamine oxidase inhibitors (MAOIs)**

1. **Bupropion** is sometimes used to treat depressed patients in whom sexual dysfunction is a significant problem. It causes minimal sedation, hypotension, cardiac effects, or sexual dysfunction; however, seizures are more likely to occur.

2. **Nefazodone** is a moderately sedating antidepressant with minimal effects on sexual functioning. It may be useful in depressed patients with associated anxiety and insomnia.

3. **Trazodone** is often used to treat depressed patients who have severe insomnia. It is markedly sedating and causes minimal anticholinergic effects.

4. **Venlafaxine** is a reuptake inhibitor of both norepinephrine and serotonin. It has no effect on cholinergic, histaminergic, or α-adrenergic receptors. It may be useful for patients who are unresponsive to SSRIs and cannot tolerate orthostatic hypotension, sedation, or adverse anticholinergic effects that are associated with TCAs.

G. **MAOIs**

1. **General considerations.** MAOIs are a group of drugs that inhibit MAO-A and -B in the CNS and have antidepressant efficacy.

   a. MAOIs were developed in the early 1950s, but they are currently used less frequently than other antidepressants.

   b. Their lack of popularity may involve an early reputation for less overall efficacy in the treatment of major depressive disorder. Also, there is a risk for hypertensive crisis associated with patients who consume tyramine-rich foods.

   c. Recent studies suggest that at appropriate doses, MAOI efficacy equals that of other antidepressants, and that the associated dietary restrictions do not need to be as stringent as once believed.

2. **Specific medications.** MAOIs differ by the type of inhibition (i.e., reversible or irreversible), the severity of adverse effects, and the specificity of inhibition (MAO-A or -B).

   a. **Hydrazines** (e.g., phenelzine, isocarboxazid) are more sedating. They should be used cautiously in individuals who metabolize these medications less efficiently. These so-called slow acetylators represent about 50% of the population.

   b. **Tranylcypromine** is more activating, perhaps because it is structurally similar to amphetamine.

   c. **Selegiline.** This medication is a selective inhibitor of MAO-B. It is currently approved by the Food and Drug Administration only for treatment of Parkinson disease; however, it may be useful at higher dosages for treating depressive disorders. It may be associated with relatively less risk for hypertensive crisis because it does not inhibit MAO-A, the enzyme that catabolizes tyramine in the gut.

      d. Reversible MAOIs (RIMAs). These medications reversibly bind MAO instead of destroying it. Complete MAO activity is regained less than 1 week after a course of a RIMA ends. RIMAs are not yet available in the United States.

   3. Efficacy

      a. Major depressive disorder. MAOIs are most commonly used by patients with major depressive disorder who do not respond or have contraindications to other antidepressants.

      b. Depressive disorders with atypical features. Some patients with "atypical depressions," which are characterized by mood reactivity, increased appetite, leaden paralysis, and hypersomnia, may respond more favorably to MAOIs than to other antidepressants.

      c. Anxiety disorders. Some patients with panic disorder, social phobia, and posttraumatic stress disorder (PTSD) may respond well to MAOIs.

   4. Adverse effects

      a. These effects include changes in arousal (e.g., sedation, agitation), weight gain, orthostatic hypotension, liver toxicity (with hydrazine MAOIs), hypertensive crisis if tyramine-rich foods or certain other medications are ingested, and sexual dysfunction.

      b. Drug interactions. Concurrent use of MAOIs with certain antihypertensive medications, meperidine, and other psychoactive medications should generally be avoided.

         (1) The individual must wait up to 6 weeks between treatment with SSRIs and MAOIs, because of the risk for "serotoninergic syndrome," which is characterized by tremor and delirium.

         (2) Concurrent use of MAOIs and meperidine has been associated with delirium and fatalities and is absolutely contraindicated.

         (3) Concurrent use of MAOIs with nasal decongestants, antiasthmatic medications, and amphetamines is associated with hypertensive crisis.

III. Indications

   A. Mood disorders. Antidepressants are indicated for the treatment of major depressive disorder; dysthymic disorder; bipolar disorders, depressed phase; mood disorders due to a general medical condition; and substance-induced mood disorders (see V A).

   B. Adjustment disorder with depressed mood (see V B)

   C. Schizoaffective disorders (see V C)

   D. Anxiety disorders. Some antidepressants are indicated for the treatment of panic disorder and obsessive-compulsive disorder (see V D).

   E. Other indications. Some antidepressants are also indicated for the treatment of eating disorders, attention deficit hyperactivity disorder, childhood enuresis, and parasomnias (see V E).

IV. Adverse Effects of Antidepressants

   A. Sedative effects are most severe with doxepin, amitriptyline, and trazodone; they are least severe with desipramine, protriptyline, and SSRIs.

B. Hypotension is more severe with tertiary amine TCAs and phenelzine than with antidepressants.

C. Anticholinergic effects are most severe with amitriptyline and doxepin. SSRIs and trazodone do not cause anticholinergic effects.

D. Cardiac conduction. Cardiac arrhythmias are most likely to occur with use of TCAs.

E. Seizures are more common with TCAs, maprotiline, and bupropion. Seizures are rarely associated with SSRIs.

F. Sexual dysfunction. Many antidepressants, particularly SSRIs, may cause anorgasmia, changes in libido, and other sexual dysfunctions. Trazodone may cause priapism. Bupropion may cause fewer adverse sexual effects.

G. Drug interactions. Antidepressants, by virtue of their effect on various neurotransmitters, receptors, and metabolic pathways, interact with many other medications.

1. **Interactions among different antidepressants** (see II G 4 b)
2. **Anticholinergic medication.** Tertiary TCAs should be used cautiously with patients who are taking other anticholinergic medications, such as antiparkinsonian (e.g., benztropine, trihexyphenidyl) and antipsychotic (e.g., chlorpromazine, thioridazine) medications.
3. **Antihypertensive medication.** Some antihypertensive medications (e.g., clonidine) are affected by TCAs.

V. Treatment Guidelines for Antidepressants

A. Mood disorders

1. **Major depressive disorder.** Antidepressants are the treatment of choice for most types of this disorder, with overall treatment response approaching 70% of cases. However, when psychosis is present, the overall probability of treatment response decreases to 30%, and may necessitate concomitant use of antipsychotic medication or ECT.

   a. Clinicians select an antidepressant based on the previous history of response in the patient or family members or the adverse effects profile. For example, a patient with severe insomnia may benefit from a more sedating antidepressant.

   b. The clinician must assess lethality carefully throughout the period of treatment.

   c. **Dosage.** Antidepressants are often initiated at a low dose, which is increased as rapidly as possible, depending on the patient's tolerance to adverse effects.

      (1) It is essential to reach a **therapeutic dose**; if adverse effects preclude this, another antidepressant should be attempted.

      (2) Elderly individuals are more sensitive to anticholinergic and hypotensive effects of antidepressants but are responsive to lower doses.

   d. **Lag time.** Therapeutic effects are usually observed 2 to 6 weeks following initiation. Different symptoms of depression respond at different times (e.g., insomnia and fatigue respond earlier and subjective sense of mood improvement occurs later).

e. Response

(1) If there is no response to a given antidepressant in 4 to 6 weeks, it should be discontinued. A different antidepressant should then be initiated after a period of time sufficient to prevent adverse drug interactions.

(2) There is some evidence that treatment response can be augmented in some cases with various adjunctive medications, including lithium and thyroid hormone.

f. Prophylaxis. Treatment with antidepressants should continue prophylactically for 6 months after favorable response, possibly at a lower dose.

2. Dysthymic disorder

a. Although the treatment of choice for dysthymic disorder is psychotherapy, clinical studies indicate that about 30% of these patients may respond well to antidepressants.

b. Treatment guidelines are similar to those for major depressive disorder (see V A 1).

3. Mood disorders due to a general medical condition may respond to antidepressants.

a. Common indications include depressive symptoms following **left-sided cerebral strokes** and **early neurodegenerative diseases** with depressive symptoms.

b. Patients with neurodegenerative diseases and other general medical conditions often are of advanced age and have cognitive impairment, impulsivity, and metabolic compromise, which mandates cautious use of antidepressants at the lowest effective doses.

4. Substance-induced mood disorders with depressive symptoms may respond to antidepressants.

a. Antidepressants should be used very carefully in these patients because of their history of drug misuse, the potential for interactions with abused medication, and the possible metabolic compromise associated with the abused drugs.

b. Cocaine- and alcohol-induced mood disorders are most commonly treated with antidepressants, in addition to abstinence from the offending substance.

B. Adjustment disorder with depressed mood. The mainstay of treatment is short-term psychodynamic or cognitive psychotherapy, but antidepressants may also be useful. Treatment guidelines for this indication are identical to those for major depressive disorder (see V A 1).

C. Bipolar and schizoaffective disorders

1. Antidepressants are the treatment of choice for depressive episodes that occur during the course of bipolar and schizoaffective disorders.

2. Because antidepressants can precipitate a manic episode in individuals with bipolar disorder, the clinician must closely monitor treatment response for manic symptoms and discontinue antidepressant treatment if they occur. Mood-stabilizing medication is often prescribed concurrently.

3. When using concomitant antipsychotic medication, the clinician must select combinations of antipsychotic and antidepressant medications that minimize additive anticholinergic, hypotensive, and sedative effects.

D. Anxiety disorders

1. **Panic disorder**. Some antidepressants, particularly imipramine, are useful for treatment of this disorder in patients in whom benzodiazepines are contraindicated or poorly tolerated.

2. **Obsessive-compulsive disorder**. Clomipramine and SSRIs, particularly fluoxetine and fluvoxamine, have efficacy in treatment of this disorder.

3. **Social phobia**. MAOIs, particularly phenelzine, may be useful adjuncts for treatment of this disorder.

4. **PTSD**. Individuals with PTSD, particularly those who have depressive symptoms, may respond to antidepressant treatment.

E. Other indications

1. **Sleep disorders**. Trazodone or other sedating antidepressants may be used to treat insomnia, particularly when it accompanies depressive disorders. Desipramine is occasionally combined with amphetamines to treat narcolepsy, particularly when cataplexy does not respond to amphetamines alone.

2. **Bulimia nervosa**. Individuals with this disorder often respond to treatment with SSRIs. Individuals with anorexia nervosa and depressive symptoms may also benefit from SSRIs.

3. **Pain disorders** are often ameliorated with antidepressant treatment. Some antidepressants, particularly TCAs, may have a specific analgesic effect and are used to treat migraine and peripheral neuropathies.

4. **Personality disorders**. Some studies suggest that antidepressants, particularly SSRIs, may be useful in treating individuals with borderline personality disorder. The favorable response to antidepressants in these disorders is specific or may be caused by a general lessening of associated depressive symptoms.

VI. Electroconvulsive Therapy

A. Overview.
Electroconvulsive therapy (ECT) was originally used to treat psychosis but is now used mainly to treat major depressive episodes, occasionally to treat manic episodes, and rarely to treat schizophrenia with catatonic features.

1. **Description**. ECT is a series of electrically induced generalized tonic–clonic seizures. It is generally administered about 3 times weekly for a 2-week period. The ECT seizure is induced through electrodes placed on the scalp and equipment that determines precisely the intensity and duration of the electrical pulse.

2. **Administering ECT**

   a. Treatments are always **preceded by medication-induced anesthesia** and **muscle paralysis** to block motor manifestations and complications of the tonic–clonic seizure and to eliminate the severe anxiety caused by paralysis.

   b. ECT must be given by specifically trained psychiatrists and anesthesiologists.

3. The **antidepressant effect** of ECT is usually evident after 1 to 3 treatments. Relapse often occurs rapidly unless several additional treatments are administered.

4. Limitations. ECT is used less frequently than other forms of antidepressant treatment for several reasons:

   a. ECT and associated hospitalization are **costly.**

   b. The patient experiences a period of **transient confusion** during a course of ECT treatment.

   c. There are **negative perceptions** of ECT, which were generated by early ECT practices.

   d. There are significant **legal requirements** and **restrictions** associated with ECT.

B. Types

1. Bilateral and unilateral ECT. Electrodes are placed either bitemporally or unilaterally across the nondominant cerebral hemisphere. Although unilateral placement may cause less cognitive problems, it may not be as effective.

2. Multiple monitored ECT (MMECT). ECT may be administered as several seizures in one session, which may hasten therapeutic response and decrease risks associated with repeated use of anesthesia. However, MMECT is associated with more cognitive confusion.

C. Indications

1. Major depressive episodes. ECT is used to treat major depressive episodes (and occasionally manic episodes) that have not responded to antidepressant or mood-stabilizing medication.

   a. ECT is used for major depressive episodes in which the individual's risk for suicide is too severe to wait for antidepressant medication to lessen self-destructive symptoms.

   b. ECT is used for major depressive episodes in patients with **contraindications to antidepressant medication**.

   c. ECT is used in patients who have responded well previously to ECT.

   d. Occasional single ECT treatments may be used prophylactically in patients with ECT-responsive depressive episodes who are at high risk for relapse.

2. Schizophrenia, catatonic type and major depressive episodes with catatonic features. ECT is used in patients with these disorders who have not responded to antipsychotic medication and are at risk for complications caused by not eating, moving, or maintaining personal hygiene.

D. Adverse effects include:

1. Complications of associated anesthesia and induced paralysis, most commonly involving difficulties maintaining an adequate airway

2. Transiently increased intracranial pressure. The presence of space-occupying intracranial lesions usually precludes the use of ECT because of an increased risk of herniation.

3. **Transient postictal asystole.** ECT must be used with caution in patients with cardiac problems.

4. **Transient memory disturbance.** This adverse effect increases in severity during the course of ECT and gradually resolves during the several weeks after treatment ends.

5. **Drug interactions.** Drugs that increase seizure threshold should not be administered during a course of ECT. Lithium should be withheld during a course of ECT because it is associated with postictal delirium.

6. **Seizure-induced bone fractures** (see VI E 1 d). If the patient is not adequately paralyzed before ECT is administered, muscle contractions can cause vertebral fractures.

E. **Treatment guidelines.** Clinicians must carefully evaluate patients and educate them about ECT. Extensive, legally required documentation must be completed.

1. **Before each ECT treatment.** The patient is restricted from oral food intake, receives several medications, and undergoes several procedures.

   a. **Anticholinergic medication** (e.g., atropine) decreases airway secretions. The vagolytic effect reduces the bradycardia that follows ECT.

   b. **General anesthesia** (e.g., methohexital) prevents the patient from experiencing panic associated with being conscious during subsequent paralysis.

   c. **Airway placement** allows manual breathing during paralysis.

   d. **Paralytic agents** (e.g., succinylcholine) induce complete muscle relaxation and eliminate complications of the motor components of tonic–clonic seizures.

2. Electrocardiogram, electroencephalogram, and breathing are closely monitored during ECT and the subsequent recovery period for several minutes to verify the seizure activity and detect response.

3. After a brief recovery period of about 30 minutes, the patient can resume usual activities.

4. ECT treatments are usually given several times a week for several weeks, or a total of 6–12 treatments.

5. Because of the underlying illness and transient cognitive impairment, hospitalization is usually indicated for a course of ECT and for several days afterward.

6. After a course of successful ECT, patients usually receive maintenance antidepressant medication for several months, even if they had no beneficial response from antidepressants before ECT. Some patients receive maintenance ECT (single treatment) monthly.

Review Test

Directions: Each of the numbered items or incomplete statements in this section is followed by answers or by completions of the statement. Select the ONE lettered answer or completion that is BEST in each case.

1. A 31-year-old woman with a history of major depressive disorder and an excellent response to amitriptyline develops a recurrent major depressive episode and extremely disturbing delusions that her flesh is rotting. Based on her previous response, amitriptyline is reinitiated. Which of the following medications is the most appropriate additional agent to administer?

(A) Clonazepam
(B) Clozapine
(C) Low-potency antipsychotic medication
(D) Risperidone
(E) Valproate

2. A 33-year-old man with major depressive disorder, single episode, is started on 20 mg/day of fluoxetine. After 3 days, he develops severe nausea and epigastric distress. Which of the following is the most appropriate next step in management?

(A) Continue the fluoxetine for at least 3 weeks at the current dose and advise the patient to take an over-the-counter antacid
(B) Continue the fluoxetine for at least 3 weeks at the current dose and advise the patient to try a different diet
(C) Discontinue the fluoxetine and initiate electroconvulsive therapy
(D) Discontinue the fluoxetine and initiate imipramine
(E) Decrease the dose of fluoxetine to 10 mg/day

3. A 41-year-old woman with dysthymic disorder is started on phenelzine, a monoamine oxidase inhibitor. Which of the following should the woman be advised to avoid?

(A) Antihistamines
(B) Caramel syrup
(C) Pseudoephedrine
(D) Fresh red meat
(E) White wines

4. A 43-year-old woman with depressive rumination, hypersomnia, hyperphagia, and a subjective sense of heaviness in her limbs has not responded to trials of fluoxetine and nortriptyline. Which of the following would be the most appropriate next step in management of her case?

(A) Initiate desipramine
(B) Initiate methylphenidate
(C) Initiate sertraline
(D) Initiate tranylcypromine
(E) Initiate trazodone

5. A 50-year-old man complains of severe depression. He is especially sensitive about his sexual performance, which he perceives as being affected by his age. Which of the following antidepressants is the best choice for initial treatment?

(A) Bupropion
(B) Fluoxetine
(C) Imipramine
(D) Sertraline
(E) Venlafaxine

6. A 54-year-old hospitalized woman who has severe recurrent major depressive disorder improves dramatically after her first two treatments with bilateral electroconvulsive therapy (ECT). After the fourth ECT treatment, she is disoriented to the date. Which of the following is the best choice for further treatment?

(A) Administer two more ECT treatments and then initiate antidepressant medication
(B) Discontinue ECT and treat with antidepressant medication
(C) Discontinue ECT until her cognitive status improves and then resume ECT
(D) Initiate a mood stabilizer and continue ECT
(E) Switch to unilateral ECT for four additional treatments

7. A 71-year-old man with carotid artery stenosis develops severe depression with anergy and hypersomnia. Which of the following antidepressants is the best choice for initial treatment?

(A) Amitriptyline
(B) Doxepin
(C) Nortriptyline
(D) Phenelzine
(E) Trazodone

Answers and Explanations

1–D. The patient's symptoms suggest mood congruent psychosis and may respond to the addition of an antipsychotic medication. Because amitriptyline has significant anticholinergic effects, an antipsychotic agent with minimal additional anticholinergic effects, such as risperidone or another high-potency medication, should be used. Low-potency antipsychotic medication has significant anticholinergic effects. Clonazepam or valproate is unlikely to alleviate the patient's psychotic symptoms.

2–D. A significant number of individuals develop intolerable nausea and other gastrointestinal symptoms when taking fluoxetine and other selective serotonin reuptake inhibitors. This patient would probably be most comfortable and most likely to continue his course of antidepressant treatment if he is switched to another medication, such as imipramine, which is less likely to cause gastrointestinal distress. Another reasonable treatment choice may be to divide the dose of fluoxetine and instruct the patient to take it with food. The patient's distress is less likely to be relieved by an antacid or a change in diet. Electroconvulsive therapy may be considered for this patient if he is unable to tolerate or does not respond to several different antidepressant medications. Lowering the dose of fluoxetine may relieve the patient's gastrointestinal symptoms but decrease the likelihood of therapeutic response.

3–C. Pseudoephedrine and other nasal decongestants, bronchodilators, and amphetamines can cause severe hypertension when monoamine oxidase is inhibited. Antihistamines do not have this effect. Foods that contain tyramine (e.g., smoked meat, aged cheese, and red wine) may also cause hypertension when ingested during treatment with a monoamine oxidase inhibitor. Caramel syrup, fresh red meat, and white wine do not contain high levels of tyramine.

4–D. The patient's symptoms suggest major depressive disorder with atypical features. This subtype of major depressive disorder may respond particularly well to a monoamine oxidase inhibitor, such as tranylcypromine. Another reasonable treatment choice for patients who do not adequately respond to several antidepressant trials is to try to augment the response with lithium or thyroid hormone.

5–A. This patient is particularly concerned with sexual performance. Of the antidepressants listed, bupropion has the fewest adverse effects on sexual performance. Selective serotonin reuptake inhibitors, such as fluoxetine and sertraline, imipramine, venlafaxine, and many other antidepressants are associated with changes in libido as well as erectile and orgasmic disturbances.

6–A. The patient is responding well to electroconvulsive therapy (ECT) but needs at least two additional treatments to minimize the risk of a quick relapse. Some degree of transient cognitive impairment is common with ECT and often becomes more severe as treatment progresses. It usually resolves within weeks following the conclusion of a course of ECT and, in this case, does not preclude two additional treatments. After conclusion of treatment, antidepressant medication is usually continued for 6 months to lessen the chance of relapse. Mood-stabilizing medication is not indicated for this patient. Unilateral ECT is associated with less cognitive impairment than bilateral ECT; however, unilateral ECT is less effective and is often reserved for patients at special risk for severe cognitive compromise, such as elderly individuals. It is not indicated in this case.

7–C. Elderly patients are often sensitive to the hypotensive, sedative, and anticholinergic effects of antidepressant medication. This patient is at special risk for hypotension because of his carotid artery stenosis. Of the antidepressants listed, nortriptyline is the least likely to cause sedation, hypotension, and anticholinergic effects. Additional good treatment choices include using other secondary tricyclic antidepressants or selective serotonin reuptake inhibitors. Tertiary tricyclic antidepressants, such as amitriptyline and doxepin, have marked hypotensive, sedative, and anticholinergic effects. Phenelzine has marked hypotensive effects. Trazodone is highly sedating.

29

Lithium and Other Mood-Stabilizing Medications

I. Overview. Lithium, valproate, carbamazepine, and clonazepam are used to treat mood disorders.

    A. Lithium (see II). In the form of a charged ion, lithium is a **first-choice drug for the treatment of bipolar disorder.**

    B. Anticonvulsants. Valproate is also a first-choice drug for treating bipolar disorder, particularly when lithium use is contraindicated or difficult to adequately monitor. **Carbamazepine** is also efficacious but causes more serious adverse effects.

    C. Clonazepam may also have some efficacy for this indication, and other medications have also been used occasionally.

II. Lithium

    A. The **mechanism of action** is unknown but may involve changes in ion transport at cell membranes.

    B. Efficacy. Approximately 70% of individuals with bipolar I disorder respond to lithium. Lithium may be less effective in individuals with rapid-cycling bipolar disorders.

    C. Indications

        1. The major therapeutic indications are for **bipolar** and **schizoaffective disorders**, including the treatment of manic, hypomanic, and mixed episodes and prophylaxis against mood episodes (see II E 1, 2).

        2. Lithium is also used as adjunctive treatment of major depressive disorder. It may augment response to antidepressant medication in some patients (see II E 3).

    D. Adverse effects. Because lithium has a low therapeutic index, close monitoring of the patient's plasma lithium levels is essential.

        1. Dose-related toxicity. As plasma lithium levels increase to greater than 1.5 mEq/L, the patient may experience tremor, nausea, vomiting, and diarrhea. Delirium may occur.

      a. Dehydration and hyponatremia increase plasma lithium levels and may predispose the patient to toxicity.

      b. At therapeutic levels, tremor may occur.

      c. Divided doses and slow-release preparations decrease peak plasma levels, which may minimize dose-related adverse effects.

   2. Polyuria. Diabetes insipidus is a common adverse effect and may be troublesome to patients.

   3. Hypothyroidism develops in approximately 5% of patients.

   4. Leukocytosis usually occurs and appears to be a benign condition.

   5. Renal damage. Interstitial nephritis develops, although rarely.

   6. Cardiac conduction. Electrocardiogram (ECG) changes may be noted and are usually benign.

   7. Dermatologic problems. Acne may develop. Sometimes the cosmetic impact of the acne interferes with patient compliance.

   8. Weight gain may interfere with patient compliance.

   9. Teratogenicity. Lithium is associated with cardiac abnormalities, particularly atrial–septal defects, and therefore is contraindicated if the patient is in the first trimester of pregnancy.

E. Treatment guidelines

   1. Treatment of manic, hypomanic, and mixed episodes in bipolar and schizoaffective disorders

      a. The **target symptoms** are mood pathology and associated psychological and physiologic changes.

      b. Baseline laboratory studies must be obtained before initiation of lithium. These studies should include complete blood count, electrolytes, blood urea nitrogen and creatinine, thyroid function tests, ECG, and a pregnancy test.

      c. Dose. The usual starting dose for lithium is about 300 mg three times daily. The typical dose required to reach therapeutic levels is 900 to 1500 mg/day, but the actual dose required to reach therapeutic level varies significantly among patients.

      d. Lag time. Target symptoms are affected about 1 week after initiating lithium. Because of the lag time, an antipsychotic medication is almost always initiated concurrently to acutely decrease psychomotor activity and psychosis.

      e. Plasma lithium levels are drawn every 5 days—more often if toxicity is suspected—and should always be drawn in the trough period before the first morning dose.

         (1) The only use of stat lithium levels is to investigate possible toxicity or to determine whether lithium ingestion has occurred.

         (2) Plasma lithium levels of 1.0 to 1.2 mEq/L are necessary for an adequate trial and must be maintained for 2 weeks before effectiveness is evaluated.

         (3) A plasma lithium level of greater than 1.0 mEq/L should be maintained for at least several weeks after a satisfactory response to prevent acute relapse.

f. Therapeutic lithium level. After 10 days at a therapeutic lithium level, antipsychotic medication is generally tapered to assess the effectiveness of the lithium.

(1) If lithium alone is ineffective for treatment of mood symptoms in bipolar disorder after an adequate trial, there is usually no reason to continue it while using other medication.

(2) Use of lithium alone may be effective in treating schizoaffective disorder, but the concurrent use of antipsychotic medication is often necessary to control the patient's psychosis completely.

2. Prophylaxis against manic, hypomanic, and depressive episodes in bipolar and schizoaffective disorders

a. Plasma lithium levels of 0.6 to 1.0 mEq/L are usually adequate for prophylaxis. Patients should be maintained at the lowest effective level to minimize adverse effects.

b. Prophylactic treatment is usually continued for about 6 months. It may need to be continued indefinitely, particularly in rapid-cycling patients.

c. Plasma levels should be checked every 2 months.

d. Blood urea nitrogen and creatinine levels should be checked every 6 months, and thyroid function tests should be performed at least once yearly.

3. Adjunctive treatment of major depressive disorder

a. Lithium may be used as prophylaxis against recurrent depressive episodes in all mood disorders; it is used less commonly for this purpose in unipolar depressive disorders.

b. Lithium may be used to augment an inadequate response to antidepressant medication in major depressive disorder. Its effectiveness for this purpose is uncertain.

III. Anticonvulsants.

The overall efficacy for treatment of bipolar disorder with anticonvulsants is 50% to 70%. Some patients who do not respond to lithium will respond to anticonvulsants.

A. Valproate is an alternative treatment of choice for patients with bipolar disorder, manic episode.

1. Valproate may be particularly useful in treating patients in emergency settings, where close laboratory monitoring may be difficult. Treatment response may occur within several days.

2. Valproate is also useful for patients who cannot tolerate or are unresponsive to lithium. It may be more effective than lithium for patients with rapid-cycling bipolar disorder.

3. Common **adverse effects** include sedation and tremor. Ataxia, alopecia, and hepatotoxicity occur infrequently.

B. Carbamazepine. Rare but serious hematologic and hepatic adverse effects (e.g., agranulocytosis) and significant sedation make carbamazepine a second-choice drug. Monitoring of plasma levels, complete blood count, and liver function tests are necessary for these patients.

C. Clonazepam. There is some evidence of efficacy of clonazepam for treating agitation during manic episodes.

IV. Other Treatments for Bipolar Disorder

A. Antipsychotic medication is often effective for treatment of manic episodes when other mood-stabilizing medications are ineffective or contraindicated.

B. Combinations of mood-stabilizing medications (e.g., lithium and valproate) are occasionally effective when neither medication has worked alone.

C. Electroconvulsive therapy, in refractory cases of bipolar and schizoaffective disorders, may be useful.

Review Test

Directions: Each of the numbered items or incomplete statements in this section is followed by answers or by completions of the statement. Select the ONE lettered answer or completion that is BEST in each case.

1. A 19-year-old woman with two previous episodes of mania develops a major depressive episode. Which of the following is the most appropriate initial pharmacologic management?

(A) Initiate imipramine
(B) Initiate lithium
(C) Initiate valproate
(D) Initiate venlafaxine
(E) Initiate venlafaxine and valproate

2. A 23-year-old man who is currently on maintenance lithium therapy presents to the emergency room complaining of tremulousness, nausea, dizziness, and diarrhea. A stat laboratory examination reveals an undetectable plasma lithium level. Which of the following statements about the patient is most accurate?

(A) He probably has a viral infection
(B) He is malingering
(C) He is not taking his lithium as prescribed
(D) His symptoms are likely caused by lithium toxicity
(E) His dose of lithium should be increased

3. A 25-year-old woman with recurrent bipolar I disorder, manic phase, has a resolution of her manic symptoms with lithium treatment. One month later, she complains of weight gain, disrupted sleep due to nocturnal polyuria, and acne. Her plasma lithium level is 0.7 mEq/L. She states that she will no longer take the lithium. Which of the following is the most appropriate next step in management?

(A) Caution the patient that failure to comply with lithium treatment will result in involuntary psychiatric hospitalization
(B) Discontinue lithium and reinitiate a mood stabilizer if her symptoms recur
(C) Discontinue lithium and initiate valproate
(D) Lower her dose of lithium
(E) Refuse to treat her unless she complies with pharmacotherapy

4. A 35-year-old man with bipolar I disorder, manic phase, has not responded to adequate trials of lithium, valproate, or carbamazepine. High doses of haloperidol barely control his hyperactivity and cause effectual blunting and drooling. Which of the following is the most appropriate next step in management?

(A) Administer electroconvulsive therapy
(B) Initiate chlorpromazine
(C) Initiate clozapine
(D) Initiate diazepam
(E) Initiate phenobarbital

5. A 49-year-old woman with bipolar I disorder who is on maintenance lithium therapy has recurrence of a manic episode. Her plasma lithium level is 0.7 mEq/L. Which of the following is the most appropriate next step in management?

(A) Continue lithium and also initiate valproate
(B) Continue lithium and also initiate haloperidol
(C) Discontinue lithium and initiate electroconvulsive therapy
(D) Discontinue lithium and switch to valproate
(E) Increase the dose of lithium

Answers and Explanations

1–E. The patient's symptoms most suggest bipolar disorder, depressed phase. The depressive episode should be treated with an antidepressant (venlafaxine), and a mood-stabilizing agent (valproate) should also be initiated to minimize the risk of inducing a manic episode. A mood-stabilizing agent initiated alone is less likely to treat the depressive episode effectively.

2–C. The undetectable stat lithium level suggests that the patient is not taking lithium. A high stat lithium level would suggest that his symptoms may be caused by lithium toxicity. In this case, the patient's symptoms are likely caused by another factor. There is little evidence that he is malingering. Raising the patient's dose of lithium would not address the issue of patient compliance and is potentially dangerous if he begins taking his lithium again.

3–C. The patient is at high risk for relapse if treatment is discontinued. Her physical symptoms are likely caused by the lithium. Switching her mood stabilizer to valproate will lessen her discomfort and prevent relapse. Threatening the patient with involuntary hospitalization or discharge from care are less effective ways of ensuring compliance. Lowering the dose of lithium will likely result in a subtherapeutic lithium level.

4–A. Electroconvulsive therapy is often an effective treatment for manic episodes that are refractory to treatment with mood-stabilizing medication. Another reasonable treatment choice may be to initiate clonazepam to reduce the patient's agitation. Chlorpromazine, clozapine, diazepam, and phenobarbital are not appropriate treatments for this man.

5–E. To maximize the chance of therapeutic response, a patient being treated for manic episodes should have a plasma lithium level of 1.0 mEq\L or greater. Increasing this patient's dose is likely to bring her level into this range. If she remains unresponsive to treatment after this plasma level is attained, the physician may appropriately attempt a trial of valproate.

Part Four

Psychotherapies

30

Psychotherapy

I. Overview

A. Definition. Psychotherapies are theories and techniques designed to improve the way an individual feels, thinks, and behaves.

B. Classification. Psychotherapies are often classified as "schools" and are distinguished by different behavioral theories and psychotherapeutic techniques.

1. **Types.** Current psychotherapies include:
   a. Somatic psychotherapy (see II)
   b. Psychodynamic psychotherapy (see III)
   c. Behavioral psychotherapy (see IV)
   d. Cognitive psychotherapy (see V)
   e. Humanistic psychotherapies (see VI)

2. Each psychotherapy in this chapter is described based on its theory, technique, and the tools that are used. It is also described according to the setting, cost, and duration of the therapy as well as the characteristics of the patients and indications.

C. Recent clinical interest in psychotherapy focuses on determining which psychotherapeutic techniques are most efficacious for a given problem. Less emphasis has been placed on theory.

II. Somatic Psychotherapy

A. Definition. Somatic psychotherapy involves physical interventions designed to improve psychological functioning.

B. Types

1. **Body manipulation** involves many forms of movement, exercise, and massage techniques, including tai chi, rolfing, sensory awareness training, and sensate focus.

2. **Psychosurgical procedures** include leukotomy and ablative techniques. Psychosurgical intervention for behavioral problems is a controversial issue.

3. Electroconvulsive therapy (ECT) involves the electrical induction of generalized seizures (see Chapter 28 VI).

4. Psychiatric medication includes antidepressant, antipsychotic, anxiolytic, and mood-stabilizing agents.

C. **Theory.** The physical configuration of the body, including the central nervous system (CNS), determines behavior; therefore, changing body configuration changes behavior.

1. **Explanation for efficacy of other psychotherapies.** Human experience, including psychotherapeutic experiences, alters the structure of the CNS through the physical changes caused by learning.

2. **Limitations of theory**

a. Somatic theories of behavior have limited use in describing environmental effects on behavior.

b. There are imprecise relationships between specific physical and behavioral changes.

D. **Technique**. Various physical interventions, including medication, ECT, massage, or movement are employed. The patient is often not required to participate in complex therapeutic relationships or learning for the treatment to be effective.

1. **Tools** that are used may include a variety of machines and psychoactive medications. Also, the therapist's or patient's physical strength and skills may be used.

2. **Setting.** These types of therapy may be administered in a hospital, office, or nonmedical settings.

3. **Duration.** Some types of somatic therapies produce effects within hours, days, or weeks.

a. Movement therapy and use of anxiolytic medication may relax the individual almost immediately.

b. ECT and antipsychotic and antidepressant medications may be effective within a few days or weeks.

c. Maintenance therapy may be prolonged.

4. The financial **cost** of somatic therapy is variable, but it is often a cost-effective modality.

E. **Patient characteristics**. A broad range of patients receive somatic therapy. Some studies suggest that patients in lower socioeconomic groups are more likely to receive somatic therapy than psychodynamic psychotherapy.

F. **Indications**

1. **Body manipulation** is often used for stress relief and generalized anxiety disorder.

2. **Psychosurgery** currently has no clear-cut indications. However, intractable obsessive-compulsive disorder is sometimes ameliorated by cingulotomy.

3. **ECT** is indicated for individuals with major depressive disorder, bipolar mood disorders, and schizophrenia when chemotherapy is contraindicated or ineffective.

4. **Medication** may be the treatment of choice or an adjunct in treatment of schizophrenia, bipolar mood disorders, depressive disorders, anxiety disorders, some cases of adjustment disorders, and sleep disorders. Some childhood disorders, including attention deficit hyperactivity disorder, may also respond to medication.

III. Psychodynamic Psychotherapy

A. **Definition.** Psychodynamic psychotherapy is a form of talking and relational therapy, involving techniques based on psychodynamic theory.

B. **Types.** Psychodynamic psychotherapies may be subclassified according to duration, focus of treatment, format (i.e., group or individual treatment), and the tools or theories emphasized.

1. **Long-term psychotherapy** (e.g., psychoanalysis, psychoanalytic psychotherapy) focuses on significantly changing the patient's personality or fostering self-understanding.

2. **Crisis** or **brief psychotherapy** focuses on dealing with acute stressors or problem solving.

3. **Group psychotherapy** focuses on interrelationships among individuals and groups.

C. **Theory**

1. **General considerations.** Behavior is strongly influenced by previous experience, much of which is no longer conscious.

   a. When people talk or behave, information may be inferred about their unconscious mentation.

   b. Bringing unconscious emotional conflicts and thinking styles to the patient's attention gives the patient insight into his thoughts, feelings, and behavior.

   (1) **Insight** allows a patient to change his behavior.

   (2) Patients resist insight, and this **resistance** must be **worked through** (i.e., approached from many different perspectives).

   c. Behavior may also change through a **corrective emotional experience**—the reexperiencing of earlier emotional conflicts in a therapeutic situation in which these conflicts are resolved.

2. **Specific theories**

   a. **Freudian theory.** Classic psychodynamic theory focuses on unconscious and unresolved childhood conflicts and defense mechanisms.

   b. **Jungian theory** focuses on unconscious symbolism in dreams.

   c. **Kleinian theory** focuses on early (i.e., pre-oedipal) unconscious conflicts.

   d. **Object relations theory**, including self-psychology and ego psychology, focuses on the patient's history of relationships with other individuals.

3. **Explanation for efficacy of other psychotherapies.** All forms of psychotherapy alter a patient's unconscious mentation.

4. **Limitations of theory**. Psychodynamic theory provides limited explanations for current environmental effects on behavior.

a. Social and emotional competencies that may develop later in life are difficult to fully describe within a classic psychodynamic framework.

b. Behavioral and emotional changes produced by medication and other somatic interventions are also difficult to describe with psychodynamic theory.

D. **Technique**. One or more patients talk with a therapist who listens, facilitates discussion by asking questions, and provides feedback by clarifying and interpreting the patient's speech and behavior.

1. **Tools.** The patient is usually instructed to make free associations (i.e., to say whatever comes to mind). These associations often include descriptions of current and past experiences, emotions, and dreams. The therapist listens carefully, asks questions, and makes clarifications to develop the patient's psychological insight. The therapist may also encourage the patient's emotional release (i.e., catharsis) when describing events or experiences that elicit strong emotional reactions.

2. The **setting** is usually in an office.

3. **Duration.** This form of psychotherapy usually lasts several months to several years.

4. The **cost** is variable but often relatively expensive when compared with pharmacotherapy.

E. **Patient characteristics.** Verbal, stable, and motivated patients have the best prognosis.

F. **Indications.** Psychodynamic psychotherapy is indicated for the treatment of adjustment disorders, personality disorders, depressive disorders, dissociative disorders, somatoform disorders, and eating disorders. It is also used for self-discovery.

IV. Behavioral Psychotherapy

A. **Definition**. Behavioral psychotherapy, sometimes referred to as behavior modification, involves changing the patient's responses to the environment or altering aspects of the environment that influence (i.e., reinforce) the patient's behavior.

B. **Terminology**

1. A **stimulus** is a cue for a particular response.

2. A **response** is a behavior that occurs on presentation of a particular stimulus.

3. **Conditioning.** A therapist creates a new pattern of responses in a patient by associating original stimuli with new stimuli.

4. An **unconditioned stimulus** is a naturally occurring stimulus that produces a particular response (e.g., an electrical shock is an unconditioned stimulus that produces distress).

5. An **unconditioned response** is a naturally occurring response to a given stimulus (e.g., distress is an unconditioned response to an electrical shock).

6. A **conditioned stimulus** is a new stimulus that is made to elicit a particular response by pairing it with an unconditioned stimulus (e.g., a buzzer is a conditioned stimulus that elicits distress if it has been repeatedly paired with an electrical shock in the past).

7. A **conditioned response** is a new response that is created to a particular stimulus by pairing that stimulus with an unconditioned stimulus (e.g., distress is a conditioned response to a buzzer that has been repeatedly paired with an electrical shock).

8. A **positive reinforcer** is an aspect of the environment that increases the frequency of a behavior. For example, money may be a positive reinforcer for working.

9. A **negative reinforcer** is an aspect of the environment that increases the frequency of behavior when it is removed. For example, a bonus paid to an employee for perfect attendance may be a negative reinforcer for staying home when one is sick.

10. A **reward** is any aspect of the environment that increases the frequency of behavior. For example, money may be a reward for working.

11. A **punishment** is any aspect of the environment that decreases the frequency of behavior. Poverty may be a punishment for not working.

C. **Types**

1. **Relaxation training.** Relaxation techniques, such as guided imagery breathing exercises, are taught and reinforced.

2. **Systematic desensitization.** Relaxation techniques are practiced as a patient is repeatedly exposed to anxiety-provoking stimuli.

3. **Aversive conditioning** combines an aversive stimulus (e.g., nausea-producing medication) with a stimulus that indicates undesirable behavior (e.g., the odor of an alcoholic beverage that initiates drinking).

4. **Operant conditioning.** The frequency of target behavior is changed by altering rewards and punishments in the environment.

5. **Biofeedback training.** Physiologic parameters, such as blood pressure and heart rate, are presented to the patient and used to reinforce particular behaviors, such as relaxation.

D. **Theory**

1. An individual's behavior is produced in response to the environment through conditioning and reinforcement involving rewards and punishments. Through conditioning and by altering reinforcement from the environment, an individual learns to produce different behavior.

2. **Explanation for efficacy of other psychotherapies.** Conditioning and reinforcement are implicit in all forms of psychotherapy.

3. **Limitations of theory**

   a. It is difficult to fully account for the effects of pharmacologic and other somatic interventions on behavior in the framework of behavioral theory.

   b. Behavioral theory provides limited explanations for the frequency of behaviors that are less obviously reinforced, such as curiosity and creativity.

E. **Technique.** Behavioral therapists carefully detail the nature of the patient's behavioral pathology, its frequency, and its relationship to the environment. Then, the therapist systematically alters environmental stimuli and the reinforcements that affect the frequency of the pathologic behavior.

1. In **classic behavioral conditioning,** an individual's pattern of responses to environmental stimuli is systematically modified, often by temporally associating stimuli. For example, if a stimulus that produces a feeling of discomfort (e.g., an electrical shock) is paired with a new stimulus (e.g., a cigarette), the new stimulus may begin to produce a feeling of discomfort.

2. In **operant conditioning,** reinforcers (i.e., rewards and punishments) are used to alter the frequency of behavior. For example, a child may use the word *please* more frequently when making a request if he is rewarded with verbal approval each time he does so. Or, an adult may speak less frequently if he is punished with ridicule each time he does so.

3. **Tools** include pairing environmental stimuli, altering the nature of available reinforcers, teaching, modeling, shaping (i.e., incrementally changing behavior), biofeedback, and guided imagery.

4. The **setting** is extremely variable. Therapy may occur in a hospital or an office. Also, it may occur in the setting in which the behavioral pathology occurs, such as at school or work.

5. The **duration** is usually a few weeks.

6. Because it is brief, behavioral psychotherapy is often **less expensive** than other forms of psychotherapy.

F. **Patient characteristics.** Patients with a wide range of pathology, intelligence, maturity, and level of motivation may respond to behavioral psychotherapy.

G. **Indications.** Behavioral psychotherapy is indicated for the treatment of many childhood psychiatric disorders, anxiety disorders, substance abuse, and somatoform disorders.

V. Cognitive Psychotherapy

A. **Definition.** Cognitive psychotherapy is designed to change the way a patient looks at the world, thereby changing the patient's response to problems.

B. **Types**

1. **Generic cognitive therapy** (Beck) uses classic cognitive theory and techniques and is often used to treat depressive disorders.

2. **Assertiveness training** is a series of cognitive and behavioral techniques that decrease social anxiety.

3. **Dialectical behavior therapy** (Linehan) is a cognitive–behavioral psychotherapy designed to reduce suicidal gestures in patients with borderline personality disorder.

4. **Rational emotive psychotherapy** (Ellis) involves cognitive techniques that emphasize aggressive confrontation of a patient's cognitive distortions.

5. **Neurolinguistic programming** emphasizes the relationship of speech to cognition.

6. **Teaching.** All forms of education potentially alter an individual's subsequent behavior by presenting new information that changes the way the environment is perceived.

C. **Theory**

1. Behavior and emotion are determined by an individual's perception of the environment, not by the "real" environment.

   a. An individual's perception of the environment is learned, creating unique cognitive patterns, or frameworks.

    b. Cognitive frameworks determine the way individuals interpret things and give stability to their behavior.

  2. Maladaptive behavior and emotional distress are caused by "faulty" cognitive frameworks. Changing an individual's cognitive frameworks may increase adaptive behavior and lessen emotional distress.

  3. Explanation for efficacy of other psychotherapies. Other forms of psychotherapy alter cognitive frameworks.

  4. Limitations of theory

    a. As with behavioral theory, it is difficult to fully account for the effects of pharmacologic and somatic intervention on behavior in the framework of cognitive theory.

    b. Cognitive theory provides limited descriptions of unconscious mental activity that may affect behavior.

D. Technique. A therapist and a patient meet to discuss the patient's cognitions and how to change them.

  1. Tools used include teaching and behavioral reinforcement. Patients may be given assignments, such as maintaining a notebook of observations about their behavior.

  2. The **setting** is usually an office. Cognitive psychotherapy may also be conducted without a therapist; the patient uses a written manual or recordings.

  3. The **duration** of most forms of cognitive therapy is usually several weeks or months.

  4. The **cost** of cognitive therapy is comparable with that of other psychotherapies of similar duration. "Self-help" books and recordings that are based on cognitive principles are inexpensive.

E. Patient characteristics. Highly motivated patients often have a good treatment response.

F. Indications. Cognitive psychotherapy is indicated for the treatment of major depressive disorder, dysthymic disorder, adjustment disorders, social phobia, substance abuse, and impulse-control disorders.

VI. Humanistic Psychotherapies

A. Definition. Humanistic psychotherapies emphasize the relationship of an individual to those around him, to society as a whole, and, occasionally, to the natural environment.

B. Types

  1. Generic humanist psychotherapy (Fromm) emphasizes the individual's need to establish a meaningful relationship with the world and to transcend personal concerns.

  2. Transpersonal psychology (Maslow) focuses on **achieving full human potential** by expanding ideas of consciousness, using techniques such as **meditation** and **trance states**.

  3. Gestalt therapy (Perls) emphasizes a "here-and- now" experience of the relationship between the individual and the environment, using dramatic **role-playing** techniques.

4. **Sensitivity training** focuses on developing increased awareness of the physical and interpersonal environment through group experiences, physical techniques, and experiences in natural settings (e.g., mountains, beach).

5. **Encounter groups,** or T-groups (Tavistock), focus on group processes, which are the collective behaviors of individuals within groups.

C. **Theory**

1. **General considerations.** Much individual unhappiness is caused by faulty relationships among the individual, significant others, society, and the natural environment.

   a. Improving the way an individual relates to her environment decreases her emotional distress and improves her adaptive behavior.

   b. Many problems of society in general are attributable to the psychopathology of individuals. Therefore, decreasing an individual's emotional distress may improve the well-being of society.

2. **Explanation for efficacy of other psychotherapies.** The curative potential of all psychotherapies lies in their ability to transform relationships.

3. **Limitations of theory.** Humanistic psychotherapies are sometimes based on moral or ethical precepts that are not universally accepted.

D. **Technique.** Humanistic psychotherapy usually involves discussions among patients and a humanistic psychotherapist. Sensory awareness techniques may also be used.

1. **Tools** include group experiences, discussion, study, and sensory awareness techniques, such as measured breathing, touching, and visualization.

2. **Settings** may include traditional offices or nonmedical settings, such as resorts or retreats.

3. The **duration** is variable. Group experiences may last one to several days.

4. The **cost** of humanistic psychotherapy often includes expenses for travel, lodging, and time missed from work.

E. **Patient characteristics.** Higher levels of patient motivation and intelligence predict a greater subjective benefit.

F. **Indications.** This therapy is useful for ameliorating existential unhappiness and encouraging self-discovery. It is also used in commercial settings to improve employees' abilities to work together.

VII. Common Features Among Psychotherapies

A. **Common features among schools of psychotherapy.** According to Jerome Frank, all effective psychotherapies provide an emotionally charged, confiding therapeutic relationship; a therapeutic rationale; hope; and new information for patients through precept, example, or self-discovery.

B. **Common features of effective psychotherapists**

1. Studies suggest that effective psychotherapists tend to have experience with personal emotional conflict.

2. Effective psychotherapists tend to be more empathic and tolerant of deviant behavior when compared with the general population.

3. Many effective psychotherapists have undergone long, rigorous training in fields such as medicine, psychology, teaching, or religion.

VIII. Recent Trends in Psychotherapy

A. Technique

1. Psychotherapeutic technique is becoming increasingly universal and theory is being de-emphasized.
2. Current studies of psychotherapy attempt to discover more systematically which psychotherapeutic techniques are most effective in promoting therapeutic change; however, universally accepted outcome measures for many psychological problems are difficult to devise.

B. Cost-effectiveness. Managed health care systems are increasingly interested in psychotherapies that produce the best results at the lowest cost.

C. Therapist qualifications and training. Both quality management and cost-effectiveness issues direct attention to determining the optimum training and certification for psychotherapists.

Review Test

Directions: Each of the numbered items or incomplete statements in this section is followed by answers or by completions of the statement. Select the ONE lettered answer or completion that is best in each case.

1. A 26-year-old man is told that the reason he always fails college classes is because he believes that he will fail and then acts accordingly. He is instructed to tell himself daily that he is a highly competent individual who can master his studies with honest effort. From which of the following schools of psychotherapy are this explanation and treatment most closely derived?

(A) Behavioral psychotherapy
(B) Cognitive psychotherapy
(C) Humanistic psychotherapy
(D) Psychodynamic psychotherapy
(E) Somatic psychotherapy

2. A 28-year-old woman complains of being unable to fly on airplanes. She says that her fear of flying is irrational, but it keeps her from traveling conveniently. Which of the following psychotherapies would be the most appropriate initial treatment?

(A) Brief cognitive therapy
(B) Psychodynamic group therapy
(C) Rational emotive therapy
(D) Sensitivity training
(E) Systematic desensitization

3. A 32-year-old executive, adopted at 2 years of age after being abandoned by his biologic parents, seeks treatment for problems with maintaining close personal relationships. He says that whenever he feels a growing sense of dependence on another person, he terminates the relationship. He wonders if this may be associated with his early childhood experiences. Which of the following psychotherapies is the most appropriate initial treatment?

(A) Assertiveness training
(B) Encounter group therapy
(C) Initiation of lorazepam
(D) Psychoanalytic psychotherapy
(E) Systematic desensitization

4. A 37-year-old woman participating in group therapy expresses guilt for not meeting the sometimes unreasonable expectations of her husband, who is not in the group. The group leader points out that her hands are clenched into fists, and then instructs her to imagine that her husband is sitting in the empty chair across from her and to express her feelings to him. As she speaks, her apologies become expressions of anger at his overbearing demands. From which of the following psychotherapies is this technique most closely derived?

(A) Assertiveness training
(B) Cognitive therapy
(C) Gestalt therapy
(D) Systematic desensitization
(E) Tavistock group therapy

5. A 46-year-old woman says that she has difficulty staying in a crowded room and within minutes must flee the room. She associates this difficulty with a belief that those around her are reading her thoughts and forcing her to mutter obscenities. She also complains of visions of "holy men" that no one else can see. Which of the following therapies would be the most appropriate initial treatment?

(A) Assertiveness training
(B) Biofeedback training
(C) Initiation of haloperidol
(D) Psychoanalytic group psychotherapy
(E) Transpersonal psychology

Answers and Explanations

1–B. Cognitive theory suggests that behavior in a given situation is determined by the individual's perception of the circumstances. In this case, the individual perceives himself as an incompetent student. If he changes this perception, his behavior may also change.

2–E. The woman's symptoms suggest a specific phobia. The treatment of choice is systematic desensitization. During this treatment, the patient may first be trained in relaxation techniques. She would then be instructed to imagine situations that are increasingly anxiety provoking. With each situation, she would practice relaxation techniques until the scene no longer produced anxiety. For her case, the scenes may progress in the following sequence: being outside an airport terminal; being in a passenger lounge; boarding an airplane; staying in the airplane for the duration of a flight. In some cases, the patient is exposed to the anxiety-provoking situation.

3–D. The patient presents with long-term symptoms that suggest personality pathology that may be rooted in early childhood losses. Psychodynamic psychotherapy, including psychoanalytic psychotherapy, may be the most useful way to approach this problem. The patient demonstrates insight into his problem, a substantial level of motivation, and stability. These factors suggest he is a good candidate for psychoanalytic therapy.

4–C. Gestalt therapy emphasizes spontaneous and genuine expression in the "here-and-now" to develop insight into an individual's psyche. Attention is paid to emotion, physical activity, and thoughts in the immediate environment.

5–C. The woman's symptoms suggest psychosis. Delusions are most likely to respond to antipsychotic medications, such as haloperidol. Her interpersonal difficulties may be more amenable to psychotherapy after the psychotic symptoms are controlled.

31

Psychodynamic Theory and Techniques

I. **Overview.** Psychodynamics refers to three separate but related entities:

   A. **Metapsychology.** Psychodynamic theory is an explanation of human consciousness, both normal and pathologic.
   B. **Vocabulary.** Psychodynamic terminology is a common language used to describe behavior and personality.
   C. **Technique.** Psychodynamic psychotherapy is a set of techniques designed to improve psychological health.

II. **Psychodynamic Principles: Applications to General Clinical Practice**

   A. **General considerations**

      1. Psychodynamic theory, terminology, and techniques are particularly applicable to the description and management of stressed individuals, such as those with general medical conditions.
      2. Clinicians should know the following psychodynamic concepts:

         a. The nature of coping and defense mechanisms (see II B, C)
         b. The types of defense mechanisms (see II D)
         c. The distinction between useful and pathologic defense mechanisms (see II C 5)
         d. Indications for psychodynamic psychotherapy (see Chapter 30 III F)

   B. **Coping mechanisms** are **conscious attempts to cope with stress** and decrease anxiety. Clinicians may need to explain to patients which coping mechanisms are useful and which are destructive.

      1. Examples of **useful** coping mechanisms are learning about one's illness to manage it better or arranging one's finances before dying.
      2. Examples of **destructive** coping mechanisms are drinking alcohol to relieve stress or maintaining one's daily routine despite having an illness that requires hospitalization.

C. **Defense mechanisms** are an individual's **unconscious intrapsychic adjustments to the perception of internal or external reality** that decrease anxiety.

1. Defense mechanisms have **two major results**:

   a. They **decrease anxiety.**
   b. They **influence adaptation** to stressful situations.

2. Defense mechanisms are interrelated, may contain common elements, and may build on each other.

3. **Origin of defense mechanisms.** During psychosocial development, anxiety is caused by conflict between instinctual drives (located in the id) and learned strictures (located in the superego).

   a. To minimize the conflict and decrease anxiety, the developing ego learns to distort internal reality (instinctual drives and fantasies) or the perception of external reality.
   b. During psychosocial development, the specific defense mechanisms an individual learns become the basis of adult personality traits.
   c. In adulthood, defense mechanisms are activated when current situations reactivate childhood conflicts.
   d. Ego psychologists believe that some defense mechanisms may be unrelated to specific childhood conflicts and instead are part of innate adaptive capacity.

4. Defense mechanisms are classified according to **maturity level** (Table 31-1).

   a. **Immature defense mechanisms** are generally learned during early childhood. They involve significant distortion of the individual's perception of external reality and therefore are limited in helping an individual adapt to stressful situations.
   b. **More mature defense mechanisms** are learned in later childhood and adulthood. These defense mechanisms provide more adaptive potential, because they involve less distortion of perceptions of external reality.
   c. Under severe stress, an individual's mature defense mechanisms may be insufficient to manage his anxiety, and he may regress to using immature defense mechanisms.

5. Defense mechanisms are pathologic when:

   a. They do not sufficiently decrease anxiety. For example, a woman uses humor as a defense mechanism in a dangerous situation, but she becomes increasingly panicky and erratic.
   b. They decrease anxiety for a short term but actually increase it in the long term. For example, a man suppresses anxiety about being rejected for overeating, but he becomes increasingly worried about being ostracized for being obese.
   c. The distortion of external reality prevents the individual from adapting adequately. For example, a woman uses projection to attribute her own unacceptable thoughts to others, but then she has difficulty making friends.

Table 31–1. Common Defense Mechanisms by Increasing Level of Maturity

Less mature	Repression
	Fantasy
	Regression
	Splitting
	Denial
	Resistance
	Conversion
	Dissociation
	Isolation
	Projection
	Undoing
	Symbolization
	Displacement
	Distortion
	Reaction formation
	Introjection
	Suppression
	Compensation
	Idealization
	Identification
	Rationalization
	Intellectualization
	Sublimation
More mature	Humor

D. Common defense mechanisms

1. **Altruism** involves decreasing one's own internal fears or anxiety by caring for others. For example, a patient with a rare but serious illness devotes himself to a self-help group for others with the same illness.

2. **Compensation** is an effort to use skills or competencies in one area to counterbalance self-perceived deficiencies in other areas. For example, a patient with a gait disturbance becomes an expert on the history of dance.

3. **Conversion.** Emotional conflicts are transformed into physical symptoms. For example, a patient who is obviously angry about being subtly insulted denies that he has feelings other than concern about his sudden gastric distress.

4. **Denial** is a failure to acknowledge a disturbing aspect of external reality. For example, a patient with a grim medical prognosis states that he will get better because he "just knows it."

5. **Displacement** occurs when the emotions associated with a psychologically unacceptable object, idea, or activity are transferred to another object or situation. The new object or situation is often symbolically related to the original. For example, a patient who was badly injured in an accident becomes angry with his surgeon for leaving a small scar during reconstructive procedures.

6. **Dissociation** involves sealing off disturbing thoughts or emotions from consciousness. For example, a few hours after a patient is in a terrible accident, she says that she has no memory of the event.

7. **Distortion.** An individual distorts his perception of disturbing aspects of external reality to make it more palatable. For example, a patient who is permanently disabled because of his careless driving views himself as a victim of bad traffic laws.

8. **Fantasy** is the substitution of reality with a less disturbing view of the world. For example, a terminally ill patient states that she is sure she will survive because her long-deceased mother assured her in a dream.

9. **Humor** is the use of amusing thoughts to decrease anxiety. For example, a patient with a severe motor disability tells droll stories about his attempts to cope with airport facilities.

10. **Idealization** occurs when an individual unrealistically attributes only excellent characteristics to another person or situation. For example, an elderly man fondly but unrealistically describes the town where he grew up as the most wonderful place to have lived.

11. **Identification** involves identifying oneself with another person who is perceived as better or more powerful. For example, a hospitalized child decides that she wants to be a doctor and asks for a stethoscope of her own.

12. **Intellectualization** is the transformation of an emotionally disturbing event into a simple cognitive problem. For example, a patient who is also a physician is consumed with reading all available clinical research reports about his illness.

13. **Introjection.** An individual absorbs aspects of another person into her own self-image. For example, a victim of spousal abuse absorbs negative opinions about her worth and adamantly defends the right of her husband to batter her.

14. **Isolation** describes the separation of a thought from its attached emotional tone, thereby making it tolerable. It is often employed during extremely stressful events. For example, hours after a serious accident involving the death of a family member and injury to himself, a patient discusses in a mechanical way the various financial and legal steps that must be initiated.

15. **Projection** is the attribution of uncomfortable internal feelings or thoughts, especially anger and guilt, to other individuals. As a result, the individual transforms anger at himself into anger toward others. These people often seem bitter or suspicious. For example, a disabled patient who is applying for compensation accuses other patients of manipulating the "system."

16. **Rationalization** is a distortion of reality that makes an undesirable act or event seem more desirable. It is often employed when individuals cannot accept the implications or outcomes of an event. For example, a patient who lost his leg in a motorcycle accident states that the accident was "a blessing in disguise," because otherwise he would have ended up in a motorcycle gang.

17. **Reaction formation** occurs when an unacceptable thought or feeling is transformed into its opposite. Often, anger is transformed into love, or fear is transformed into bravado. For example, a parent whose child was killed by a drunk driver becomes involved with alcohol rehabilitation counseling.

18. **Regression** is characterized by an individual's return to more immature levels of functioning. It occurs when high anxiety levels are not alleviated by more mature defense mechanisms, such as intellectualization and humor. For example, patients presented with a poor medical prognosis often manifest regression through denial or fantasy.

19. **Repression.** Aspects of reality (e.g., memories, cognitions, impulses) are completely separated from conscious awareness. For example, a patient is

not consciously aware that he is terminally ill, although the situation is obvious.

20. **Resistance** is active opposition to bringing unconscious thoughts to consciousness. For example, a patient continually misses her psychiatrist appointments to discuss emotional problems associated with her medical illness.

21. **Splitting** occurs when an individual psychologically separates positive qualities into one individual or group and negative qualities into another. Splitting occurs because the individual is unable to tolerate ambivalent feelings toward a particular individual or group. For example, a patient in the care of both a neurologist and a neurosurgeon unrealistically considers the neurologist completely incompetent and considers the neurosurgeon caring and skilled.

22. **Sublimation** occurs when unacceptable impulses are channeled into more acceptable activities. For example, a patient with cardiovascular disease who must maintain a limited diet focuses on elaborate recipes.

23. **Suppression** involves forcing anxiety-provoking thoughts or feelings into unconsciousness, often by substituting them with other thoughts or feelings. For example, a patient repeatedly misses his doctor's appointments by becoming involved with a work project immediately before he should leave for the doctor's office, claiming he "forgets about the time."

24. **Symbolization.** An individual substitutes one aspect of internal or external reality for another. For example, a woman's overconcern about her small breasts actually represents her insecurity about her sexuality.

25. **Undoing** involves performing an activity that symbolically reverses a previous behavior or thought. It is commonly present in individuals who feel either conscious or unconscious guilt. For example, a person recently diagnosed with a malignancy becomes excessively concerned with nutrition, exercise, and a healthy lifestyle.

E. **Managing defense mechanisms.** There are several responses that a physician may give to patients with recognizable defense mechanisms.

1. **Do nothing.** Many defense mechanisms, including immature ones, are healthy and effective in helping an individual cope with stressful circumstances.

2. **Recognize that the patient is under too much stress to function adaptively,** and take any possible action to decrease the stress.

3. Consider referring the patient for **psychiatric consultation,** which may determine the nature of the patient's untoward reaction to stress and may suggest therapeutic interventions.

III. Psychodynamic Psychotherapy (see Chapter 30)

A. **General considerations.** Psychodynamic psychotherapy is usually practiced by a therapist and one or more patients in an office setting and is characterized by discussion and explorations of a patient's thoughts, feelings, perceptions, and behavior. The **goal** is to improve a patient's functioning and sense of well-being by decreasing anxiety that is caused by unconscious emotional conflicts.

1. Psychodynamic psychotherapy can decrease anxiety by:

   a. **Changing a patient's coping and defense mechanisms** to more adaptive patterns (crisis or brief psychotherapy)

   b. **Resolving a patient's unconscious emotional conflicts** that arose in childhood, thereby eliminating both the anxiety and defense mechanisms they engendered (psychoanalytic psychotherapy or psychoanalysis)

2. **Mechanisms.** Psychodynamic psychotherapy works through three mechanisms.

   a. It provides the patient with **insight.** If the patient understands his behavior in psychodynamic terms, he can change it.

   b. It provides an opportunity for **"working through"**—with newly gained insight, a patient explores his behavior in different situations.

   c. It provides a **corrective emotional experience.** In the therapeutic relationship, a patient may reexperience childhood emotions and conflicts, resolving them in a healthier manner.

3. Psychodynamic psychotherapy may also use **healing factors** common to other forms of psychotherapy. These healing factors include the provision of hope, the comfort of a confiding relationship, the creation of success experiences, and the provision of an explanation for emotions and behavior.

B. **Role of the psychotherapist.** A psychodynamic psychotherapist discovers a patient's defense mechanisms and unconscious conflicts and then gives the patient this insight and the opportunity to work through them.

1. The psychotherapist has several clues to learn about a patient's unconscious mental processes, including:

   a. What the patient chooses to talk about (e.g., recurrent themes, free associations, specific events)

   b. What a patient dreams about and how he presents these dreams

   c. How the patient relates to the therapist. Therapy is often emotionally charged, and the way a patient interacts with the therapist can reveal much about the patient's interactions with others.

   d. What is actually happening in the patient's life (e.g., problems, successes)

2. **Psychotherapeutic techniques.** A therapist provides a safe and accepting environment conducive to self-disclosure.

   a. By **listening** and **observing**, a psychotherapist comes to understand a patient in ways the patient may not understand himself.

   b. **Maintaining therapeutic distance.** A therapist does not disclose much information about herself or her feelings toward the patient. The rationale for this approach is that transference—the patient's attitudes and interactions with the therapist based on past experience with others—is more difficult for the therapist to interpret if it is colored by real issues in a personal relationship.

   c. **Avoiding countertransference.** A psychotherapist must carefully avoid confusing her own feelings and conflicts with those of her patients. She must also be particularly careful to avoid acting on her own feelings, such as anger or romantic attachment, toward the patient.

    d. Questions are used in psychotherapy to direct a patient's attention to important issues.

    e. Clarifying. The therapist may attempt to clarify a patient's statements to make issues clear to both the patient and therapist.

    f. Confronting. The therapist may confront the patient with evidence of behavior or thoughts that the patient has been avoiding or denying.

    g. Interpreting. The therapist's interpretations of the patient's thoughts and behavior—often discussed in terms of unconscious conflicts and defense mechanisms—are important for providing the patient with insight.

C. Uses of psychodynamic psychotherapy

1. Psychodynamic psychotherapy can help an individual cope more effectively with a life stressor.
2. It can provide an individual with greater understanding and knowledge of potential sources of satisfaction.
3. It can ameliorate personality disorders by improving an individual's understanding and control of his interpersonal relationships.

D. Limits of psychodynamic psychotherapy

1. Psychodynamic psychotherapy cannot cure psychiatric disorders that involve biologic thought disturbances, although it can ameliorate some of the associated emotional consequences.
2. It cannot force an individual to change; the individual must already be dissatisfied with his current emotional state.

Review Test

Directions: Each of the numbered items or incomplete statements in this section is followed by answers or by completions of the statement. Select the ONE lettered answer or completion that is BEST in each case.

1. A 27-year-old man sustains severe facial disfigurement during an industrial accident in which he was burned with acid. Since his recovery, he has avoided meeting people and drinks heavily every night. Which of the following words of advice are best for his development of a better coping mechanism?

(A) Donate time to helping pediatric burn victims
(B) Join Alcoholics Anonymous
(C) Join a self-help group for individuals who have difficulty addressing audiences
(D) Read literature about the dangers of alcoholism
(E) Rehearse a statement to say to new acquaintances that will put them at ease about the facial scars

2. A 35-year-old man is discussing memories of his uncle with his psychotherapist and presses the therapist for details of the therapist's relationships with his own family. When the therapist is not forthcoming, the patient becomes angry and states, "This is unfair. Why can't you ever tell me anything about yourself? I think you are hiding something, and I'm tired of this." Which of the following responses by the therapist is likely to be the most useful to this patient?

(A) Angry outbursts are not something that we can tolerate in psychotherapy. Take a few deep breaths and get a grip on your emotions. Now, what were you saying about your uncle?
(B) I can't tell you anything about myself. We are here to discuss your life, not mine. Let's get back to your memories of your uncle. Have you had any more thoughts about this person?
(C) I sense that you are angry. I must explain that your thoughts and feelings about me are much more important than any details of my own life. What do you think I might be hiding from you?
(D) You believe that you are angry with me about hiding my life from you. You are really angry at your uncle. Let's look at that more closely.
(E) You seem angry. I wonder why.

3. A 36-year-old woman who is hospitalized in a psychiatric unit following a suicide gesture complains unrealistically that nurses from the night shift are lazy, inconsiderate, and abusive toward her. She says that she feels very comfortable with the excellent nursing care she receives during the day, but she will sign out of the hospital against medical advice unless she is guaranteed that the nursing supervisor for the night shift receives disciplinary action. Which of the following defense mechanisms is most likely responsible for this patient's statements?

(A) Dissociation
(B) Distortion
(C) Projection
(D) Rationalization
(E) Splitting

4. A 44-year-old physician says that he feels guilty and ambivalent about arranging vacation plans that will take him from his practice for any extended period. As a result, he puts off making hotel or airline reservations until it is too late to get discounted rates, which angers his spouse. His therapist suggests that he regularly read travel novels and brochures about exotic vacation destinations to whet his appetite to travel. Which of the following defense mechanisms is suggested by the therapist's advice?

(A) Intellectualization
(B) Reaction formation
(C) Rationalization
(D) Sublimation
(E) Suppression

5. A 45-year-old woman feels guilty and ashamed of her anger toward her adolescent children. She does not discuss her anger with anyone, because she thinks it will shock and repel others. Her own parents had always demanded that she suppress expressions of anger. During an emotional psychotherapy session, she describes her anger to her therapist. The therapist is sympathetic and points out that her anger is reasonable and is not unusual. After the session, the woman feels greater self-acceptance. Which of the following terms best describes the source of the patient's improved sense of well-being?

(A) Corrective emotional experience
(B) Insight
(C) Reaction formation
(D) Sublimation
(E) Transference

6. During the last few sessions of a course of psychoanalytic psychotherapy that lasted several years, a 58-year-old man reminisces about a pet dog that was put to sleep after years of faithful companionship. The therapist states, "Perhaps your sadness about giving up your dog is similar to the sadness that you feel about having to give up therapy." Which of the following techniques best describes the therapist's statement?

(A) Clarification
(B) Confrontation
(C) Countertransference
(D) Interpretation
(E) Therapeutic distance

7. A 64-year-old woman recently forgot her adult daughter's birthday until the day before the event. She hastily bought a blouse as a present. During a psychotherapy session, the woman expresses great remorse that she did not choose the best color blouse for her daughter. Her psychotherapist interprets this as displaced remorse about forgetting the daughter's birthday. The patient replies, "That is ridiculous. Let's drop the whole subject." Which of the following most likely accounts for the patient's statement?

(A) Reaction formation
(B) Regression
(C) Resistance
(D) Transference
(E) Working through

Answers and Explanations

1–E. Rehearsing a statement that will make social interactions easier is a conscious attempt at managing anxiety. Donating time to children suggests the defense mechanism of altruism. Joining Alcoholics Anonymous or reading about alcoholism may be good medical advice. Joining a self-help group for individuals who have difficulty addressing audiences suggests the defense mechanism of reaction formation.

2–C. To be most effective, the psychodynamic therapist must avoid influencing transference with excessive self-disclosure. This patient is owed some acknowledgment of his anger and a clear explanation for the therapist's technique. The patient's belief that the therapist is hiding something is probably a manifestation of transference and should be explored through further questioning. Suggesting that some statements or emotions are off-limits in psychotherapy usually compromises its effectiveness. Prematurely interpreting the patient's anger before the patient has explored it is also less likely to be effective.

3–E. The patient has unrealistically identified one group of the nursing staff as excellent and another as unacceptable, avoiding experiencing conflicting feelings about the entire group. Splitting is common in individuals with borderline personality disorder and may lead to serious conflicts within treatment teams.

4–B. The therapist is suggesting that the patient replace his aversion to traveling with the opposite emotion. An example of intellectualization would be the patient analyzing the pros and cons of interrupting a medical practice. An example of rationalization would be the patient contemplating the idea that he can provide better care to his patients if he is relaxed and well rested. An example of sublimation would be the therapist suggesting that the patient take frequent day trips. An example of suppression would be exactly what the patient complains that he does—i.e., finding other tasks to concentrate on until it is too late to make travel reservations.

5–A. The patient suffered because she could not express her anger. The therapist's acceptance of the anger helped correct the patient's difficulties with her own emotions. An example of insight would be the patient developing an understanding that her problems with expressing emotion originated from parental restraints. An example of reaction formation would be the patient giving gifts to her children. An example of sublimation would be the patient criticizing a minor aspect of her children's performance at school. An example of transference would be the patient's belief that the therapist secretly disapproves of her angry outburst.

6–D. By interpreting the patient's fond memories about his dog as sadness about the present situation, the therapist is attempting to give the patient insight into his feelings about giving up relationships. An example of clarification would be the therapist saying, "So you have never fully accepted the loss of your dog." An example of confrontation would be the therapist saying, "You are sad about losing your relationship with me." An example of countertransference would be the therapist saying, "It is irritating to be compared to a dog."

7–C. The therapist's interpretation is plausible. The patient's active refusal to acknowledge it is most likely a manifestation of resistance, an active refusal to deal with unconscious conflict.

Part Five

Special Issues

32

Psychiatric Emergencies

I. Overview

A. **Psychiatric emergencies** are a significant part of medical practice. They may involve imminently life-threatening behavior and often raise medicolegal issues (e.g., involuntary treatment, liability, clinician duties to warn and protect others).

B. **Examples.** Psychiatric emergencies include patients with acute psychosis, violent or suicidal behavior, emotional trauma and acute anxiety, psychological and physical abuse, problems with psychoactive drugs (e.g., intoxication, dependence), and patients who refuse lifesaving treatment.

II. The Psychotic Patient

A. **General considerations**

1. Psychosis becomes a psychiatric emergency when it causes severe agitation or disorganized behavior, violence, self-destructive acts, or renders the patient unable to care for himself.

2. Psychosis also implies the presence of a severe psychiatric disorder, which is often assessed or treated on an emergency basis to prevent further exacerbation.

3. The **principles of emergency treatment** of psychosis are to stabilize behavior, perform comprehensive diagnostic assessment, and institute specific interventions based on etiology.

B. **Emergency assessment**

1. **Guidelines.** The clinician should:

a. Consider the patient's ability to care for himself or to accept treatment voluntarily

b. Assess the patient's potential for violence or suicide

c. Consider the patient's need for involuntary detention, restraint, or medication

2. **Determine psychopathology.** It is often critically important to diagnose rapidly the cause of psychosis to determine further assessment and treatment.

a. Quality of the psychosis. The particular features of psychosis in any given patient may suggest certain disorders, but it is easy to misdiagnose—many psychotic disorders have atypical presentations.

(1) **Hallucinations** or **delusions** with strong mood components (e.g., self-condemnation, grandiosity) suggest a mood disorder.

(2) **Bizarre delusions** and **auditory hallucinations** suggest schizophrenia.

(3) **Visual hallucinations** suggest delirium.

(4) **Prominent delusions** and an absence of other disturbances suggest delusional disorder.

b. Other associated diagnostic mental status findings in a psychotic patient include:

(1) Impaired sensorium, cognition, or memory, which suggests delirium or dementia

(2) Prominent mood symptomatology (e.g., depression or mania), which suggests mood disorders

c. Relevant history includes the onset, duration, and clinical course of symptoms.

(1) A history of physical symptomatology suggests psychosis due to a general medical condition.

(2) A history of drug abuse suggests substance-induced psychotic disorder.

(3) A history of a psychiatric disorder suggests an exacerbation of a chronic psychotic disorder.

(4) A recent, severe environmental stressor suggests brief psychotic disorder with marked stressors.

(5) The **premorbid adjustment** of the patient may distinguish between a brief psychotic disorder and exacerbation of a chronic psychotic disorder.

(6) **Medication.** If the patient takes medication, it may suggest a substance-induced psychotic disorder. Also, use of psychiatric medication may suggest that the individual is receiving ongoing treatment for a chronic psychotic disorder.

d. Physical examination. Specific signs suggest that the mental disorder may be due to a general medical condition or substance.

(1) **Focal neurologic deficits** suggest central nervous system (CNS) pathology.

(2) **Peripheral neuropathies** suggest metabolic or nutritional disorders.

(3) Signs of hyper- or hypothyroidism or Cushing syndrome suggest endocrinopathies or use of exogenous thyroid hormone or steroids.

(4) **Evidence of trauma** suggests psychosis due to CNS dysfunction or metabolic disturbance.

(5) **Evidence of substance use** (e.g., needle marks) suggests substance-induced psychotic disorder or the possibility of a general medical condition associated with substance abuse.

e. **Laboratory studies** should include routine tests and toxicology screens for substances of abuse, psychotherapeutic drugs, and toxins. Imaging studies and electroencephalogram may be indicated when there is evidence of neurologic dysfunction or cognitive impairment.

3. **Mental disorders in which psychosis occurs** (Table 32-1)

C. **Emergency management**

1. **Control anxiety.** Psychotic symptoms are anxiety provoking, and this anxiety should be treated.

a. Simple and repeated **reassurance** is essential.

b. **Antipsychotic medication** is often useful for decreasing anxiety. However, these agents often do not immediately alleviate hallucinations, delusions, or illogical thinking.

c. **Benzodiazepines**, alone or combined with high-potency antipsychotic medication, are also useful for this indication.

Table 32-1. Mental Disorders in Which Psychosis Occurs

Mental Disorders	Comments
Psychotic disorders	
Brief psychotic disorder	Most often seen by physicians in the context of medical trauma; may involve severe agitation and paranoia; usually lasts 1 or 2 days
Delusional disorder	Patients often present emergently because of severe agitation or threats that stem from plausible delusions
Schizoaffective disorder	Patients may present primarily with psychosis or with psychosis during a mood episode
Schizophrenia	Psychosis occurs during active phase of the illness, characterized by specific types of bizarre delusions, prominent hallucinations, marked loosening of associations, catatonic behavior or grossly inappropriate affect
Schizophreniform disorder	Presentation is similar to that of schizophrenia, but the course lasts less than 6 months
Shared psychotic disorder	Psychotic symptoms develop in the context of a close relationship with another person(s) who already has established delusions
Psychotic disorders due to a general medical condition	Seen particularly in endocrinopathies
Cognitive disorders	Psychosis may be part of delirium or dementia
Mood disorders	Psychosis may be present in bipolar and major depressive disorders; may be mood congruent or incongruent
Autistic disorder	Symptoms may be suggestive of psychosis

2. **Treat severe agitation.** Agitation and occasional violence can occur in the presence of psychosis.

   a. **Physical restraint** should be used if a psychotic patient becomes severely agitated or violent and cannot be calmed with less restrictive measures.

   b. **High-potency antipsychotic medication** (e.g., haloperidol) is effective in rapidly controlling agitation, although the antipsychotic effect may occur hours or days later.

      (1) Five milligrams of haloperidol or fluphenazine should be administered intramuscularly.

         (a) The dose can be repeated hourly until agitation is controlled and physical restraint is no longer necessary.

         (b) Two or three doses usually suffice.

      (2) The patient should be monitored for extrapyramidal syndromes and hypotension.

   c. **Low-potency, sedating antipsychotics** are less efficacious for this indication.

      (1) Frequently repeated doses of low-potency antipsychotic medications (e.g., chlorpromazine) are more likely to cause hypotension and anticholinergic effects.

      (2) Severe sedation may complicate diagnosis, particularly when delirium or dementia is present.

3. **Ensure a safe environment.** Psychotic patients have a higher risk for self-injury.

   a. **Close observation** in a controlled environment is essential and often helps alleviate the patient's anxiety.

   b. **Involuntary detention** may be necessary if an acutely psychotic individual wants to leave the treatment facility.

4. **Treat any underlying psychiatric disorder or general medical condition.**

   a. Psychosis is often caused by an underlying **physiologic disturbance** that requires acute treatment.

   b. **Mood disorders** presenting with psychosis may require preliminary physical and laboratory assessments (e.g., plasma electrolytes, complete blood count, electrocardiogram) before initiating medication (e.g., lithium or antidepressants).

   c. Psychosis due to **severe emotional stress** (e.g., brief psychotic disorder with marked stressors) [see V A] may require specific psychological and social interventions, such as crisis psychotherapy or placement in a sheltered setting.

5. If the patient is not admitted to a psychiatric unit, the clinician must ensure that the patient can manage in another setting (e.g., home, medical unit).

D. Medicolegal implications

1. Acute, **involuntary detention** and **treatment** are often indicated for individuals with acute psychosis and are usually legal pending psychiatric consultation.

2. Involuntarily administering antipsychotic medication is usually permissible if the purpose is to prevent imminent harm to the patient or others.

III. The Combative Patient

A. General considerations

1. Few clinical situations are as unpleasant or dangerous as treating a combative patient.
2. Managing combative behavior involves clear limit-setting, physical restraint, appropriate use of antipsychotic medication, diagnosis of underlying psychopathology, and careful disposition.

B. Emergency assessment

1. The clinician should assess the patient's potential for harming himself or others, noting the patient's level of agitation, his physical strength, and the presence of weapons.
2. A past history of violence is the most valuable clue for predicting future violent behavior, so patients with a known history of violence should be cautiously managed in any setting.
3. **Determine the reason for combativeness.** The clinician should determine if the patient has general anger or anger toward a specific person, or if the patient is attempting to frighten or manipulate.
4. It is critically important to determine whether the patient has a particular victim in mind or a specific violent plan (see Chapter 33 VII D).
5. **Determine stressors.** If a patient's combative behavior is in response to a discrete stressor (e.g., the physical presence of particular individuals or some erroneous perception of the environment), the patient may be calmed by removal of the stressor.
6. **Determine psychopathology**
   a. Many severe psychopathologies, including delirium and dementia, psychotic disorders, substance intoxications and withdrawals, mental retardation, and intermittent explosive disorder, predispose an individual to combative behavior.
   b. Antisocial and borderline personality traits also predispose an individual to violent behavior.
7. The clinician should **delay physical examination of combative patients until the behavior is controlled.** Physical diagnosis is particularly difficult if the examiner is trying to prevent personal injury.

C. Emergency management

1. **Guidelines**
   a. The clinician should **set clear limits** of tolerance for the patient's agitation, threats, and violent acts. For example, the clinician may say, "I cannot complete this examination unless you stop shouting." The clinician should not make threats. For example, the clinician should not say, "If you don't stop shouting, I will call security."
   b. **Verbal interventions are rarely effective** at controlling combative patients and often further enrage the patient.
   c. The safety of patients, medical personnel, and visitors should be protected by immediately warning others of violent patients and giving per-

sonnel a chance to remove potential weapons or delicate equipment from the room.

    (1) If physical restraint is necessary, an adequate number of appropriately trained personnel should be used.

    (2) Hospital personnel should search for concealed weapons and put the patient in a hospital gown.

    (3) The clinician should try to establish some rapport with a restrained combative patient by acknowledging the patient's anger or fear and by reassuring the patient that the intent is to help.

  2. Use of medication

    a. Antipsychotics are usually the medication of choice to control agitation in the medical emergency setting.

      (1) High-potency antipsychotics (e.g., haloperidol) are preferred.

      (2) Medication used for this purpose is usually administered intramuscularly.

    b. The use of **benzodiazepines** to control agitation is controversial, because these agents can cause additional disinhibition and violence. Benzodiazepines also can cloud the patient's consciousness, making diagnosis difficult.

    c. Treatment of chronically combative patients may involve the use of propranolol, carbamazepine and other anticonvulsants, and lithium. However, these medications play almost no role in emergency intervention.

  3. Inform others at disposition. An important part of managing a combative patient is warning those who will receive the patient at disposition. This may include ambulance personnel, staff at a receiving facility, or family members.

D. Medicolegal implications

  1. Treatment of combative patients often requires involuntary restraint, detention, and treatment with medication, all of which are usually legal in emergency medical situations.

  2. The clinician must **carefully document the situation,** including the exact nature of the combative behavior and the steps taken to control it.

  3. After the acutely dangerous behavior is controlled, involuntary treatment of the underlying psychopathology may be limited by mental health laws.

  4. Combative behavior often involves infractions of law; thus, law enforcement personnel are often involved in these cases.

  5. In many cases involving combative patients who make threats, the clinician has a duty to warn and protect potential victims, as outlined in the *Tarasoff* decision (see Chapter 33 VII D).

IV. The Suicidal Patient

A. General considerations. Suicidality is a transient emotion, and suicide is almost always preventable.

  1. Suicidal patients are those who have recently made a suicide attempt, complain of suicidal thoughts, admit to suicidal thoughts when questioned, or demonstrate suicidal behavior.

2. Some suicidal behavior is overt, but some attempts are covert. Patients presenting with drug overdose, single-car auto accidents, and "accidental" self-inflicted trauma should be routinely evaluated for suicidality.
3. It is often difficult to distinguish between suicidal ideation or behavior intended to communicate the individual's unhappiness and suicide attempts meant to end life, because both motivations are often present.
4. **United States statistics**
   a. One million people attempt suicide yearly.
   b. Twenty-five thousand to fifty thousand people commit suicide yearly.
   c. The overall suicide rate is about 15 in 100,000.
   d. The suicide rate in individuals who have previously presented to a psychiatric emergency room is 150 in 100,000.
5. In minors and adolescents, suicidal thoughts are common and actual suicides are uncommon but increasing in frequency. Clustering (i.e., a rash of suicide attempts within a peer group) is an occasional phenomenon.

B. **Emergency assessment**
   1. **Guidelines**. Any potentially suicidal patient should be detained until emergency assessment is completed.
      a. Clinicians should take all suicide threats seriously.
      b. **Gathering information.** The clinician should establish rapport with the patient and gradually approach the question of suicidality.
         (1) A patient with a serious psychiatric disorder should be questioned about suicide, because these patients are more likely to attempt suicide.
         (2) Patients presenting with a drug overdose should be questioned about suicide, because some overdoses are deliberate suicide attempts.
         (3) The clinician should ask the patient about demoralization (i.e., lack of hope), because this can lead to suicide.
         (4) The clinician should attempt to gather information from third parties, such as family, friends, and field personnel.
      c. The clinician should not identify with the patient. It is rarely therapeutic for a stranger to agree that suicide is a good option.
      d. Suicide prevention measures should be based on the patient's clinical picture.
   2. **Assess lethality**. The physician must assess the potential lethality of the patient's suicidal ideation or behavior and the availability of environmental means to prevent suicide. The clinician should:
      a. Determine the presence and practicality of a patient's suicidal thoughts and plans
      b. Obtain a history of past suicidality
      c. Elicit the patient's view of the future
      d. Be suspicious of a sudden lifting of depression in an individual with a hopeless view of the future, because it may indicate a decision to commit suicide
      e. Search for key mental status findings— depression, demoralization, psychosis, or cognitive impairment

f. Assess the patient's underlying psychopathology, environmental support system, and risk factors for suicide (see IV B 4)

3. **Assess any underlying psychopathology.** Patients with mood disorders, psychotic disorders, and borderline personality disorder often present with suicidal thoughts or plans, and they may need specific therapeutic intervention.

4. **Risk factors** do not accurately predict suicide in a given individual. However, the following factors are useful in assessing the risk.

   a. **History of suicide threats and attempts** is the single most important risk factor for future suicide attempts and completed suicide.

   b. **Perceived hopelessness** (i.e., demoralization) is a major risk factor.

   c. **Presence of psychiatric illness**, particularly mood disorders, substance abuse, and schizophrenia. The rate of suicide in psychiatric patients is at least ten times that of the general population.

   d. **Gender.** Twice as many females attempt suicide, whereas twice as many males complete it.

   e. **Age.** The highest rate of suicide attempts is in young adults; the rate of completed suicide increases with age.

   f. **Social isolation.** Isolated individuals have a higher rate of both attempts and completed suicides.

   g. **Low job satisfaction.** Underemployed individuals have higher suicide rates.

   h. **Chronic illness.** Individuals who are chronically ill have higher suicide rates.

5. **Factors that decrease the probability of future suicide attempts**

   a. The patient took steps to ensure rescue.

   b. The patient is now happy to be alive and is remorseful about the suicide attempt.

   c. The patient has no future suicide plans.

   d. The patient's family shows concern about the patient's welfare.

C. **Emergency management.** Suicidal patients may be passive-aggressive and manipulative. Clinicians must avoid making treatment decisions based on anger or dislike.

1. **Hospitalization.** If the risk of further suicidal behavior is uncertain or high, the patient should be hospitalized involuntarily.

   a. If the patient's physical safety is assured by family or friends who are willing and capable of monitoring the patient, emergency psychiatric hospitalization, which can be costly and stigmatizing, should be avoided. Outpatient crisis intervention can be initiated.

   b. After a suicidal patient is detained or hospitalized, the hospital staff must take precautions to prevent suicide attempts or elopement. Patients should be searched for dangerous objects and should not be left alone.

2. **Crisis psychotherapy** for suicidal behavior usually addresses common issues, including feelings of hopelessness, low self-esteem, and anger.

3. **Treatment of underlying psychopathology**

a. **Psychoactive medications** (e.g., antidepressants) are often effective in treating underlying depressive psychopathology in suicidal patients. However, patients may also use them in suicide attempts.

b. **Electroconvulsive therapy** is sometimes the treatment of choice for severely depressed patients who are actively suicidal.

c. **Longer-term psychotherapy** for chronically suicidal patients is often challenging. It may involve cognitive techniques (e.g., changing the patient's perception of his situation) and exploring the patient's ambivalent feelings and covert anger.

D. Medicolegal implications

1. The common use of involuntary detention during treatment of a suicidal patient raises civil commitment issues.

2. Patients who commit suicide are a source of significant professional liability if they did not receive a complete and well-documented assessment, or if failure to hospitalize or treat was not based on clinical indications.

3. If a patient's medical record indicates a high risk for suicide, it must explain (by every treating clinician with responsibility) why the patient was not hospitalized. The decision not to hospitalize cannot be based on health care rationing, such as lack of hospital space.

4. If a patient commits suicide while hospitalized in either a general or psychiatric institution, liability issues are raised.

V. Emotional Trauma

A. General considerations.
Highly stressful events, including natural disasters, accidents, and violence, are often emotionally traumatizing to victims and observers.

1. Medical emergencies are especially likely to produce emotional trauma.

2. Emotional trauma can cause psychopathology, including acute stress disorder, posttraumatic stress disorder, adjustment disorders, brief psychotic disorder, and exacerbation of schizophrenia.

3. **Principles of treatment** include recognition of emotional trauma, support and reassurance, and protection from further trauma.

B. Emergency assessment

1. **Determine the presence of emotional trauma.** Medical and social history may suggest emotional trauma, and anxiety and dissociative symptoms may be prominent.

2. **Determine the cause of trauma.** Some sources of emotional trauma may be obvious from history or physical examination (e.g., a close brush with death during a disaster, a physical wound), but others may be more covert (e.g., guilt about having caused a traffic accident in which a bystander was killed).

3. Any associated psychopathology (e.g., acute stress disorder) should be diagnosed.

C. Emergency management

1. **Provide reassurance and supportive psychotherapy.** Giving patients the opportunity to talk about a traumatic situation is often dramatically effective in ameliorating distress.

   2. **Protect the patient from further trauma.** If the source of emotional trauma is known (e.g., spousal abuse), clinicians have an ethical and sometimes legal responsibility to intervene if possible.

   D. **Medicolegal implications.** If a patient's emotional trauma is caused by physical or sexual abuse, society increasingly assigns health care personnel a legal obligation to report the abuse and intervene (see VI).

VI. Psychological, Sexual, and Physical Abuse

   A. **General considerations.** Abuse often causes medical and psychological complications, and is therefore a factor in medical emergencies.

   1. Children, the elderly, and disabled individuals are at significantly greater risk for abuse.
   2. Individuals with cognitive impairment (e.g., mental retardation, dementia) or dependent personality disorder are at greater risk for abuse.

   B. **Emergency assessment.** Abuse may be obvious from history or physical examination (e.g., complaint of rape), or it may be covert (e.g., a child with long-bone fractures from physical abuse whose parents say he received them from falling out of bed).

   1. Abused patients often try to hide the abuse or protect the abuser from consequences.
   2. Because psychologically healthy individuals are often targets of abuse, attributing the trauma to the victim's psychiatric problems may trivialize the magnitude of the event or shift blame from the abuser.
   3. Underlying psychopathology in an abused patient never justifies the abuse. "Blaming the victim" must be carefully avoided.
   4. Emotional trauma caused by abuse can cause psychopathology (see V A 2). Physical trauma caused by abuse can also cause psychopathology, including delirium and dementia.

   C. **Emergency management.** The clinician should:

   1. Protect the patient from further abuse
   2. Provide reassurance and supportive therapy
   3. Treat resultant psychopathology and underlying psychopathology, if present

   D. **Medicolegal implications.** Most states have mandatory reporting requirements for health care personnel.

VII. Substance-Related Psychiatric Emergencies

   A. **Overdose**

   1. **General considerations.** Overdose of prescribed medications or abused substances is often diagnosed in emergency settings.

   a. Deliberate overdose may represent a suicide attempt.
   b. Overdose may be an attempt to self-treat withdrawal from a variety of medications.
   c. Drug overdose often involves multiple substances.
   d. Overdose can cause substance-induced mental disorders, particularly delirium.

2. Emergency assessment

    a. For all patients presenting with delirium, the clinician should investigate the possibility of a drug overdose and consider the possibility that multiple drugs are involved.

    b. Clinicians should evaluate suicidality as well as the possibility of substance abuse or dependence.

3. Emergency management. Specific medical intervention depends on the offending substances. The clinician should:

    a. Manage suicidality (see IV C)

    b. Carefully manage resultant substance-induced mental disorders, particularly those that increase likelihood of severe agitation, anxiety, or disorganized behavior

    c. Address underlying substance abuse, if present, by making plans for detoxification and drug rehabilitation

B. Substance-induced mental disorders

    1. General considerations. Many substances, including drugs of abuse, medications, and environmental toxins, can alter mental status (Table 32-2).

        a. Substances can induce a wide range of psychopathology, including delirium, dementia, amnesia, psychosis, mood changes, anxiety, sleep problems, and personality change (see Chapter 12).

        b. Patients or their caregivers (e.g., parents, nursing home staff) may not associate substances with a change in mental status.

        c. Exposure to substances

            (1) Patients may be exposed to substances by deliberate use for recreational purposes, self-prescription for physical or psychological distress, orders of a physician, mistaken use due to confusion, or accidental ingestion or absorption from the environment.

Table 32-2. Common Causes of Substance-Induced Mental Disorders

Substance	Examples
Recreational drugs	Alcohol, amphetamines, cannabis, cocaine, hallucinogens, inhalants, nicotine, opioids, phencyclidine, benzodiazepines and other sedative-hypnotics
Over-the-counter medication	Analgesics; antiasthmatics, including epinephrine; antipruritics including antihistamines and steroids; cold preparations, including antihistamines, pseudoephedrine, and dextromethorphan; "energy pills" (caffeine); hypnotics, including antihistamines; weight reduction medication, including caffeine and pseudoephedrine
Home remedies	Household chemicals, herb extracts
Prescribed medication	Opioid analgesics and antitussives, antihypertensive medication, antitubercular medication, steroid preparations, amphetamines, benzodiazepines, antiparkinsonian medication, antidepressant medication, anticonvulsant medication, antipsychotic medication
Environmental toxins	Food additives (e.g. caffeine) and contaminated food, industrial chemicals, waste storage by-products

(2) It is common for patients to be exposed to a number of substances simultaneously, either by design or if one or more substances (e.g., adulterated recreational drugs) are unknowingly present.

d. Identifying a substance as an etiology of a mental disorder affects both acute and long-term treatment.

(1) Substances should be a suspected etiology in any acute alteration in mental status, even when there is no obvious history of substance ingestion.

(2) Laboratory testing for certain substances should be routinely performed in any sudden onset of delirium, dementia, or other cognitive disorder; psychosis; or mood episode.

2. Emergency assessment

a. The clinician should **obtain a complete history of possible recent substance exposure** in any patient presenting with a changed mental status, specifically asking about:

(1) Recreational drug use, including nature of use [e.g., continuous, episodic (binge)], type and amount of substance used, form of substance (e.g., vegetable matter, extract, solution), route of administration (e.g., oral, intranasal, intravenous), duration of use, most recent use, and previous adverse reactions

(2) Self-prescribed medications, including brand names and sources, reasons for use, amounts used, duration of use, most recent use, and previous adverse reactions

(3) Prescribed medications, including types, name and contact number of prescribing physician, reasons for use, amounts used, duration of use, most recent use, and previous adverse reactions

(4) Environmental exposure, including unusual foods or substances recently ingested; recent visits to industrial chemical process, waste storage, or contamination sites; recent exposure to pesticides; and recent exposure to volatile substances, such as paints or solvents

b. The clinician should also obtain a substance abuse history.

c. Depending on the circumstances, the clinician should perform some or all of the toxicologic examinations to detect presence and concentrations for alcohol, amphetamines, barbiturates, cannabis, cocaine, heavy metals, opioids, organophosphates, and phencyclidine.

3. Emergency management. Specific emergency supportive measures may depend on the offending substances and their concentration, the metabolic status of the patient, and the nature of the induced mental disorder. The clinician should:

a. Ensure the safety and comfort of patients who are agitated, disorganized, or psychotic

b. Provide patient education to prevent repeat exposure

c. Notify the prescribing physician if prescribed medication is the offending substance

d. Notify public health authorities if an environmentally acquired toxin is the offending substance

C. Substance abuse emergencies

1. **General considerations.** Substance abuse or dependence should be considered a possible etiology or contributing factor in almost all psychiatric emergencies. Substance use can lead to a variety of psychiatric emergencies, including:

    a. Acute onset of self-destructive behavior, combativeness, or agitation during intoxication, withdrawal, or a substance-induced mental disorder

    b. Acute depressive symptoms or suicidal ideation due to distress or guilt about substance abuse or its consequences (e.g., loss of money, employment, or relationships with significant others)

    c. Marital or **family disturbances**

2. **Emergency evaluation**

    a. The clinician should obtain a substance use history in almost all psychiatric emergency situations (see VII B 2 a).

    b. If substance abuse is present, further evaluation may be warranted after the patient is stabilized.

3. **Emergency management.** The clinician should:

    a. Provide substance-specific management for acute intoxication or withdrawal symptoms (see Chapter 12 IV)

    b. Initiate patient education about acute and long-term adverse psychological and physical consequences of substance abuse as soon as possible

    c. Initiate counseling of family members

    d. Initiate plans for **drug rehabilitation** as soon as possible

D. Acute toxicity caused by psychotherapeutic medication (see Chapters 26–29)

1. **General considerations.** Psychotherapeutic medications may cause acute adverse effects.

    a. These adverse effects include sedation, agitation, anticholinergic effects, motor problems, hypotension, and cognitive impairment.

    b. Recognition and management of these adverse effects are essential to prevent further physiologic compromise, relieve discomfort, and improve medication compliance.

    c. Diagnosis and treatment of patients who are taking psychotherapeutic medication are often complicated by the underlying psychopathology.

2. **Emergency assessment**

    a. Third-party information is particularly useful for emergency assessment, because the patient's psychopathology or medication toxicity may impair his ability to relate history.

    b. Patients taking psychiatric medication who have a sudden change in behavior should be suspected of having an acute toxic reaction.

    c. The clinician should **determine the reason for the toxic reaction:**

        (1) Was there a deliberate overdosage?

        (2) Are there possible drug interactions?

        (3) Are underlying general medical conditions present, and are they influencing the toxicity or treatment?

d. Determine the underlying psychopathology

   (1) It may be difficult to distinguish symptoms caused by medication toxicity from symptoms caused by the underlying psychopathology.

   (2) The decision to discontinue the offending medication, reinstate it at a different dosage, or substitute or add other medication is influenced by the patient's psychiatric diagnosis.

3. **Emergency management.** The clinician should:

   a. Immediately institute necessary medical supportive measures

   b. Quickly obtain, evaluate, and act on the results of toxicologic investigation

   c. Institute specific intervention based on the offending medication. For example, a clinician should give anticholinergic medication to a patient with a dystonic reaction caused by an antipsychotic medication.

   d. Manage suicidal behavior if deliberate overdose is involved (see IV C)

   e. Manage the behavioral manifestations of the underlying psychiatric disorder

   f. Prevent repeat episodes of toxicity by appropriately altering the psychiatric medication regimen and treating related general medical conditions

VIII. Refusal of Lifesaving Treatment

A. **General considerations.** The clinician's role in forcing patients to undergo emergency lifesaving treatment has profound ethical implications and is circumscribed by law.

B. **Reasons for refusal of treatment**

   1. A patient's refusal of treatment may be based on **religious, ethical, financial,** or **utilitarian beliefs.**

      a. The refusal may represent a wish to die or simply a wish to avoid a particular medical intervention.

      b. The patient's reason for treatment refusal may appear based on ignorance or poor judgement; however, this situation does not necessarily permit coercion from the clinician.

   2. A patient's refusal of treatment may be **based on psychopathology**.

      a. The patient may **fail to comprehend the situation** because of delirium or dementia.

      b. Individuals with a depressive episode (e.g., with major depressive disorder or bipolar disorders) or with personality pathology (e.g., borderline personality disorder) may have **suicidal intentions**.

      c. Individuals with a psychotic disorder may have **delusional beliefs** about treatment.

C. **Involuntary lifesaving treatment.** Emergency lifesaving treatment is generally provided involuntarily only in the following situations:

   1. **Conservatorship.** The patient's legal status is such that others are empowered to make medical decisions for him.

   2. The refusal of treatment is because of the patient's cognitive failure to comprehend the nature of the problem or the treatment.

3. The refusal of treatment represents a self-destructive wish that is a direct result of a mental disorder for which involuntary treatment has already been approved.

4. Treatment of the acute life-threatening condition also treats a mental disorder for which involuntary treatment has already been approved.

5. It is almost never legal to initiate involuntary lifesaving treatment to pre-empt the onset of a condition that will interfere with cognitive capacity. For example, in a cognizant patient who foolishly refuses antibiotics for systemic infection, a clinician cannot force treatment to forestall the onset of delirium.

D. Emergency assessment. The clinician should:

1. Determine precisely the patient's reason for treatment refusal

2. Obtain psychiatric assessment. This assessment is almost always indicated to determine the circumstances of treatment refusal and its relationship to possible psychopathology as well as the patient's cognitive capacity.

E. Emergency management

1. Sensitive discussion and education with the patient and significant others are often dramatically effective in convincing the patient to allow lifesaving medical interventions.

   a. When these interventions are refused, the clinician should exhaustively explore alternatives that are acceptable to the patient.

   b. If a patient continues to refuse treatment, the clinician should continue to make the patient comfortable. The clinician should not let her own frustration or anger with the patient become the basis for management decisions.

2. The actual evaluation and documentation necessary to initiate involuntary treatment vary by locality.

3. Determining an individual's competency to refuse treatment for nonemergent conditions is made by judicial authority and may be based on psychiatric assessment of cognitive capacity.

Review Test

Directions: Each of the numbered items or incomplete statements in this section is followed by answers or by completions of the statement. Select the ONE lettered answer or completion that is BEST in each case.

1. A 26-year-old man is brought into the emergency room for the fourth time in 1 week for making superficial lacerations on his wrists. His other three presentations were similar; each time, he was discharged with a referral to an outpatient mental health clinic. He states that he will jump off an ocean pier if he is not admitted to the hospital. Which of the following is the most appropriate intervention?

(A) Admit the patient to a medical ward pending routine psychiatric consultation
(B) Inform the patient that his superficial wrist cuts are unlikely to result in death, and explain to him that his actions are a "cry for help"
(C) Order emergency psychiatric assessment
(D) Order hospital security to escort the patient off hospital grounds
(E) Refer the patient again to the mental health clinic

2. A 26-year-old woman is brought to the emergency room for a leg fracture she sustained when she ran into traffic. She is highly agitated, has disorganized speech, and shouts that demons are pursuing her. She refuses any treatment. Attempts to verbally reassure and calm her are unsuccessful. Which of the following is the most appropriate next step in management?

(A) Administer a benzodiazepine involuntarily
(B) Administer an analgesic medication involuntarily
(C) Administer a high-potency antipsychotic medication involuntarily
(D) Allow the patient to leave the emergency room
(E) Restrain the patient and set her leg fracture

3. A 29-year-old woman comes into the emergency room with severe facial bruises. Only on direct questioning does she admit that the bruises were inflicted by her husband. She says that they had an argument and both of them "got physical." She begs the clinician not to inform police, saying that both partners were "in the wrong." Which of the following is the most appropriate intervention?

(A) Inform the patient that you are obligated to file a report of spousal abuse with the proper authority, and offer her information about assistance for battered spouses
(B) Inform the patient that you are obligated to file a report of spousal abuse with the proper authority, and involuntarily detain her for her own safety
(C) Insist that the patient remain in the emergency room until her husband is arrested
(D) Insist that the patient remain in the emergency room until her spouse returns for conjoint counseling, but do not inform civil authorities
(E) Reassure the patient that confidentiality will be maintained, but educate her about the dangers of spousal battery

4. A 39-year-old man threatens an emergency room clinician with bodily harm if he is not immediately given an analgesic medication. Which of the following is the most appropriate initial response?

(A) The clinician should ask another clinician to join him while completing the patient assessment
(B) The clinician should immediately order an analgesic medication for the patient
(C) The clinician should say, "Sir, if you threaten me again, I will summon security"
(D) The clinician should tell the patient that an analgesic will be ordered only if it is indicated after a complete physical examination
(E) The clinician should leave, telling the patient that he will return in a moment, and then immediately summon hospital security

5. An 89-year-old man who lives in a nursing home is brought to the emergency room because of fever and lethargy. He refuses physical examination and says, "Get away from me or I'll sue." Which of the following is the most appropriate initial intervention?

(A) Allow the patient to return to the nursing home
(B) Ask the patient why he is refusing treatment
(C) Attempt to cajole the patient into accepting assessment
(D) Obtain a second concurring opinion regarding the need for emergency medical care, and involuntarily treat
(E) Order a psychiatric consultation

Answers and Explanations

1–C. This patient has a behavioral disturbance, has made repeated suicide gestures, and continues to voice suicidal plans. Although he may not be at high risk for suicide, he is at risk for harming himself and should be detained for psychiatric assessment. Admitting him to a general medical ward does not ensure adequate monitoring of his behavior. Referrals to outpatient treatment and crisis counseling have not been effective for this patient. Escorting the patient off hospital grounds is unlikely to guarantee that he will not return, and it may compromise his safety.

2–C. The patient's symptoms suggest psychosis. Her agitation should be treated immediately with a high-potency antipsychotic medication to ensure her safety and decrease her psychosis. In an emergency situation, it is permissible to involuntarily administer antipsychotic medication for this purpose. A benzodiazepine may cause disinhibition or oversedation. Analgesic medication should be used after her behavior is stabilized. The clinician is obligated to ensure the patient's safety; allowing her to leave the emergency room in her current condition exposes the patient to unacceptable risk. The leg fracture should be set when the patient has been calmed.

3–A. In most states, the clinician has a mandatory responsibility to report spousal abuse. The abused spouse should be offered counseling and assistance. However, there are no grounds for involuntary detention in this case. This woman is at high risk for further battering, especially because she believes that she is partially to blame.

4–E. This patient is threatening and potentially combative. His verbal threat is not acceptable behavior in a medical setting; personal safety and the safety of others are the primary initial considerations, and further assessment should not occur until safety is assured by the presence of appropriate personnel.

5–B. In cases of treatment refusal, the most important initial intervention is to determine the precise reason for treatment refusal. Often, other treatment alternatives will become apparent. This patient may wish to die, be afraid of pain, not comprehend the situation, or mistrust others. After the reason for treatment refusal is known, it may be useful to obtain psychiatric assessment of the patient's capacity to refuse treatment.

33
Law and Ethics in Psychiatry

I. Overview

A. **Forensic issues.** Psychiatric practice and theory involve a number of important forensic issues, including patient rights, confidentiality, competency, involuntary treatment, guardianship, and professional duties to patients and society. Legislation and jurisprudence in these areas are evolving and vary from one jurisdiction to another.

B. **Practicing psychiatry**

1. To practice legal and ethical psychiatry, an individual must possess a fairly comprehensive knowledge of the law as it applies to medicine and psychiatry, a knowledge of professional ethics, and common sense.

2. **Minimizing litigation.** To minimize the risk of litigation because of liability or criminal responsibility for untoward results of psychiatric treatment, a clinician should conform with good medical practice and the law, carefully document facts and decision-making processes in the patient's medical record, seek timely consultation with colleagues about difficult cases, and communicate effectively with patients.

II. Patient Rights. Certain patient rights pertain to psychiatric treatment.

A. **The right to treatment.** Involuntarily hospitalized psychiatric patients have a right to a minimum standard of care directed at curing or improving their mental disorder.

B. **The right to refuse treatment.** Except in limited circumstances (see VI), patients have the absolute right to refuse treatment.

C. **The right to the least restrictive alternative.** Psychiatric patients have the right to an effective treatment intervention that is least restrictive of the individual's behavior or requires the least amount of physical confinement.

D. **Personal rights.** Psychiatric patients who are hospitalized are entitled to acceptable standards for decent surroundings, privacy, confidentiality, freedom to wear personal clothing and communicate with others, and visitation.

E. **Rights of minors.** Certain rights, particularly those pertaining to confidentiality and treatment refusal, of psychiatric patients who are minors may be assigned to a legal guardian.

III. Confidentiality

A. **Confidentiality is implicit** in the clinician–patient relationship and can be ethically breached only in specific circumstances. The following are appropriate breaches of confidentiality:

1. Essential information can be released during an emergency (e.g., contacting a relative to get critical medical information about an incoherent patient).
2. Patients can request the release of information.
3. Clinical information can be discussed among designated treatment personnel.
4. The judiciary can subpoena clinical information.
5. The state can mandate that clinicians report certain types of information.

   a. Mandated reporting of abuse of spouses, children, the elderly, and the disabled is common.
   b. The evolving obligation of health care professionals to "warn and protect" others may mandate disclosure of a patient's violent threats (see VII D).

B. Patients should always be informed when confidentiality has been breached.

IV. Competency. Psychiatrists may assess a patient's competency in relation to several issues.

A. **Competency to give informed consent.** To give informed consent for a medical procedure, a patient must be able to understand the nature of a procedure, the alternative procedures, the consequences of not having the procedure, and the fact that consent is voluntary.

B. **Competency to enter into contracts.** To enter into a contract, an individual must be able to comprehend the nature, significance, and effects of the agreements.

C. **Competency to stand trial.** To be competent to stand trial, a defendant must be able to understand the charges against him and rationally consult with an attorney.

D. **Determining an individual's responsibility for criminal acts** is closely associated with competency issues.

1. An individual is not responsible for criminal acts if, as a result of a mental disorder other than "antisocial conduct," he lacks the ability to understand the wrongfulness of his conduct or conform his conduct to the law.
2. **Historic rulings**

   a. *M'Naghten* **rule** (1843). A person is not criminally responsible if, as a result of a mental disorder, he is unable to understand the nature of the act and understand "right from wrong."
   b. **Irresistible impulse** (1922). A person is not criminally responsible if, as the result of a mental disorder, he cannot resist impulses under which the criminal act was committed.
   c. *Durham* **(product) rule** (1954). A person is not criminally responsible if the act was the product of a mental disorder. This rule was impractical because determining a causal link was difficult.

E. Competency and age

1. As a direct consequence of chronologic age, minors may not be considered legally competent for many purposes, including the ability to consent to or refuse some psychiatric treatments.
2. Legal guardians often must make many decisions about psychiatric treatment for minors.

V. Guardianship

A. Adults. When judicial proceedings determine that an adult patient is incompetent in certain capacities (e.g., managing finances or health care), legal guardians may be appointed to act for the patient in these capacities, usually for a maximum of one year.

1. Psychiatrists may assess competency for the purpose of considering commencement or renewal of guardianship.
2. Guardianship may be assigned for the purpose of consenting to or refusing psychiatric treatment. In these cases, the guardian must give informed consent for the patient's treatment.

B. Minors are usually under the general guardianship of their parents, unless the court assigns guardianship to other parties.

VI. Involuntary Treatment

A. Involuntary psychiatric treatment. Although laws about involuntary psychiatric treatment vary among states, they have some common features.

1. **Involuntary psychiatric hospitalization** for limited periods, subject to judicial review, is usually permissible if qualified clinicians determine that the patient is suicidal, homicidal, or gravely disabled (i.e., unable to provide for food, clothing, or shelter) because of a mental disorder.
2. **Other forms of involuntary treatment.** Administration of psychiatric medication, seclusion, or physical restraint is often permissible only during immediate psychiatric emergencies (e.g., when violent behavior must be controlled) or when a specific court order is obtained through a judicial decision that treatment is in the best interests of the refusing patient.

B. Involuntary medical treatment

1. **Informed consent** must be obtained from the patient or guardian before patients can be given even lifesaving medical treatment, except in limited cases. However, if the patient cannot give informed consent because of unconsciousness or other severe cognitive impairment, most states allow emergency medical treatment.
2. Nonemergency medical treatment for a patient who cannot give informed consent usually requires judicial permission.
3. Psychiatrists may evaluate a patient's capacity to give informed consent (see IV A).

VII. Professional Responsibilities

A. Suicide. In most cases, health care professionals are obligated to take steps to prevent a patient's suicide that may occur because of a mental disorder (see Chapter 32 IV).

1. Potentially suicidal patients may be involuntarily detained for brief periods pending psychiatric evaluation.
2. In potentially suicidal patients, reasonable steps must be taken to prevent self-injury during treatment. For example, a hospitalized suicidal patient may need close observation by a nursing staff.

B. Duty to treat

1. Psychiatrists and other clinicians have a duty to evaluate and provide acute treatment during psychiatric emergencies.
2. Clinicians are not legally obligated to accept patients for nonemergent psychiatric treatment.
3. **Abandonment.** A clinician cannot arbitrarily terminate necessary psychiatric treatment without providing the patient with a treatment alternative.

C. Negligence. Psychiatrists and other clinicians have a duty to provide patients with conscientious evaluation and treatment and to respect patient rights.

1. Failure to provide appropriate diagnostic or therapeutic interventions, failure to use diagnostic or therapeutic interventions correctly, and failure to monitor treatment response are the most common sources of clinical negligence.
2. *Respondeat superior.* A psychiatrist is obligated to assume responsibility for the quality of care delivered by anyone who works under his direction.

D. *Tarasoff* warnings. Clinicians have a duty to "warn and protect" others of possible harm by patients under their care.

1. This rapidly evolving area of jurisprudence started with the *Tarasoff* decisions (1976, 1981), in which a California psychiatrist was held liable by the court for failing to take steps personally to warn and protect an individual threatened by his patient.
2. Although the parameters of the rulings are ambiguous, the courts view clinicians as having a duty to make reasonable attempts to warn identifiable persons of potential physical injury from a patient who the clinician believes may pose a serious threat.
3. Also, the court views clinicians as having a duty to take steps to protect identifiable potential victims from their patients (e.g., by detaining the patient).

E. Boundary violations. Psychiatrists and other mental health care professionals have a duty to maintain the personal and social boundaries that are appropriate to good treatment of patients.

1. **Sexual relations** with psychiatric patients are considered harmful and unethical in all circumstances and are often illegal. Also, sexual relations with former patients are often considered unethical.
2. **Other forms of nonclinical interaction** (e.g., physical contact, financial dealings, social engagements) between psychotherapists and their patients may also be considered harmful or unethical.

F. Professional ethics. Many important ethical obligations are generally recognized in psychiatry and the mental health field.

1. Act in the best interests of the patient.
2. Avoid doing harm.
3. Maintain confidentiality as much as possible.
4. Inform patients about all aspects of treatment and foster patient autonomy.
5. Do not engage in sexual relationships or other inappropriate relationships with patients (see VII E).
6. Avoid conflicts of interest in treating patients.
7. Document treatment accurately and thoroughly in the medical record.
8. Take steps to prevent grossly inappropriate or harmful treatment of patients by colleagues.

VIII. Psychiatric malpractice claims

A. Psychiatric malpractice claims usually involve patient suicide, failure to properly diagnose or treat conditions, untoward effects of a prescribed medication, or inappropriate sexual behavior with patients.

B. **"The four Ds."** The establishment of liability for medical malpractice requires four conditions:

1. **Duty.** The clinician owed a duty of care to the patient.
2. **Deviation.** The clinician deviated from this duty of care.
3. **Damages.** The deviation resulted in damages to the patient.
4. **Direct causation.** The deviation was the direct cause of the damages.

Review Test

Directions: Each of the numbered items or incomplete statements in this section is followed by answers or by completions of the statement. Select the ONE lettered answer or completion that is BEST in each case.

1. A 19-year-old man with mild mental retardation who was asking strangers for money impulsively strikes a man who refuses to give any to him. The young man is arrested and charged with battery. Which of the following is most important for determining his responsibility for the criminal act?

(A) Because of his mental disorder, he is unable to understand the nature of the act and "right from wrong"
(B) Because of his mental disorder, he cannot resist impulses under which the act was committed
(C) He is unable to understand the charges against him and rationally consult with an attorney
(D) He lacks the ability to understand the wrongfulness of his conduct or to conform his conduct to the law
(E) His act was the product of a mental disorder

2. A 28-year-old man with a history of assaultiveness is evaluated in a psychiatric emergency room. A clinician assesses that he suffers from persecutory delusions and auditory hallucinations. The patient says that he plans to kill his mother if she does not stop using "mental telepathy" to interrupt his thoughts. Which of the following is the most appropriate action by the clinician who has evaluated the patient?

(A) Administer antipsychotic medication and reevaluate the patient in several hours
(B) Inform the police of the patient's statement, and request that he is arrested
(C) Inform the police of the patient's statement, and involuntarily admit the patient to a psychiatric hospital
(D) Offer the patient voluntary hospitalization, and inform the police if he refuses and leaves the emergency room
(E) Telephone the patient's mother and inform her of the threat, and involuntarily admit the patient to a psychiatric hospital

3. A 31-year-old man with schizophrenia is admitted to a medical ward for treatment of abdominal injuries he sustained in a fight. The local law enforcement contacts the physician treating the patient, requesting information about the patient's condition. The patient states that he does not want information released to anyone. Which of the following is the most appropriate course for the clinician to take?

(A) The clinician should acknowledge that he is treating the patient but refuse to divulge any medical information
(B) The clinician should deny any knowledge of the patient
(C) The clinician should discuss the medical status of the patient with the law enforcement official, document the discussion in the patient's medical record, and notify the patient of the discussion
(D) The clinician should discuss the medical status of the patient with the law enforcement official and document the discussion in the patient's medical record, but the clinician should not notify the patient of the discussion
(E) The clinician should refer the law enforcement official to the hospital administrative staff for any information

4. A 50-year-old woman expresses suicidal ideation to a police officer and is taken involuntarily to a busy emergency room. Because the waiting time for evaluation will be several hours, she is placed in restraints and put in a curtained booth to ensure that she does not harm herself. Which of the following rights is most compromised by this action?

(A) Right to decent surroundings
(B) Right to effective treatment
(C) Right to have personal effects
(D) Right to least restrictive effective alternative
(E) Right to refuse treatment

5. A 71-year-old man develops tardive dyskinesia after being treated with chlorpromazine for 35 years. He sues his current psychiatrist for alleged negligence in prescribing the medication. To establish liability, which of the following factors must be demonstrated?

(A) Clozapine was not considered as an alternative treatment
(B) The medication was used in inappropriately high doses
(C) The patient has suffered damages
(D) The patient was not informed of all the possible adverse effects of chlorpromazine
(E) The psychiatrist was insufficiently trained in prescribing antipsychotic medication

Answers and Explanations

1–D. The widely accepted standard for determining an individual's responsibility for criminal behavior is the individual's ability to understand the wrongfulness of his conduct and to conform his conduct to the law. Previous standards for criminal responsibility include the ability to distinguish "right from wrong" (*M'Naghten* rule), the presence of an "irresistible impulse" arising from a mental disorder, and behavior that is the product of a mental disorder. Competency to stand trial is determined by the individual's ability to understand the charges against him and rationally consult with an attorney.

2–E. The *Tarasoff* decision established that mental health clinicians are obligated to warn and protect identifiable persons believed to be at risk for physical harm from a patient that the clinician has evaluated. In an emergency room, the warning is usually delivered by telephone or telegram. Protecting the potential victim often involves involuntary hospitalization of the patient based on the patient's danger to others.

3–E. Medical confidentiality precludes discussion of medical information about the patient without the patient's permission, except in very specific situations. In some cases, information can be divulged in response to a judiciary request, but the facts in this case are unclear. The best course of action is for the clinician not to divulge information, but to refer the matter to the institution's administration for further clarification of the potentially complex issues involved.

4–D. Patients have a right to the least restrictive effective treatment. Although placing this patient in restraints may be expeditious and effective in preventing suicide, other less restrictive treatment, such as closer observation, seclusion, or quicker assessment, may accomplish the same goal in a less restrictive manner. Because this patient is not receiving treatment on a voluntary basis, she does not have the right to refuse treatment.

5–C. To establish medical negligence, four conditions must exist, including damage to the patient. The other conditions are a clinician's duty to the patient, a deviation from that duty, and a direct causal link between the clinician's deviation from duty and the damage to the patient.

34

Geriatric Psychiatry

I. Overview

A. Statistics. The elderly are the fastest growing portion of the population. It is projected that the percent of the United States population 65 years of age and older will grow from 12% to 21% by the year 2030.

B. Aging individuals may face unique psychological challenges, including increasing physical limitations, status and role changes, increased medical disability, decreased income because of illness or retirement, and disruption of interpersonal relationships through death, retirement, and so on.

C. The epidemiology, presentation, complications, evaluation, and treatment of mental disorders in elderly patients are modified by the physiologic changes associated with aging, intercurrent general medical conditions, and social factors.

II. Geropsychiatric Assessment

A. General considerations. Elderly individuals are often troubled by specific psychiatric complaints, particularly memory difficulties, insomnia, anxiety, depression, and hypochondriasis.

  1. Some of these complaints are the result of normal aging processes and social attitudes toward the elderly. In some cultures, elderly individuals may be marginalized, excluded, or derided.

  2. To recognize symptoms that represent psychopathology, a clinician must have knowledge of the normal physiology and psychology of aging and age-related psychopathology. The clinician must also carefully assess the patient's history and mental status.

B. History

  1. History-taking in elderly patients should be more leisurely if possible, because older patients may have slower recall and verbal performance.

  a. The clinician should give special attention to a patient's sensory limitations, particularly hearing problems.

  b. The clinician should avoid using current jargon, because older patients often do not use contemporary jargon.

2. **Medical history.** The clinician should obtain a detailed history of the patient's general medical conditions and the current medications the patient is taking. Also, it is particularly important to obtain a careful review of systems, because psychiatric problems in the elderly are more likely associated with physiologic compromise.

3. **History from other individuals** (e.g., spouse, family, caregivers) is also valuable when evaluating elderly patients, because behavioral changes may not be subjectively obvious to the patients themselves.

C. **Mental status.** Because there is a significantly higher prevalence of cognitive impairment in the elderly, a clinician should carefully assess cognitive functioning.

1. The **mini-mental state examination** is commonly used. It consists of questions that measure orientation, registration (i.e., naming), attention and calculation, recall, language comprehension and expression, and form construction.

2. **Sensory** and **motor impairments** that may interfere with performance on mental status examination must be explored.

D. **Physical examination.** The elderly must be routinely evaluated for age-related general medical conditions that interfere with psychological function or complicate psychiatric treatment.

E. **Diagnostic formulation.** The clinician's diagnostic formulation must account for the general medical conditions and psychosocial stressors that are more common in the elderly.

1. **Cognitive function.** Any changes in cognitive function should be regarded as abnormal and potentially requiring treatment.

2. Because the elderly have more concurrent general medical conditions, the psychiatric diagnostic assessment involves discrimination of those conditions that are contributory to changes in mental status.

III. Geropsychiatric Treatment

A. **General considerations**

1. The **therapeutic relationship** must be carefully maintained with respect and empathy, because the age disparity between patient and clinician may make communication more difficult.

2. It is particularly important to advise caregivers about potential adverse effects of psychiatric treatment, and ask that they report any adverse effects to the clinician.

3. There must be close collaboration with physicians treating other general medical conditions, especially when pharmacotherapies are involved.

4. **Office visits** may need to be brief, and appointment reminders may be necessary.

B. **Geriatric psychopharmacology.** Judicious use of pharmacologic therapies is often extremely useful for elderly patients. However, excessive use of medications for sedation of elderly individuals in group settings (e.g., nursing homes) is particularly dangerous and must be avoided.

1. Pharmacotherapy in the elderly is modified by age-related pharmacokinetic factors, the presence of general medical conditions, and the concomitant use of other medications.

2. **Administering psychiatric medication.** The elderly generally metabolize drugs more slowly, are more sensitive to adverse effects of psychopharmacologic agents, and respond to lower doses.

    a. Pharmacotherapy in the elderly usually involves lower dosages and slower titrations—i.e., "Start low, go slow."

    b. Clinicians may have to monitor adverse effects and patient response to treatment more frequently.

3. **High-potency antipsychotic medications** that have minimal anticholinergic, hypotensive, and sedating effects are usually preferred, but patients must be closely monitored for the development of medication-induced movement disorders.

4. **Antidepressant medications** that have minimal anticholinergic and cardiovascular effects are usually preferred, especially nortriptyline, trazodone, and less-activating selective serotonin reuptake inhibitors, such as sertraline and paroxetine.

5. **Benzodiazepines** are the most frequently misprescribed and abused drugs in elderly populations. They should be prescribed with extreme caution, because the elderly have a slower metabolism and because of the risk of cognitive impairment.

6. **Lithium** must be used cautiously in elderly patients because there is a greater prevalence of impaired renal function; lower plasma levels are often therapeutic.

C. **Geriatric psychotherapy**

1. **Focus of treatment.** Psychotherapeutic intervention in the elderly often focuses on issues involving multiple losses (e.g., of relationships, health, work-related identity), a decreased ability to control the environment, and challenges to self-esteem. Adjustments to new roles in late life (e.g., grandparenthood, retirement, advisor, invalid) are also common issues.

    a. **Insight-oriented psychotherapy** often centers on resolving losses, improving self-esteem, and clarifying identity and life purpose.

    b. In elderly individuals, anxiety about death is not as common as the fear of disability, pain, and dependency.

    c. According to **Erikson** (1968), a central task of psychological development in the last phase of life is attaining ego integrity, characterized by an understanding and acceptance of one's life and purpose. Failure to attain this integrity causes a state of despair and disgust.

2. **Modifications of technique.** Psychotherapy may need to proceed slowly; the clinician needs to provide clear explanations, repeat therapeutic interventions (e.g., questions, clarifications, confrontations, insights), and speak with sufficient volume to compensate for the patient's potential hearing impairment.

3. Elderly individuals may face challenges in obtaining psychotherapy. These challenges include their own negative perceptions about psychotherapy,

which is common in the elderly cohort; family resistance; disinterest by psychotherapists in treating the elderly; and financial limitations.

IV. Psychiatric Disorders in the Elderly

A. Psychopathology and general medical conditions in the elderly

1. General medical conditions are more common in the elderly, and the senescent brain is sensitive to physiologic stress.

2. Changes in the mental status exam of elderly patients can be caused by physiologic changes of normal aging, the onset of acute general medical conditions, or progression of chronic general medical conditions (see Chapter 9).

B. Substance-induced psychopathology.
Substances (e.g., medications, recreational drugs, toxins) adversely affect mental status more often in the elderly because of age-related changes in central nervous system susceptibility, pharmacokinetics, and drug interactions.

1. Substance-induced mental disorders in the elderly may be caused by misprescription, patient errors in compliance, or a patient's increased sensitivity to adverse effects. Medications that are commonly involved include:

   a. **Analgesics** (e.g., opioids, indomethacin)

   b. **Anticonvulsants** (e.g., phenytoin, phenobarbital, carbamazepine)

   c. **Antihypertensives** (e.g., propranolol)

   d. **Antineoplastic medication** (e.g., methotrexate, fluorouracil)

   e. **Psychoactive medications.** Benzodiazepines are the most common offending agents. Antidepressants and other sedatives, anxiolytics, and hypnotics may also cause cognitive impairment and mood pathology in the elderly.

   f. **Other medications** (e.g., L-dopa, steroids)

2. **Metabolic disturbances.** Medications may indirectly lead to psychopathology by causing metabolic disturbances.

   a. **Diuretics** may induce dehydration and electrolyte imbalance.

   b. Oral **hypoglycemic medication** may lower blood sugar excessively and may induce the syndrome of inappropriate secretion of antidiuretic hormone (SIADH).

   c. **Antineoplastic medication** may lead to metabolic disturbances by causing diarrhea and vitamin deficiencies.

3. **Drug** and **alcohol abuse** are also more likely to cause substance-induced mental disorders in the elderly than in younger populations.

C. Cognitive disorders
in the elderly mandate careful evaluation and treatment for general medical conditions that may be responsible.

1. **Dementia.** Dementia of the Alzheimer type is the most common dementia in the elderly, followed by vascular dementia (see Chapter 10).

   a. Although an elderly patient may have an irreversible dementing illness, improving concurrent medical or psychiatric illnesses may substantially improve the patient's cognitive functioning and quality of life.

   b. In patients with irreversible dementia, family education and emotional and social support are useful.

    2. Clinicians should be particularly attentive to the cognitive problems associated with use of pharmacologic agents in the elderly. Clinicians should attempt to use the lowest effective doses of medications for the shortest possible period of time.

D. Schizophrenia and other psychotic disorders

    1. Epidemiology

        a. The prevalence of persecutory ideation in the elderly is elevated (about 4%), and the prevalence of schizophrenia is 1%.

        b. Women have a higher frequency of late-onset psychotic disorders.

        c. Psychotic symptoms in the elderly may be associated with sensory impairments.

    2. Etiology. The late onset of psychosis is highly suggestive of psychosis due to a general medical condition.

    3. Differential diagnoses of psychotic symptoms include delirium or dementia with psychotic features, psychotic disorder due to a general medical condition, substance-induced psychotic disorder, mood disorders with psychotic features, schizophrenia, schizoaffective disorders, delusional disorders, brief psychotic disorder, and senile reclusiveness.

    4. Clinical course. Both positive and negative symptoms of schizophrenia may improve with aging.

    5. Treatment

        a. All patients with **persecutory delusions** should be evaluated for sensory impairment, which should be corrected.

        b. Delusional symptoms in elderly individuals may remit in structured and supportive environments, particularly those with psychosocial interventions.

        c. Antipsychotic medication is useful, but the need for maintenance treatment must be measured against the higher incidence of adverse effects.

E. Depressive disorders

    1. Epidemiology

        a. In the elderly population, 15% may have depressive symptoms, and 4% have major depressive disorder.

        b. As many as 50% of the elderly who have a serious, symptomatic general medical condition also have mood disorder due to a general medical condition, substance-induced mood disorder, major depressive disorder, dysthymic disorder, or adjustment disorder with depressed mood.

        c. The incidence of depressive disorders in elderly men and women is similar.

        d. Family history. There is a greater prevalence of mood disorders in relatives of elderly patients with major depressive disorder. However, this increased prevalence is less than that in relatives of younger individuals with major depressive disorder.

    2. Etiology

        a. Stressful life events contribute significantly to the risk for depression in the elderly.

    b. Depressive symptoms may be caused by a dementia or mood disorder due to general medical conditions or a substance-induced dementia or mood disorder.

  3. Diagnosis and symptomatology

    a. The symptoms of major depressive disorder may be characterized by worry about physical problems ("depressive equivalents") and by the patient's reluctance to admit feeling depressed.

    b. Neurovegetative symptoms, such as lack of energy, decreased motor activity, and somnolence, may be difficult to distinguish from frailty.

    c. In the elderly, psychotic features are more common in major depressive disorder.

  4. Differential diagnoses for depressive disorder in the elderly include personality changes due to general medical conditions, impairment in affective expression due to Parkinson disease or other motor disorders, and loss of energy due to sleep disorders.

  5. Clinical course

    a. Major depressive disorder in the elderly is associated with a higher degree of mortality. However, mortality is decreased in patients who receive successful treatment.

    b. Suicide rates increase as individuals age.

      (1) In elderly white males, 50 in 100,000 commit suicide yearly.

      (2) In the general elderly population, 10 in 100,000 commit suicide yearly.

      (3) The suicide rate for elderly men is five times that for elderly women.

      (4) The ratio of suicide attempts to actual suicides in individuals younger than 40 years of age is 20:1, whereas this ratio in the elderly is 4:1.

      (5) Risk factors for suicide in the elderly include physical illness, previous attempts or gestures, bereavement, isolation and loneliness, and mental disorders.

      (6) Fifty to seventy percent of individuals who commit suicide in late life have had depressive symptoms.

    c. Recurrent depressive episodes are common in the elderly.

    d. Factors that suggest a poor prognosis for depressive disorders in the elderly include the presence of delusions during the initial depressive episode, poor health, and continuing psychosocial stressors.

  6. Treatment

    a. Psychotherapy is useful in elderly patients.

    b. Pharmacotherapy. The clinician must carefully select medication and closely monitor effects, because the elderly are particularly susceptible to adverse effects of antidepressant medication (see III B 2).

    c. Electroconvulsive therapy (ECT) is the most effective treatment for severe depressive episodes in the elderly.

    d. Psychotic depression may necessitate use of antidepressant and antipsychotic medication or ECT.

F. Bipolar disorders

1. **Diagnosis and symptomatology.** Manic episodes in the elderly present with less euphoria, hyperactivity, and grandiosity and more irritability, suspiciousness, and confusion.
2. **Differential diagnoses** include mood disorder due to general medical conditions and substance-induced mood disorders.
3. **Clinical course.** Mood episodes in bipolar disorders may occur more frequently with aging.
4. **Treatment**

   a. **Lithium** is a treatment of choice, but elderly patients must be carefully monitored for confusion, ataxia, and decreased renal functioning.

   b. **Antipsychotic medications** are useful for the acute management of manic episodes.

G. Anxiety disorders

1. **Epidemiology.** About 20% of the elderly population have clinically significant anxiety symptoms, but phobic and obsessive-compulsive disorders are less common.
2. **Diagnosis and symptomatology**

   a. **Somatic symptoms** of anxiety, such as tremulousness, tachycardia, dizziness, and dyspnea, may be difficult to distinguish from general medical conditions.

   b. Anxiety associated with hypochondriacal symptoms is common.

   c. Dissociative anxiety symptoms are uncommon.
3. **Differential diagnosis** is anxiety associated with other mental disorders.
4. **Clinical course.** Elderly individuals with anxiety disorder have frequently been symptomatic for many years. Anxiety disorders that begin in late life frequently become chronic.
5. **Treatment.** The elderly are at increased risk for adverse effects from benzodiazepines, especially long-acting agents.

H. Sexual disorders

1. **Age-related physiologic changes in sexual response**, such as decreased vaginal lubrication and erectile ability, occur in both sexes, and may lead to sexual dysfunction.
2. General medical conditions that interfere with sexual function, such as genitourinary neoplasms and neuropathies, are more common in the elderly.
3. Social attitudes that equate healthy sexuality exclusively with youthfulness may also lead to sexual disorders in the elderly.

I. Substance-related disorders

1. **Epidemiology.** The prevalence of alcoholism in the elderly population is 2%–10%, and the prevalence of alcoholism in the elderly seeking medical care is 15%. Benzodiazepine abuse may be common in the elderly.
2. **Diagnosis and symptomatology.** Signs and symptoms of substance dependence, intoxication, and withdrawal are often more subtle in the elderly than in the younger population.

   a. Elderly individuals with alcoholism may have a clinical picture characterized by confusion, poor hygiene and nutrition, incontinence, and myopathy. They also may sustain falls or accidental hypothermia.

    b. Functional impairment may be more difficult to diagnose because of the absence of work responsibilities and increased care provided by others.

  3. Clinical course

    a. Alcohol dependence in late life is characterized by exacerbations and remissions.

    b. Elderly alcoholics exhibit increased mortality with risk for gastrointestinal, cardiac, and pulmonary diseases; falls; and dementia.

  4. Treatment of adverse physical consequences is often more important in the elderly than in younger populations during management of substance use disorders. Treatment in residential settings is often necessary.

J. Sleep disorders. Both sleep complaints and disorders are more frequent in the elderly (see Chapter 21).

Review Test

Directions: Each of the numbered items or incomplete statements in this section is followed by answers or by completions of the statement. Select the ONE lettered answer or completion that is BEST in each case.

1. A 68-year-old man without a history of psychiatric disturbances complains of seeing the spirits of his deceased friends peering at him from windows. He also complains that his coffee tastes strangely bitter and is probably poisoned. He has no history of substance abuse. He says that he has been taking ibuprofen daily for about 3 months for headaches; he takes no other medications regularly. He is completely oriented to time and place. Which of the following is the most likely diagnosis?

(A) Dementia due to Parkinson disease
(B) Psychotic disorder due to a general medical condition
(C) Schizoaffective disorder
(D) Schizophreniform disorder
(E) Substance-induced psychotic disorder

2. A 77-year-old woman complains of increasing constipation that is not responsive to laxatives. Most of her conversation concerns this problem and the discomfort that it causes. She also admits to difficulty concentrating, a lack of energy, and disinterest in pursuing other activities. She denies feeling depressed, but she asks, "How can I visit friends or go shopping if my bowels don't function?" Which of the following is the most useful intervention?

(A) Inform her that constipation is common in elderly individuals
(B) Initiate amitriptyline
(C) Initiate a selective serotonin reuptake inhibitor
(D) Advise her to begin psychotherapy
(E) Initiate a more potent laxative

3. A 79-year-old man, widowed for 10 years, seeks psychotherapy for depression. He says that he was recently diagnosed with prostate cancer, and he is now concerned that he will not have an opportunity to help raise his 3-year-old grandson and pass on family stories to him. He believes that his own son is uninterested in his family's experiences. The man wonders where he "went wrong" in raising his children. Which of the following issues is likely to dominate psychotherapeutic exploration?

(A) Clarification of life's meaning
(B) Fear of death
(C) Fear of pain
(D) Loss of spouse
(E) Need to accomplish goals

4. An 83-year-old man complains of severe insomnia. He has taken flurazepam nightly for 1 year without subjective relief. He says that sleep deprivation has made him forgetful and has caused him difficulty focusing his thoughts during the day. Mental status examination shows mild memory deficits. Which of the following is the most useful initial intervention?

(A) Continue the flurazepam and add trazodone
(B) Gradually taper the dosage of flurazepam
(C) Immediately discontinue the flurazepam
(D) Increase the dosage of flurazepam
(E) Switch to lorazepam

5. A 91-year-old woman is admitted to a group residential care facility after she becomes too frail to manage alone in the house she has lived in for 55 years. During her first week in the facility, she is noted to be occasionally disoriented to time and place. She becomes extremely anxious, irritable, and verbally threatening. She complains of a subjective sense of confusion and says that she wants to be left alone. Which of the following is the most appropriate initial intervention?

(A) Allow the patient to gradually establish new relationships with others at her own pace
(B) Initiate crisis psychotherapy
(C) Initiate frequent supportive interaction
(D) Initiate haloperidol
(E) Initiate lorazepam

Answers and Explanations

1–B. The onset of psychotic symptoms in late life suggests psychotic disorder due to a general medical condition. Assessment of these patients requires comprehensive physical examination and laboratory studies. The patient is well oriented, so dementia is unlikely; however, he may have an underlying general medical condition (e.g., normal pressure hydrocephalus) that will cause dementia if it progresses further. Schizoaffective disorder and schizophreniform disorders usually begin earlier in life. Substance-induced psychotic disorders caused by prescribed medication are relatively more common in the elderly than in younger individuals; however, this patient is not taking medication that is associated with psychosis.

2–C. The patient's lassitude, disinterest, and difficulty with concentrating suggest depression. Elderly individuals who are depressed may focus primarily on somatic complaints and may deny a subjective depression. A selective serotonin reuptake inhibitor (SSRI) may alleviate her depression and obsessive rumination. SSRIs are usually well tolerated in the elderly. Amitriptyline is more likely than an SSRI to cause adverse effects, including a worsening of her constipation. Telling the patient that constipation is more common in her age-group is unlikely to comfort her. Initially engaging her in psychotherapy may be difficult, because the patient does not believe that she is depressed. Initiating a more potent laxative is unlikely to solve the patient's depressive symptoms.

3–A. Psychological issues in late life often focus on resolving life's purpose. This patient seems to believe that his task is to transmit the family story as his grandson matures, and he may be prohibited from doing this because of an intercurrent illness. Helping the man assess his life from other perspectives may be therapeutic. Fear of death and pain and the need to accomplish goals are issues more common in younger individuals. Loss of a spouse is often a focus of psychotherapy in the elderly; however, there is limited information to suggest that it is the central issue in this case.

4–B. The patient's memory deficit is probably caused or exacerbated by using a benzodiazepine as a hypnotic agent. Even moderate doses of benzodiazepine may cause memory impairment in elderly individuals. Tapering the flurazepam may improve his cognitive status and prevent potential withdrawal symptoms caused by immediately discontinuing it. Adding trazodone to the patient's regimen or switching to another benzodiazepine is unlikely to improve his memory. Education in sleep hygiene may be important for elderly individuals with sleep complaints. If hypnotics are necessary, they should be used very briefly and at a low dosage.

5–C. The individual's symptoms suggest fear and irritability associated with memory disturbances and possibly mild dementia. It is likely that new and unfamiliar surroundings have exacerbated her deficits. Frequent supportive interaction and the placement of familiar objects,
calendars, and clocks in her immediate vicinity may be helpful interventions. A comprehensive
assessment and treatment for underlying medical or psychiatric conditions (e.g., depressive disorders) may also be useful in decreasing her confusion. Emotional support should be actively offered, because she may withdraw further if left alone. Psychotherapy may be useful with elderly
patients; however, it is usually most effective when it proceeds slowly. Haloperidol may be useful if nonpharmacologic treatment does not successfully decrease her agitation. Lorazepam may
exacerbate her memory deficits.

Comprehensive Examination

Directions: Each of the numbered items or incomplete statements in this section is followed by answers or by completions of the statement. Select the ONE lettered answer or completion that is BEST in each case.

1. A 10-year-old girl awakes almost every night 2 hours after going to sleep. According to her parents, she screams, sits up in bed, and appears to be confused and frightened. After 2 or 3 minutes, she goes back to sleep. She has no memory of these events the following morning. Which of the following is the most likely diagnosis?

(A) Circadian rhythm sleep disorder
(B) Narcolepsy
(C) Nightmare disorder
(D) Sleep terror disorder
(E) Sleepwalking disorder

2. A 15-year-old girl presents with loquacity, hypervigilance, tachycardia, and pupillary dilation after ingesting an unknown drug at a party 3 hours ago. Her coordination appears unimpaired, and her mucous membranes are moist. Which of the following substances is the most likely cause?

(A) Amphetamine
(B) Cannabis
(C) Lysergic acid diethylamide (LSD)
(D) Phencyclidine
(E) Psilocybin

3. A 16-year-old boy has an 8-year history of intermittent motor tics, which are sometimes accompanied by grunts, and cause him significant social embarrassment. After inhaling methamphetamine supplied by a friend, his tics suddenly became severe. Which of the following is the most likely diagnosis?

(A) Amphetamine-induced movement disorder
(B) Huntington disease
(C) Stereotypic habit disorder
(D) Sydenham chorea
(E) Tourette disorder

4. A 17-year-old boy has an 11-year history of motor tics that are accompanied by grunts and occasional coprolalia. Which of the following disorders most likely accompanies his primary disorder?

(A) Generalized anxiety disorder
(B) Obsessive-compulsive disorder
(C) Panic disorder
(D) Postencephalitic dementia
(E) Schizophrenia

5. A 17-year-old boy with no previous psychiatric problems has the rapid onset of severe anxiety and agitation, vivid auditory hallucinations, and persecutory delusions that have persisted for 6 weeks. He has no history of substance abuse. Physical examination and laboratory studies, including toxicology for substance of abuse, are unremarkable. Which of the following features of this case is associated with a better prognosis?

(A) Lack of history of substance abuse
(B) Lack of associated medical conditions
(C) Relatively young age of patient
(D) Prominent psychotic symptoms
(E) Male gender

6. A 19-year-old woman presents with a history of recurrent episodes of binge eating and fasting. She seems obsessed about her weight and what she regards as her disgusting eating habits. She is very thin, but she believes that she is at significant risk for becoming obese because of her eating habits. Which of the following findings is most likely reported during a review of systems?

(A) Amenorrhea
(B) Chronic diarrhea
(C) Chronic fatigue and cold intolerance
(D) Recurrent dental caries
(E) Recurrent exercise-induced tendinitis

7. A 19-year-old man is brought to the emergency room because of severe agitation after smoking what he thought was crack cocaine. He has slurred speech, ataxia, circumoral numbness, and horizontal nystagmus. Which of the following substances most likely caused his symptoms?

(A) Cannabis
(B) Heroin
(C) Methamphetamine
(D) Phencyclidine
(E) Toluene

8. A 19-year-old man returns from college to live with his parents and three younger brothers after a 7-month episode of mental illness that culminated in psychiatric hospitalization and a diagnosis of schizophrenia. Which of the following actions on the part of the family would most likely improve his adjustment and decrease the likelihood of rehospitalization?

(A) Encourage animated discussions at dinner, with an emphasis on exploring areas of friction among family members
(B) Insist that the patient abstain from social interaction
(C) Keep family stresses and overt conflicts to a minimum
(D) Keep the patient at home as much as possible
(E) Strongly encourage the patient to return to school or get a job

9. A 20-year-old man with severe agitation during the active phase of schizophrenia is given three doses of 5 mg of haloperidol intramuscularly over a 4-hour period. He becomes rigid and diaphoretic. His oral temperature is 101°F. Which of the following adverse effects is most likely responsible for the man's symptoms?

(A) Akathisia
(B) Catatonia
(C) Neuroleptic malignant syndrome
(D) Neuroleptic-induced dystonia
(E) Pseudoparkinsonian symptoms

10. A 21-year-old woman develops mutism and immobility, interrupted only by brief episodes of peculiar grimacing. Which of the following is the most likely diagnosis?

(A) Autism
(B) Catatonia
(C) Factitious disorder
(D) Malingering
(E) Selective mutism

11. A 22-year-old man complains of seeing strange visions of angels on the walls of his bedroom as he falls asleep. Which of the following is the most likely diagnosis?

(A) Delirium
(B) Hallucinogen persisting perception disorder
(C) Hypnogogic hallucinations
(D) Hypnopompic hallucinations
(E) Occipital lobe partial seizures

12. A 23-year-old woman who is currently preparing to defend her doctoral dissertation becomes worried that grade I cells found in a routine Pap smear indicate that she has cervical cancer. Further studies are entirely negative, but she remains excessively worried and unable to concentrate on her work despite reassurance by her physician. Which of the following interventions is most likely to resolve her symptoms?

(A) Careful explanation of the benign nature of the physical complaint
(B) Discussion about current emotional stressors
(C) Skillful physician reassurance
(D) Use of a benzodiazepine
(E) Use of placebo medication

13. A 23-year-old man presents with a 4-month history of disturbing auditory hallucinations, moderately disorganized thought processes, and increasing anxiety and confusion. Which of the following factors implies an unfavorable prognosis in this case?

(A) Magnetic resonance imaging (MRI) shows no gross changes in brain morphology
(B) He has a family history of schizophrenia
(C) He has an extensive premorbid history of social withdrawal
(D) He has catatonic symptomatology
(E) There was a sudden onset of symptomatology

14. A 24-year-old woman complains of severe anxiety when she has to speak at business meetings or attend social events. She is unable to host or attend even small parties, and this has narrowed her social life and decreased her chances of networking in her career. She feels isolated and inadequate. Which of the following is the best choice of treatment?

(A) Assertiveness training and a course of phenelzine
(B) Lorazepam
(C) Psychodynamic psychotherapy and a course of imipramine
(D) Stimulus flooding and a course of low-dose lorazepam
(E) Systematic desensitization

15. A 24-year-old woman complains of an inability to reach orgasm during even passionate sexual activity. She neither takes medication nor uses drugs, and she is otherwise in good health. Which of the following statements is the most accurate about her condition?

(A) It is most likely caused by unresolved conflicts about sexual issues
(B) It is most likely lifelong and not acquired
(C) It is most likely caused by an undiagnosed medical condition
(D) It is unlikely to affect her self-esteem or the quality of her interpersonal relationships
(E) The most appropriate pharmacologic treatment would involve the use of a selective serotonin reuptake inhibitor

16. A 25-year-old man with AIDS complains of severe right upper quadrant pain. An intravenous (IV) line is established because of the likelihood that IV therapy will be initiated after laboratory studies are completed, and normal saline is started. An hour later, the patient remarks to a consulting physician, "I don't know what's in the IV, but it has really helped cut the pain." Which of the following is most likely?

(A) The pain is psychogenic
(B) The patient has factitious disorder
(C) The patient is responding to placebo
(D) The patient has a histrionic personality disorder
(E) The patient was volume-depleted

17. A 26-year-old man with alcohol dependence develops ataxia, confusion, and gaze paralysis. Which of the following is the most appropriate pharmacotherapy?

(A) Chlordiazepoxide
(B) Cobalamin
(C) Folate
(D) Lorazepam
(E) Thiamine

18. A 27-year-old man has a lifelong history of social isolation, disinterest in sexual relationships, and few sources of pleasure. On examination, he appears emotionally distant. There is no evidence of peculiar thinking or suspiciousness. Which of the following is the most likely diagnosis?

(A) Avoidant personality disorder
(B) Schizoid personality disorder
(C) Schizophreniform disorder
(D) Schizotypal personality disorder
(E) Social phobia

19. A 28-year-old man begins treatment with lithium for bipolar disorder. Which of the following changes is most likely after 6 months of lithium treatment?

(A) Decreased white cell count
(B) Decreased serum sodium
(C) Increased serum creatinine
(D) Increased serum thyroid-stimulating hormone
(E) Prolonged QRS interval

20. A 29-year-old woman is started on tranylcypromine for depression. Which of the following precautions should be given to her?

(A) Avoid heavy exercise
(B) Do not eat red meat, lima beans, or stewed tomatoes
(C) Do not use nonsteroidal anti-inflammatory analgesics
(D) Do not use oral decongestants
(E) Drink as much fluid as possible

21. A 30-year-old woman has a long history of chaotic social relationships, periods of dysphoria and anger, many suicide gestures, and a poor sense of identity. She also describes transient periods of confusion accompanied by a sense of unreality. These periods seem to be associated with threatened abandonment by others. Which of the following is the most likely diagnosis?

(A) Acute stress disorder
(B) Borderline personality disorder
(C) Depersonalization disorder
(D) Dissociative identity disorder
(E) Dysthymic disorder

22. A 31-year-old man commits suicide by shooting himself in the head with a shotgun. Which of the following cerebrospinal fluid (CSF) findings is most likely?

(A) Decreased level of 5-hydroxyindoleacetic acid (5-HIAA)
(B) Decreased level of acetylcholine
(C) Decreased level of dopamine
(D) Decreased level of γ-aminobutyric acid
(E) Decreased level of norepinephrine

23. A 31-year-old man who is being treated with an unknown medication for panic disorder decides to discontinue the medication "cold turkey." Eighteen hours later, he is brought to the emergency room after having a generalized tonic–clonic seizure and is confused. Which of the following medications was he most likely taking?

(A) Alprazolam
(B) Clonazepam
(C) Imipramine
(D) Phenelzine
(E) Propranolol

24. A 31-year-old man sustains only minor injuries in an automobile accident in which his wife was killed. Hours after the accident, he seems oddly calm and says that he feels no emotion. Which of the following psychodynamic defense mechanisms is most strongly suggested by this reaction?

(A) Depersonalization
(B) Derealization
(C) Disorientation
(D) Intellectualization
(E) Isolation

25. A 32-year-old man complains of irresistible daytime sleepiness, brief moments during which he is unable to open his eyes, and vivid dreamlike visions on awakening. Which of the following medications is most likely beneficial?

(A) Desipramine
(B) Diazepam
(C) Fluoxetine
(D) Haloperidol
(E) Methylphenidate

26. A 33-year-old woman complains of being unable to leave her home unaccompanied. She also avoids crowds and public transportation. Which of the following additional symptoms does this woman most likely have?

(A) Alcohol abuse
(B) Obsessions
(C) Panic attacks
(D) Persecutory delusions
(E) Suicide gestures

27. During her acrimonious divorce proceeding, a 33-year-old woman suddenly falls to the floor of the courtroom and is unresponsive to verbal intervention. She has no history of seizure disorder or head trauma. Physical examination and routine laboratory studies obtained in the emergency room are normal. After about 30 minutes, the patient appears normally responsive. Similar episodes occur several times during the following week. Magnetic resonance imaging (MRI) and electroencephalogram (EEG) are unremarkable. She seems peculiarly calm and unconcerned about the episodes and says that she does not think the attacks are worth worrying about. Which of the following is the most likely diagnosis?

(A) Atonic seizure
(B) Conversion disorder
(C) Factitious disorder
(D) Hypochondriasis
(E) Malingering

28. A 33-year-old man is started on 5 mg of fluphenazine twice daily, 2 mg of benztropine twice daily, and 300 mg of lithium three times daily. Twenty-four hours later, he complains of tremulousness, diarrhea, and headache. Which of the following is the most likely cause of his symptoms?

(A) Anticholinergic toxicity
(B) Lithium toxicity
(C) Neuroleptic-induced dystonia
(D) Neuroleptic-induced extrapyramidal syndrome
(E) Neuroleptic malignant syndrome

29. A 34-year-old woman becomes extremely anxious, with tachycardia, hyperventilation, and feelings of impending doom, whenever she drives across a bridge. She avoids destinations where travel over bridges is required. Which of the following is the most likely diagnosis?

(A) Avoidant personality disorder
(B) Generalized anxiety disorder
(C) Obsessive-compulsive disorder
(D) Panic disorder with agoraphobia
(E) Specific phobia

30. A 34-year-old man requests rhinoplasty from a cosmetic surgeon. The individual is convinced that his nose is grossly misshapen and that it interferes with his romantic pursuits and career advancement. Objective assessment by the cosmetic surgeon indicates that there is a barely perceptible nasal asymmetry but no other abnormality. Which of the following is the most likely diagnosis?

(A) Body dysmorphic disorder
(B) Conversion disorder
(C) Delusional disorder, somatic type
(D) Hypochondriasis
(E) Somatization disorder

31. A 35-year-old executive is devastated when he loses his job after his company is sold. Several weeks later, he states that losing his job was actually helpful because he now has more time to spend with his family. Which of the following psychodynamic defense mechanisms is most strongly suggested by this statement?

(A) Compensation
(B) Derealization
(C) Displacement
(D) Projection
(E) Rationalization

32. A 35-year-old man complains of the recent onset of neck pain, impaired vision only in his right eye, dizziness, and urinary hesitancy. He is irritable and emotionally labile. Which of the following is the most likely diagnosis?

(A) Acute intermittent porphyria
(B) Hypochondriasis
(C) Multiple sclerosis
(D) Somatization disorder
(E) Wilson disease

33. A 37-year-old man complains of severe anxiety at social functions, and he tries to avoid them at all costs. His anxiety about and avoidance of social functions have interfered with his career and social life. Which of the following is the most appropriate treatment?

(A) Assertiveness training
(B) Biofeedback
(C) Flooding
(D) Graduated desensitization
(E) Psychoanalytic psychotherapy

34. A 37-year-old man with major depressive disorder, single episode, has responded well to 50 mg/day of sertraline after 3 weeks of treatment. He has had minor nausea but has otherwise tolerated the medication without adverse effects. Which of the following is the most logical next step in management?

(A) Continue the sertraline indefinitely unless the nausea worsens
(B) Continue the sertraline for 6 months
(C) Decrease the sertraline by 10 mg weekly until he is medication free or the depression recurs
(D) Discontinue the sertraline after completing a 1-month course
(E) Switch to fluoxetine

35. Two weeks following a terrifying experience during which she was threatened by a robber, a 38-year-old woman continues to suffer from nightmares about the event. She also reports a sense of confusion about the event and increased anxiety. She feels she cannot return to the shopping mall where the event occurred. Which of the following is the most likely diagnosis?

(A) Acute stress disorder
(B) Adjustment disorder with anxious mood
(C) Panic disorder with agoraphobia
(D) Posttraumatic stress disorder
(E) Specific phobia

36. A 39-year-old man is reported missing by his wife. The next day, the police spot his car in the parking lot of a hotel in a city 200 miles away. They find him in the hotel lobby, appearing somewhat dazed and confused. He does not respond to his name, and he has registered in a different name at the hotel. Which of the following is the most likely diagnosis?

(A) Bipolar disorder, manic episode
(B) Complex partial seizure disorder
(C) Depersonalization disorder
(D) Dissociative identity disorder
(E) Dissociative fugue

37. A 39-year-old man with trisomy 21 has had increasing irritability, moodiness, and forgetfulness during the previous year. He has more difficulty communicating and is unable to manage self-care as well as he previously did. Which of the following is the most likely diagnosis?

(A) Adjustment disorder with mixed disturbance of emotions and conduct, chronic
(B) Dementia due to normal pressure hydrocephalus
(C) Dementia of the Alzheimer type
(D) Major depressive disorder
(E) Personality change due to partial complex seizures

38. A 40-year-old man is brought to the emergency room by police, who found him standing on the railing of a bridge at midnight. When they directly questioned him about suicidal intent, he stated that he was "thinking about it." Which of the following factors most increases the individual's risk for actually attempting suicide?

(A) He had a fight with his spouse
(B) He has schizophrenia
(C) He is dissatisfied with his occupation
(D) He is homosexual
(E) He is undergoing financial hardship

39. A 40-year-old man complains of a fear of snakes, which prevents him from hiking in the local mountains. He believes that his fear is unreasonable, because he recognizes that thousands of other hikers are never harmed by snakes. Which of the following is the most likely diagnosis?

(A) Acute stress disorder
(B) Agoraphobia
(C) Obsessive-compulsive disorder
(D) Panic disorder with agoraphobia
(E) Specific phobia

40. A 41-year-old man accuses his therapist of having an unreasonable fee schedule and an arbitrary and dismissive manner. This accusation occurs at the end of a psychotherapy session that focused on the patient's memories of his overbearing father. Which of the following psychodynamic concepts best describes this accusatory behavior?

(A) Cathexis
(B) Countertransference
(C) Dissociation
(D) Secondary process
(E) Transference

41. A 42-year-old man with generalized anxiety disorder stops taking his twice-daily dose of 10 mg of diazepam. He says that although diazepam at this dose partially controls his anxiety, he feels too "mentally slow" to function adequately in his job as a securities analyst. Which of the following is the most appropriate next step in management?

(A) Switch to buspirone
(B) Switch to clomipramine
(C) Switch to clonazepam
(D) Switch to imipramine
(E) Switch to zolpidem

42. A 43-year-old man with schizophrenia is describing his anxiety about others watching him. He suddenly stops talking and, after a moment of silence, he begins describing his preoccupation with identifying species of flowers. Which of the following psychodynamic terms best describes this behavior?

(A) Blocking
(B) Empathic failure
(C) Mirroring
(D) Narcissism
(E) Schizoid fantasy

43. A 44-year-old man is admitted with complaints of severe malaise, neck pain, and dizziness. Physical examination shows a maculopapular rash across a significant portion of his body. The rash appears on new areas of his body during the second day of his hospitalization. A nurse finds poison oak leaves in the patient's belongings by the bedside. When questioned, the patient angrily signs out against medical advice. Which of the following is the most likely diagnosis?

(A) Antisocial personality disorder
(B) Factitious disorder
(C) Malingering
(D) Schizophrenia
(E) Schizotypal personality disorder

44. A 44-year-old man remains severely depressed after adequate trials of three different antidepressant medications. He suffers from feelings of hopelessness, tearfulness, anorexia, and weight loss. He has had neither previous episodes of mania nor psychotic symptoms. A recent comprehensive physical evaluation, including laboratory studies of renal, liver, pancreatic, and thyroid functioning, was unremarkable. Which of the following is the most appropriate next step in management?

(A) Discontinue antidepressant medication and initiate intensive cognitive psychotherapy
(B) Prescribe a combination of an antidepressant plus an atypical antipsychotic agent
(C) Prescribe a combination of an antidepressant agent and lithium, thyroxine, or amphetamine
(D) Prescribe a combination of three antidepressants with different pharmacologic profiles
(E) Prescribe a selective serotonin reuptake inhibitor and a monoamine oxidase inhibitor

45. A 46-year-old woman believes that her habit of smoking cigarettes is medically beneficial, because it helps her avoid obesity. Which of the following psychodynamic defense mechanisms is most applicable to this case?

(A) Denial
(B) Derealization
(C) Intellectualization
(D) Rationalization
(E) Reaction formation

46. A 47-year-old man has recurrent manic episodes with grandiose delusions. He has no history of substance abuse or seizures. A 4-week trial of lithium taken orally at 300 mg three times daily produces a serum lithium level of 1.3 mEq/L, but fails to control his symptoms. Which of the following is the appropriate next step in management?

(A) Continue lithium and add a low dose of haloperidol
(B) Increase the dose of lithium to 600 mg twice daily
(C) Initiate electroconvulsive therapy
(D) Discontinue lithium and begin a trial of clonazepam
(E) Discontinue lithium and begin a trial of valproate

47. A 5-year-old boy has mental retardation, microcephaly, short stature, short palpebral fissures, hypoplastic maxillae and philtrum, and micrognathia. Which of the following is the most likely etiology?

(A) Head trauma from child abuse
(B) Intrauterine rubella infection
(C) Intrauterine exposure to alcohol
(D) Protein deficiency
(E) Trisomy 21

48. An unconscious 50-year-old patient who is dressed as a woman is discovered to have male genitalia during emergency physical examination following an automobile accident. The patient's driver license and other identification show a feminine name. Which of the following is the most likely diagnosis?

(A) Delusional disorder, somatic type
(B) Gender identity disorder
(C) Klinefelter syndrome
(D) Testicular feminization
(E) Transvestism

49. A 50-year-old woman with schizoaffective disorder, bipolar type, is treated with chlorpromazine and lithium. She complains of polydipsia and nocturia. Which of the following is the most likely cause?

(A) Chlorpromazine-induced diabetes mellitus
(B) Lithium-induced diabetes insipidus
(C) Lithium-induced syndrome of inappropriate secretion of antidiuretic hormone
(D) Psychogenic polydipsia
(E) Response to dry mouth caused by chlorpromazine-induced cholinergic blockade

50. A 51-year-old man reports that while fishing on a pier, he is bothered by the persistent and intrusive impulse to leap over the railing. He denies any desire to commit this act, but he now avoids fishing because he fears that he may actually jump. Which of the following statements about his condition is most accurate?

(A) He has a compulsion
(B) He has a delusion
(C) He has an impulse-control disorder
(D) He has a hallucination
(E) He has an obsession

51. A 52-year-old man with a long history of alcohol dependence, characterized by frequent binge drinking, is started on 50 mg/day of naltrexone and has no binges during the next 6 months. Which of the following is the most likely mechanism that decreased his binge drinking?

(A) Naltrexone functions as a partial agonist for opioid receptors and thereby lessens the craving for alcohol
(B) Naltrexone functions as a placebo by providing a sense of security and confidence that alcohol dependency can be overcome
(C) Naltrexone negatively reinforces drinking behavior by creating symptoms of opioid withdrawal
(D) Naltrexone blocks subjective sense of reward from alcohol-mediated release of endogenous opioids
(E) Naltrexone competitively inhibits metabolism of alcohol, causing subjective dysphoria at low doses

52. A 53-year-old woman with three adolescent children presents to a therapist complaining of feeling worthless and deeply unhappy. She says that she does not feel that there is any reason to continue living. Which of the following actions is the most critical during the remainder of the interview?

(A) The therapist should ask about any medications that the patient may be taking for other general medical conditions
(B) The therapist should inquire directly about suicidal thoughts and specific plans
(C) The therapist should point out that many people feel this way at some point during their lives
(D) The therapist should share the belief that the patient is a valuable human being on whom other people may depend
(E) The therapist should tell the patient honestly that she will be hospitalized because she may be a danger to herself

53. A 54-year-old man is currently taking phenelzine. While skiing, he dislocates his shoulder and is brought into the emergency room in severe pain. Which of the following analgesic medications is contraindicated?

(A) Acetaminophen
(B) Ibuprofen
(C) Meperidine
(D) Pentazocine
(E) Propoxyphene

54. A 59-year-old man is released from prison after serving a 12-year sentence for setting several destructive forest fires. He now spends time planting trees and supporting forest conservation efforts. Which of the following psychodynamic defense mechanisms is most strongly suggested by his actions?

(A) Denial
(B) Dissociation
(C) Intellectualization
(D) Sublimation
(E) Undoing

55. A 62-year-old man with a long history of alcohol dependence presents with memory impairment, which he has had for several months. He provides vague and incorrect information about his activities during the last few weeks. His speech and ability to follow directions and name objects are intact. Which of the following is the most likely diagnosis?

(A) Amnesia
(B) Delirium
(C) Dementia
(D) Dissociation
(E) Psychosis

56. A 67-year-old woman complains of having difficulties with memory and focusing attention, insomnia and rumination about having undiagnosed bowel cancer that is causing her constipation, insomnia, and weight loss. Mental status examination shows listlessness, moderate psychomotor retardation, and absence of aphasia or anomia. Which of the following is the most likely diagnosis?

(A) Age-related cognitive decline
(B) Delirium
(C) Dementia
(D) Hypochondriasis
(E) Major depressive episode

57. A 68-year-old survivor of a Nazi concentration camp complains of a recent recurrence of nightmares about horrific events that she witnessed. She relates that she has felt irrationally guilty about being alive, and she says that she has been emotionally distant from other people during her entire adult life. She has avoided discussing her wartime experiences or associating with others who experienced similar trauma. She has always had severe insomnia, an excessive startle response, and general anxiety. After viewing a cinematic dramatization of concentration camp experiences, she says that she wants to travel to the concentration camp sites and meet with other survivors at a planned reunion. Which of the following therapeutic strategies is most likely to ameliorate her symptoms?

(A) Encourage her enrollment in group therapy with a focus on assertiveness training
(B) Encourage her to avoid initially immersing herself in environments that may trigger traumatic memories and to begin psychodynamic psychotherapy to explore survivor guilt
(C) Encourage her to make the trip to the concentration camp site and meet with other survivors
(D) Initiate psychotherapy to cognitively reframe her experiences and focus on the present
(E) Initiate lorazepam or a similar benzodiazepine

58. A 78-year-old woman currently authoring successful cookbooks is given codeine for a severe toothache. After taking several doses, she is found confused, disoriented, and frightened, cowering in her bedroom and describing "huge ants" crawling on her floor. Which of the following is the most likely diagnosis?

(A) Alcohol withdrawal
(B) Brief psychotic disorder
(C) Codeine-induced delirium
(D) Codeine-induced psychotic disorder
(E) Vascular dementia

59. An 18-year-old man is brought to the emergency room in coma. He is given an intravenous injection of 1.0 mg of naloxone. Within minutes, he becomes alert, agitated, and nauseated and has tachycardia. Which of the following is the most likely etiology for his response to naloxone?

(A) Adverse interaction between phencyclidine and naloxone
(B) Anaphylactic response to naloxone or its vehicle
(C) Opioid withdrawal caused by naloxone
(D) Paradoxical excitement with increasing sedation from naloxone
(E) Placebo response to naloxone

60. An 87-year-old woman complains of hopelessness, fatigue, and hypersomnia. Mental status examination shows intact recent memory, tearfulness, and suicidal rumination. Which of the following is the most appropriate antidepressant medication?

(A) Amitriptyline
(B) Doxepin
(C) Nortriptyline
(D) Phenelzine
(E) Trazodone

61. During a 6-month course of psychotherapy, a psychotherapist and her patient gain insight about the implications of early memories the patient has of several unexpected separations from her parents and the resulting emotional turmoil. Which of the following disorders is most likely successfully treated with this intervention?

(A) Dysthymia
(B) Enuresis
(C) Obsessive-compulsive disorder
(D) Schizophrenia
(E) Social phobia

62. During the course of which of the following conditions must a disturbance of consciousness, with a reduced ability to focus, sustain, or shift attention, be present for a period of time?

(A) Delirium
(B) Dementia
(C) Dissociative fugue
(D) Dissociative amnesia
(E) Substance-induced amnestic disorder

63. In which of the following patients is methylphenidate the most logical treatment?

(A) A 12-year-old girl with motor tics and vocalizations
(B) A 15-year-old boy with a 5-year history of assaultiveness, stealing, and lying
(C) A 31-year-old woman with depressive rumination, obesity, and hypersensitivity to rejection
(D) A 42-year-old man with advanced AIDS who has difficulty concentrating, severe loss of energy, and feelings of hopelessness
(E) A 69-year-old man with agitated depression and suicidal rumination 6 months following the death of his wife

64. The prevalence of winter-type seasonal depressive episodes is highest in

(A) individuals with thiamine deficiency
(B) individuals with complete blindness
(C) individuals living in higher latitudes
(D) individuals older than 65 years of age
(E) males

65. What is the lifetime incidence for schizophrenia?

(A) 0.01%
(B) 0.05%
(C) 0.1%
(D) 0.5%
(E) 1%

66. Which of the following disorders is most likely responsive to antidepressant medications?

(A) Anorexia nervosa, restricting type
(B) Borderline personality disorder
(C) Bulimia nervosa, purging type
(D) Male erectile disorder
(E) Female orgasmic disorder

67. Which of the following is the most accurate statement about sexual sadism?

(A) Sexual excitement may be derived from purely psychological suffering of the victim
(B) Acts of sadism must be committed before a diagnosis of sexual sadism is made
(C) Sexual activity is usually considered sadistic only when the partner is nonconsenting
(D) Simulated suffering of victims is part of sexual sadism
(E) The severity of the sadistic acts is usually constant over time

68. Which of the following medications is most likely to increase a patient's plasma lithium levels?

(A) Benztropine
(B) Chlorpromazine
(C) Codeine
(D) Ibuprofen
(E) Penicillin

69. Which of the following symptoms is most likely associated with phenothiazine antipsychotic medication?

(A) Hyperreflexia
(B) Photosensitivity
(C) Diarrhea
(D) Weight loss
(E) Urinary incontinence

70. Which of the following reasons accounts for the administration of atropine before a session of electroconvulsive therapy (ECT)?

(A) to enhance the antidepressant effect of ECT
(B) to produce amnesia for the ECT treatment
(C) to reduce cognitive impairment caused by the ECT
(D) to reduce oral secretions and decrease bradycardia
(E) to reduce the danger of fractures caused by seizure

71. Which of the following age-groups has the highest prevalence of alcohol abuse?

(A) 15 to 18 years of age
(B) 18 to 22 years of age
(C) 22 to 29 years of age
(D) 30 to 45 years of age
(E) 45 to 60 years of age

72. Which of the following substances is most commonly associated with life-threatening medical complications during withdrawal?

(A) Methamphetamine
(B) Cocaine
(C) Cannabis
(D) Diazepam
(E) Pentazocine

73. Which of the following adverse effects occurs most frequently during treatment with clozapine?

(A) Seizures
(B) Renal failure
(C) Agranulocytosis
(D) Pigmentary retinopathy
(E) Anticholinergic delirium

74. Which of the following brain structures is most closely associated with sleep architecture?

(A) Hypothalamus
(B) Amygdala
(C) Dorsal raphe nucleus
(D) Hippocampus
(E) Cingulate gyrus

75. Which of the following measures is most effective for decreasing the prevalence of substance abuse among adolescents?

(A) Imposing significant and unavoidable penalties for adolescents convicted of drug-related criminal offenses
(B) Providing impartial information about the effects of substance abuse on health
(C) Providing moral messages and warnings about the danger of substance abuse
(D) Providing alternative activities and environments, such as work training programs and playgrounds
(E) Teaching social effectiveness and resistance skills against peer pressure to abuse substances

76. Which of the following features is essential to diagnose schizophrenia?

(A) Absence of mood symptoms
(B) Disorganized behavior
(C) Disorganized speech
(D) Duration of symptoms for at least 6 months
(E) Prominent auditory hallucinations

77. Which of the following statements about tacrine is most accurate?

(A) In mildly affected individuals, it has been relatively effective in reducing symptomatology
(B) In some patients, it has been remarkably effective in reversing cognitive decline
(C) It increases levels of dopamine in cerebral cortex
(D) It is contraindicated in patients with renal disease
(E) It is relatively effective only in individuals with obvious and severe memory impairment

78. Which of the following is the best example of primary process thinking?

(A) Automatisms
(B) Complaining without cause
(C) Dreaming
(D) Deductive reasoning
(E) Obsessions

79. Which of the following population groups has the highest risk for alcohol dependence?

(A) Adolescent males with social disadvantages
(B) Adult sons of alcoholic fathers
(C) Irish nationals
(D) Physicians
(E) Spouses of alcohol-dependent individuals

80. Which of the following etiologies is responsible for the highest number of cases of mild mental retardation?

(A) Fetal alcohol exposure
(B) Fragile X
(C) Perinatal anoxia
(D) Polygenetic and environmental factors
(E) Trisomy 21

81. Which of the following statements best describes the doctrine of a least restrictive alternative?

(A) In deciding a treatment course, a clinician should select a treatment that least restricts the future use of other treatment options
(B) Mentally ill patients have a right to be treated with the least restrictive treatment that is clinically effective
(C) Restricting the use of treatments for mental illness must not be based on financial or social considerations
(D) The least restrictive alternative should be avoided when treating mentally ill patients who have significant risk for self-destructive behavior
(E) The risk-benefit ratio of a proposed treatment for a mentally ill patient cannot justify restricting patient options

82. Which of the following psychodynamic defense mechanisms is considered the most mature?

(A) Displacement
(B) Dissociation
(C) Projection
(D) Splitting
(E) Sublimation

Directions: Each group of items in this section consists of lettered options followed by a set of numbered items. For each item, select the one lettered option that is most closely associated with it. Each lettered option may be selected once, more than once, or not at all.

Questions 83–84

For each case, select the most appropriate pharmacotherapy.

(A) Phenelzine
(B) Fluoxetine
(C) Electroconvulsive therapy
(D) Methylphenidate

83. A 25-year-old woman complains of binge eating and chronic depression that becomes worse when she feels rejected. She has not responded to a trial of sertraline.

84. A 46-year-old man is rescued after leaping from a bridge in a suicide attempt. Examination shows that he has severe depression with hopelessness and continued suicidal intent.

Questions 85–86

For each patient with mental status changes, select the most appropriate pharmacotherapy.

(A) Cobalamin
(B) D-penicillamine
(C) Tacrine
(D) Thiamine
(E) Thyroxine

85. A 31-year-old woman has recent onset of depression, irritability, choreoid movements, and amenorrhea

86. A 58-year-old man has the gradual onset of memory difficulties and cognitive slowing; physical examination shows positive Babinski signs bilaterally, and laboratory examination shows megaloblastic anemia

Questions 87–88

For each individual with impaired social development, select the most appropriate diagnosis.

(A) Asperger disorder
(B) Autistic disorder
(C) Childhood disintegrative disorder
(D) Rett disorder
(E) Social phobia

87. A 5-year-old boy presents with a history of social withdrawal and a failure to develop friendships with other children. He is preoccupied with ensuring that all the toys in his room are placed in exactly the same spots each day, and he eats exactly the same food for breakfast each morning. His language ability is appropriate for his age when he makes requests or answers direct questions. He is able to read simple books, dresses himself, and can operate the household television and stereo.

88. A 7-year-old girl presents with severe deficits in both receptive and expressive language, peculiar gripping hand movements, a poorly coordinated gait, and microcephaly. Her parents say that she appeared normal until she was about 1 year of age, when she stopped manipulating objects well and became increasingly socially withdrawn.

Questions 89–90

For each sexual symptom, select the most commonly associated medication.

(A) Bupropion
(B) Fluoxetine
(C) Lithium
(D) Thioridazine
(E) Trazodone

89. Priapism

90. Retrograde ejaculation

Questions 91–92

For each description, select the most applicable symptom.

(A) Alogia
(B) Ambivalence
(C) Aphasia
(D) Apraxia
(E) Auditory hallucinations

91. Negative symptom of schizophrenia

92. Positive symptom of schizophrenia

Questions 93–94

For each patient with complaints of fatigue, select the most likely polysomnographic finding.

(A) Decreased duration of sleep cycle
(B) Decreased rapid eye movement (REM) latency
(C) Decreased sleep efficiency
(D) Decreased sleep latency
(E) Sleep phase shift

93. A 29-year-old woman complains of fatigue, depressive rumination, difficulty concentrating, and loss of interest in living

94. A 70-year-old man complains of fatigue, daytime somnolence, and frequent awakenings at night

Questions 95–97

For each patient with a withdrawal syndrome, select the most likely responsible substance.

(A) Alprazolam
(B) Caffeine
(C) Cannabis
(D) Cocaine
(E) Hallucinogens
(F) Heroin
(G) Mescaline
(H) Nicotine
(I) Phencyclidine
(J) Toluene

95. Shortly after admission to the emergency room because of obtundation, a 23-year-old woman develops anxiety, vague auditory hallucinations, tremulousness, nausea, and insomnia

96. Shortly after admission to the emergency room because of persecutory delusions and belligerence, an 18-year-old man demonstrates fatigue, dysphoria, unpleasant dreams, and psychomotor agitation

97. Shortly after admission to the emergency room because of obtundation, a 19-year-old man has dysphoria, nausea, diarrhea, and piloerection

Questions 98–100

Select the most widely accepted indication for each of the following types of psychotherapy as a primary treatment modality.

(A) Bipolar II disorder, most recent episode depressed
(B) Borderline personality disorder
(C) Cognitive disorder not otherwise specified
(D) Dementia due to neurodegenerative disease
(E) Major depression, single episode, with melancholic features
(F) Obsessive-compulsive disorder
(G) Schizophrenia
(H) Social phobia, generalized type
(I) Specific phobia

98. Behavioral psychotherapy

99. Cognitive psychotherapy

100. Psychodynamic psychotherapy

Answers and Explanations

1–D. The child's symptoms suggest sleep terror disorder, which is characterized by confused awakenings accompanied by signs of anxiety. Typically, there is amnesia for the events, which occur during non-rapid eye movement (NREM) sleep. It is most common during childhood. Nightmares occur during REM sleep, and the individual usually remembers the disturbing dreams.

2–A. The girl's symptoms suggest amphetamine intoxication, which can last for several hours. Cannabis intoxication may have a similar presentation, but is more likely to be accompanied by dry mouth, impaired coordination, time distortion, and perceptual disturbances. There is no evidence of perceptual disturbances, making lysergic acid diethylamide (LSD), psilocybin, or phencyclidine less likely choices.

3–E. The boy's symptoms suggest Tourette disorder, which presents with a history of motor and vocal tics. Amphetamine commonly exacerbates tics. Because the tics were preexisting in this case, the disorder is not amphetamine induced. Huntington disease, stereotypic habit disorder, and Sydenham chorea all produce various abnormalities of movement, but are not associated with the characteristic combination of motor and vocal tics found in adolescents.

4–B. The boy's symptoms are highly suggestive of Tourette disorder. Obsessive-compulsive disorder is present in approximately 30% of patients with Tourette disorder and may be responsible for significant additional pathology.

5–D. The case suggests schizophreniform disorder. Features associated with good prognosis in schizophreniform disorder include the rapid onset of prominent psychotic symptoms, confusion during the psychotic episode, good premorbid functioning, and absence of affectual flattening.

6–A. The girl's symptoms suggest anorexia nervosa, which is characterized by failure to maintain minimal body weight, intense fear of being overweight, distortion of body image, and amenorrhea. Bingeing and fasting are often present in anorexia nervosa, but a diagnosis of bulimia nervosa is not made if the other features of anorexia nervosa are present. Diarrhea is caused by laxative abuse, and dental caries is associated with self-induced vomiting, both of which may be caused by purging. Fatigue and cold intolerance may be caused by starvation, and tendinitis may be caused by excessive exercising in an attempt to lose weight.

7–D. The man's symptoms suggest phencyclidine intoxication, which is characterized by agitation, impulsiveness, nystagmus, hypertension or tachycardia, numbness, ataxia, dysarthria, hyperacusis, and perceptual distortions. Drug users are often misinformed about which substance they have ingested.

8–C. Many studies indicate that individuals with schizophrenia who live with their families of origin maintain better adjustment and have fewer relapses when family stress and conflict are minimal. Gradual involvement with social skills training programs and a supportive but nondemanding family environment seem to produce better adjustment for the individual.

9–C. Neuroleptic malignant syndrome is characterized by the onset of muscular rigidity and hyperpyrexia following administration of antipsychotic medication. Patients who receive relatively high doses of high-potency antipsychotic medications over a short period of time are at greatest risk for this syndrome.

10–B. Catatonia is characterized by immobility, excessive purposeless motor activity, negativism, mutism, peculiarities of voluntary movement, and echolalia or echopraxia. It may be caused by a variety of general medical conditions and may be seen in schizophrenia.

11–C. The man's symptoms suggest hypnogogic hallucinations, which occur during transition to sleep and may be associated with narcolepsy. These hallucinations are believed to be associated with rapid eye movement (REM) dreaming. Hypnopompic hallucinations are similar phenomena that occur during transition from sleep to wakefulness.

12–B. The woman's symptoms suggest hypochondriasis, which is characterized by excessive worry about the meaning of a physical symptom that does not respond to physician reassurance after an adequate workup. Hypochondriacal symptoms usually become evident during periods of psychological stress. Brief psychotherapy that improves the individual's ability to cope with stressful life circumstances often leads to resolution of symptoms. By definition, reassurance and explanations are ineffective in ameliorating hypochondriasis. Benzodiazepines are occasionally useful in dealing with extreme anxiety stemming from hypochondriacal concerns but may interfere with the demanding cognitive tasks that this patient has during her doctoral work. Placebo response in hypochondriasis is usually minimal and temporary.

13–C. The man's symptoms suggest schizophreniform disorder, which is characterized by symptoms of schizophrenia that persist for longer than 1 month but less than 6 months. A premorbid history of social withdrawal is predictive of a prolonged clinical course and a resultant diagnosis of schizophrenia. A variety of magnetic resonance imaging (MRI) abnormalities, including decreased cerebral asymmetry and enlarged ventricles, are associated with more severe symptoms and course in schizophrenia. A family history of schizophrenia is commonly found in second-degree relatives and has little prognostic significance. The presence of catatonic symptomatology is not associated with any particular clinical course. A sudden onset of psychotic symptomatology has a more favorable prognosis.

14–A. The woman's symptoms suggest social phobia, which is characterized by excessive fear and avoidance of social situations. Assertiveness training is the treatment of first choice for social phobia. This variation of cognitive psychotherapy includes educating the individual about anxiety-controlling techniques, role playing, and desensitizing the individual to anxiety-provoking social stimuli. Some studies indicate that monoamine oxidase inhibitors (MAOIs), such as phenelzine, are also useful; buspirone is also occasionally used. Benzodiazepines used alone and systematic desensitization used alone have not shown consistent efficacy. Psychodynamic psychotherapy may improve the individual's self-image but does not reliably decrease phobic anxiety. Stimulus flooding, during which a patient is immersed in the feared situation, is rarely, if ever, used to treat social phobia.

15–B. Female orgasmic disorder, or anorgasmia, is usually lifelong until orgasmic capacity is achieved. This disorder contrasts with many other sexual dysfunctions, which are acquired following a period of normal sexual function. Female orgasmic disorder often affects self-image and interpersonal relationships. No specific intrapsychic conflicts have been reliably associated with this condition. Selective serotonin reuptake inhibitors can induce anorgasmia.

16–C. It is common for patients to respond to the placebo effect inherent in many medical interventions. These responses do not suggest that pain or discomfort is factitious, exaggerated, or has no physiologic basis. Although the normal saline was unlikely to have corrected the patient's underlying pathology, it may have had powerful reassuring effects that reduced the subjective experience of pain.

17–E. The man's symptoms suggest Wernicke encephalopathy, which is characterized by delirium, gait disturbance, and ophthalmoplegia; it develops during alcohol withdrawal. The condition is caused by the acute effects of thiamine deficiency on a variety of subcortical structures, including the periventricular regions. It must be immediately treated with intramuscular administration of thiamine to lessen the risk of persistent memory deficits, which are seen in Korsakoff psychosis.

18–B. The man's symptoms suggest schizoid personality disorder, which is characterized by social disinterest and withdrawal and indifference to others. The absence of peculiar thinking makes diagnoses of schizophreniform or schizotypal personality disorder unlikely. Avoidant personality disorder and social phobia are also characterized by social withdrawal, but there is usually a desire for human interaction.

19–D. Lithium causes hypothyroidism in about 20% of individuals, and levels of thyroid-stimulating hormone often increase in response. Lithium causes an increase in white cell counts. Serum creatinine is used to monitor renal function, because lithium may occasionally cause renal damage. Lithium has no clear effect on serum sodium or the QRS interval.

20–D. Similar to other monoamine oxidase inhibitors (MAOIs), tranylcypromine inhibits the metabolism of pseudoephedrine, which is found in many oral decongestants, and can lead to severe hypertension. Dietary restrictions for MAOI treatment include avoiding many aged cheeses, meats, and beverages that contain high levels of tyramine. Meperidine, and opioid analgesic, must also be avoided.

21–B. These symptoms suggest borderline personality disorder, which is characterized by conflict-ridden interpersonal relationships, impulsivity and self-destructiveness, disturbances of identity, and occasional transient dissociative experiences. Acute stress disorder follows an extreme stressor and is limited to a 1-month duration. Depersonalization disorder and dissociative identity disorder may involve transient dreamlike episodes but would not account for the identity disturbances, chaotic interpersonal relationships, and suicide gestures. Dysthymic disorder is characterized by persistent dysphoria but does not account for the other features present in this case.

22–A. Decreased levels of 5-hydroxyindoleacetic acid (5-HIAA), a metabolite of serotonin, have been found in the cerebrospinal fluid (CSF) of individuals who have committed suicide by violent measures. This implies decreased serotonin levels in the central nervous system (CNS), which suggests a rationale for use of serotonin agonists for treatment of some forms of depression.

23–A. Alprazolam, a short-acting benzodiazepine, is commonly used in relatively high doses to treat individuals with panic disorder. Abrupt cessation of alprazolam may cause significant withdrawal symptoms, including confusion and generalized tonic–clonic seizures. Clonazepam is another benzodiazepine used to treat individuals with panic disorder, but withdrawal symptoms are usually less rapid and severe. Imipramine, phenelzine, and propranolol are also used to treat individuals with panic disorder but are not associated with confusion or seizures on withdrawal.

24–E. Isolation describes the separation of a thought from its attached emotional tone. It is often apparent when an individual experiences an extremely stressful event, and it may preserve some emotional equilibrium and functioning during the emergency. Depersonalization and derealization are also defense mechanisms that involve dissociation of mental functions but are often accompanied by anxiety. Disorientation and intellectualization are not accompanied by odd calmness.

25–E. The man's symptoms suggest narcolepsy, which is characterized by irresistible attacks of refreshing daytime sleep, cataplexy, sleep paralysis, and hypnogogic and hypnopompic hallucinations. Methylphenidate is the treatment of choice for this disorder.

26–C. The woman's symptoms suggest agoraphobia. Agoraphobia is almost always associated with panic disorder and may be caused by a fear of having panic attacks in a situation in which rescue may be difficult.

27–B. The woman's symptoms suggest conversion disorder, which is characterized by sensory or motor deficits without a known physiologic basis that are associated with psychological stress. The symptoms are often associated with a striking blandness that is sometimes referred to as "la belle indifférence." Atonic seizures can present as sudden drop attacks; however, the absence of electroencephalogram (EEG) abnormalities and the patient's lack of concern make this diagnosis less likely. Hypochondriasis presents with increased worry about the meaning of physical symptoms. Factitious disorder and malingering cannot be ruled out, but the absence of external incentives and the patient's apparent avoidance of the sick role make both diagnoses less likely.

28–B. The man's symptoms suggest acute lithium toxicity, which is characterized by tremulousness, gastrointestinal distress, headache, and confusion. Lithium toxicity often occurs when serum lithium levels exceed 1.5 mEq/L.

29–E. The woman's symptoms suggest a specific phobia, which is characterized by fear and avoidance of specific objects or situations. Panic attacks that occur during the course of panic disorder are not clearly related to specific objects or events.

30–A. The man's symptoms suggest body dysmorphic disorder, which is characterized by excessive preoccupation with a defect in appearance that is in reality minor or nonexistent. Individuals with body dysmorphic disorder are often distraught about their supposed deformity, blaming it for many of their problems and for avoiding the company of others. Conversion disorder, hypochondriasis, and somatization disorder do not necessarily involve the exaggeration of a physical defect. Delusional disorder may be difficult to distinguish from body dysmorphic disorder and may become an additional diagnosis if the individual's preoccupation reaches delusional proportions.

31–E. Rationalization refers to a distortion of reality that makes an act or event more desirable. It is often employed when individuals have difficulty accepting the implications of particular outcomes of events. Compensation, derealization, displacement, and projection are other defense mechanisms.

32–C. Multiple sclerosis is characterized by episodes of widely scattered motor, sensory, and cognitive deficits and personality changes that result from transient lesions throughout the central nervous system (CNS). Acute intermittent porphyria may explain sudden personality changes, but it is usually accompanied by abdominal pain. Wilson disease may produce personality change and motor symptoms, but it would not explain pain or sensory changes. Individuals with multiple sclerosis may appear hypochondriacal; however, they have good reason to be concerned about somatic changes. Individuals with multiple sclerosis are sometimes incorrectly diagnosed with somatization disorder at first presentation, because they often have unusual and multisystemic complaints.

33–A. The man's symptoms suggest social phobia. The treatment of choice for social phobia is assertiveness training, which is a combination of cognitive and behavioral techniques that include desensitization, education, and role-playing. Other forms of behavioral and psychodynamic therapies have not been demonstrated to be as effective in treating social phobia.

34–B. The recommended maintenance therapy following response to antidepressants in major depressive disorder, single episode, is usually 6 months; there is a higher risk of quick relapse if antidepressants are discontinued sooner. Some recent studies suggest longer maintenance therapy following recovery from a depressive episode if there is a history of multiple relapses. There is little reason to gradually taper sertraline from the present dosage. Switching the individual to another selective serotonin reuptake inhibitor, such as fluoxetine, is difficult to justify in this case; the sertraline is apparently effective, and nausea is an adverse effect of all SSRIs.

35–A. The symptoms are most suggestive of acute stress disorder, which is characterized by traumatic reexperiencing of the event, dissociative symptoms, and hyperarousal. Symptoms in acute stress disorder persist for no longer than 1 month; in posttraumatic stress disorder, symptoms persist for more than 1 month. Adjustment disorder with anxious mood is not diagnosed if all features of acute stress disorder are present. Panic disorder and specific phobia do not explain all the symptoms present in this case.

36–E. The man's symptoms suggest dissociative fugue, which is characterized by sudden and unexpected travel to another location, amnesia for past events, and either identity confusion or substitution of a new identity. Although impulsivity and poor judgment may occur during manic episodes, there are no other manic symptoms in this man's case. Complex partial seizures may be accompanied by wandering and confusion, but more complex behavior, such as registering under an assumed name, is rare. Depersonalization disorder is characterized by subjective feelings of unreality. Dissociative identity disorder is characterized by the presence of two or more complete identities.

37–C. The man's symptoms suggest progressive cognitive impairment. The neuropathologic changes of Alzheimer disease in individuals with trisomy 21 approach 100% by age 30. Neither major depressive disorder nor adjustment disorder with behavioral and emotional disturbance is likely to cause forgetfulness and difficulty communicating. Complex partial seizures are a relatively less common cause for this individual's symptoms.

38–B. Schizophrenia is a significant risk factor for suicide. Other major risk factors include the presence of a mood disorder, alcohol dependence, singlehood, old age, and unemployment. A subjective feeling of hopelessness, the presence of a lethal plan, and being male are also associated with a greatly increased risk of actual suicide in those who have suicidal ideation. Sexual orientation in and of itself does not seem to predispose an individual to suicide.

39–E. The man's symptoms suggest specific phobia, animal type, which is characterized by a circumscribed and persistent fear and avoidance of an animal. The fear is perceived by the individual as unreasonable. Acute stress disorder is associated with a specific event that caused intense fear, followed by traumatic and intrusive memories, dissociative symptoms, and anxiety. In agoraphobia, obsessive-compulsive disorder, and panic disorder, the fear is not circumscribed around a particular component of the environment.

40–E. The interaction suggests transference, defined in psychodynamic terminology as the shifting of feelings originally associated with one person to another. Often, there is some real or imagined similarity between the original interpersonal situation and the new one. In this case, the patient's anger toward his father is now shifted toward his therapist. Cathexis, countertransference, dissociation, and secondary process do not describe this situation.

41–A. Buspirone is an anxiolytic medication that is not associated with cognitive impairment, the adverse effect of diazepam that is troublesome to this patient. Clomipramine, clonazepam, imipramine, and zolpidem are not indicated for treatment of generalized anxiety disorder.

42–A. The event described in this case suggests blocking, which is defined in psychodynamic terminology as the sudden repression of anxiety-provoking thoughts in midsentence. Conversation, if it resumes, is usually about an unrelated topic. Empathic failure, mirroring, narcissism, and schizoid fantasy are not characterized by this thought disturbance.

43–B. The man's symptoms suggest factitious disorder, which is characterized by the intentional production of physical or psychological symptoms to assume the sick role. Often, individuals with factitious disorder discontinue treatment or leave a medical facility when their feigning is discovered. These individuals may go from place to place in search of new health care providers. Malingering also involves the intentional production of symptoms, but the goal of the behavior is to gain tangible rewards. Individuals with factitious disorder may also have a personality disorder; however, there is no evidence of a personality disorder in this case.

44–C. Augmentation strategies are often initiated when trials of several individual antidepressants from different chemical classes are unsuccessful in treating major depressive disorder. Lithium, thyroxine, or amphetamine is added to a single antidepressant in hopes of improving efficacy, a phenomenon supported by several studies. None of the other regimens listed has been demonstrated to be more useful in nonpsychotic refractory depression. Selective serotonin reuptake inhibitors and monoamine oxidase inhibitors must never be combined. Electroconvulsive therapy may be another effective strategy.

45–D. The woman's belief suggests rationalization, which is characterized by a distortion of reality that makes an actual act or event more desirable. Similar to many other defense mechanisms, rationalization contains elements of denial. Denial, derealization, intellectualization, and reaction formation are not as applicable in this case.

46–E. The man's symptoms and treatment history suggest that he has bipolar disorder. Valproate or carbamazepine may be effective in treating some cases of bipolar disorder that are unresponsive to lithium. Increasing the dose of lithium in this case would probably only produce more adverse effects, because the serum lithium level at the current dose is already at the top of the therapeutic range. Adding haloperidol may control the patient's symptoms, but its short- and long-term adverse effects make it a less desirable choice. Electroconvulsive therapy may also be highly effective, but it is usually reserved for manic episodes that are unresponsive to a series of appropriate pharmacologic treatment strategies. Clonazepam is occasionally used adjunctively in treating manic episodes if other mood stabilizers are ineffective.

47–C. The cluster of signs suggests fetal alcohol syndrome, which is produced by intrauterine exposure to relatively high levels of alcohol. It is unknown whether there is a threshold level that produces these effects or if there is a critical exposure period. The other conditions listed can also produce mental retardation and various physical findings, but they differ from the cluster in this case.

48–B. This case suggests gender identity disorder, which is characterized by extreme discomfort with one's phenotypic gender and a desire to live as a member of the other gender. Relatively little is known about these individuals who do not come to clinical attention, because they often keep their condition secret. Gender identity disorder specifically excludes intersex conditions caused by chromosomal or genetic defects. Transvestism involves cross-dressing for sexual arousal.

49–B. The woman's symptoms are most likely caused by lithium-induced diabetes insipidus, an extremely common adverse effect of lithium treatment. Chlorpromazine can increase serum glucose but is unlikely to produce diabetes mellitus. Lithium is not associated with syndrome of inappropriate secretion of antidiuretic hormone. Although psychogenic polydipsia may produce these symptoms, it is less likely. Chlorpromazine can produce a dry mouth and a resultant desire to consume liquid, but patients usually specify this complaint.

50–E. The man has an obsession, which is defined as an intrusive and recurrent thought, idea, impulse, or image that the individual finds disturbing and irrational. Obsessions often involve themes of violence, suicide, sexuality, or forbidden or embarrassing activities. It is rare for an individual to engage in behaviors suggested by an obsession, but the thoughts are often disturbing or guilt provoking. Individuals who have obsessions may go to great lengths to ensure that they cannot act on these obsessions. Unlike obsessive thoughts, compulsions involve actual behaviors.

51–D. Naltrexone is an opioid antagonist. It is most likely effective in the treatment of alcohol dependence because it blocks the euphoric effects of alcohol-mediated release of endogenous opioids. Disulfiram, another pharmacologic treatment strategy for alcohol dependence, interferes with metabolism of alcohol by inhibiting aldehyde dehydrogenase, causing extreme physical discomfort from resultant high levels of acetaldehyde. Knowing this potential effect, patients are more likely to avoid ingesting alcohol.

52–B. Feelings of self-worthlessness, dysphoria, and a lack of motivation to live are risk factors for suicide attempts. It is critical for the therapist to ascertain if the patient has this intent. It is also critical for the therapist to determine any suicide plan, because the potential lethality of suicidal intention is closely related to the planned method. Offering emotional support and information is also important but is secondary to preventing suicide.

53–C. Phenelzine is a monoamine oxidase inhibitor (MAOI), and combining MAOIs with meperidine has reportedly led to fatalities. The mechanism of this adverse interaction is unknown, and no other opioid analgesic is known to produce it. Other drugs that should be avoided while taking MAOIs include those that contain sympathetic amines, such as nasal decongestants, asthma medications, and appetite suppressants. Amphetamines, methylphenidate, and levodopa are also contraindicated.

54–E. Undoing refers to performing an activity that symbolically reverses a previous behavior or thought. It is commonly present in individuals who suffer either conscious or unconscious guilt. Denial, dissociation, intellectualization, and sublimation are other defense mechanisms.

55–A. The man's symptoms suggest amnesia, which is characterized by memory impairment without other cognitive changes that are characteristic of dementia and without delirium. His vague and incorrect answers may represent confabulation, the substitution of imagined events for those that occurred during a period of memory impairment. A likely etiology in this case may be alcohol-induced persisting amnestic disorder, often called Korsakoff psychosis.

56–E. The woman's symptoms suggest a major depressive episode, which is characterized by depressed mood; difficulties with concentrating; decreased energy, interests, and appetite; and disturbed sleep. Subjective complaints of memory and other cognitive difficulties are common in depressed individuals and may suggest the presence of a cognitive disturbance; however, a cognitive disturbance is less likely in this case, because there is an absence of aphasia or anomia. Depressed individuals may appear preoccupied with somatic symptoms; however, these concerns are usually better explained by the depressive rumination of a major depressive episode than by a separate diagnosis of hypochondriasis.

57–C. This case suggests that the woman has posttraumatic stress disorder (PTSD), delayed onset. It is characterized by persistent reexperiencing of traumatic events, coupled with anxiety and emotional numbing. Peer support groups, during which traumatic experiences are recalled and discussed, are the most effective form of treatment, often providing significant subjective relief despite the short-term increase in stress. The use of benzodiazepines for treating symptoms of PTSD must be weighed against the increased risk of substance abuse in individuals with PTSD. Other forms of treatment have not had consistent success.

58–C. The woman's symptoms suggest delirium, which is characterized by the rapid onset of impaired consciousness and cognitive deficits; accompanying visual hallucinations and anxiety are common. Opioid analgesics are known occasionally to induce delirium in elderly individuals. Alcohol withdrawal is a less likely diagnosis, because there is no history to suggest alcohol dependence. The hallucinations are better explained in this case by delirium instead of psychosis, because a disturbance of consciousness and cognition is also present. Vascular dementia is unlikely in the absence of previous cognitive impairment.

59–C. Naloxone is an opioid antagonist and is injected as a potentially lifesaving measure when the etiology of a coma may be opioid overdose. In individuals with opioid dependence, it can produce symptoms of opioid withdrawal, such as agitation, tachycardia, and nausea.

60–C. The woman's symptoms suggest major depressive disorder, and use of an antidepressant is indicated. Elderly individuals are especially sensitive to adverse effects of antidepressants. In this case, nortriptyline is the best choice of the medications listed, because it causes fewer anticholinergic effects and relatively minimal hypotension and sedation. Sedation may be especially troublesome to this individual, because she has hypersomnia. Amitriptyline and doxepin are strongly anticholinergic. Amitriptyline, trazodone, and phenelzine can cause postural hypotension. Amitriptyline, doxepin, and trazodone can cause significant sedation.

61–A. Exploration of unconscious conflict is a major component of psychodynamic psychotherapy. Of the disorders listed, this form of psychotherapy is most often effective for patients who suffer from the chronic depression seen in dysthymia. A number of psychodynamic models of depression suggest that unresolved conflicts about early abandonment are a central component of adult depression. Although psychodynamic psychotherapy may be useful for patients suffering from many disorders, the major symptoms of social phobia, enuresis, and obsessive-compulsive disorder respond best to cognitive-behavioral therapies and some anxiolytic and antidepressant medications. Schizophrenia usually necessitates antipsychotic medication and social therapies.

62–A. Delirium is characterized by a disturbance of consciousness that may wax and wane. There is a reduced clarity of awareness, with difficulty sustaining, focusing, and shifting attention. Dementia, dissociative fugue, dissociative amnesia, and substance-induced amnestic disorder may cause various disturbances in thinking and awareness but are defined by other features.

63–D. Methylphenidate may be a useful antidepressant treatment in medically ill patients suffering from severe depression and anergia. It may also have some efficacy in treating geriatric patients with marked apathy. In most other depressed patients, treatment with more typical antidepressants is usually preferred. Methylphenidate can exacerbate tics. Although it is a treatment of first choice for attention deficit hyperactivity disorder, it has no efficacy in the treatment of unrelated behavioral problems.

64–C. The prevalence of winter-type seasonal depressive episodes is highest in higher latitudes. The prevalence is also higher in younger individuals and women. Although blind individuals may have an increased risk for disorders related to circadian rhythms, there is no evidence of increased risk for seasonal depressive episodes.

65–E. The lifetime incidence for schizophrenia is around 1%. Patients with schizophrenia occupy 50% of all psychiatric hospital beds, and account for 15% of individuals who receive psychiatric treatment. Only 50% of patients with schizophrenia receive ongoing treatment.

66–C. Of the disorders listed, bulimia nervosa has the highest rate of response to antidepressant medications. Some studies have demonstrated that antidepressant treatment for anorexia nervosa and borderline personality disorder has limited benefits. Antidepressants have not been proved useful in treatment of male erectile disorder and may inhibit orgasm.

67–A. Sadistic activities in sexual sadism can involve psychological as well as physical suffering. The diagnosis can be made based on the patient's fantasies, even if sadistic acts have not been committed. A partner's cooperation does not necessarily preclude the diagnosis of sexual sadism, but the suffering must be real and not merely simulated. The severity of sadistic acts characteristically increases during the course of the disorder, making early diagnosis and treatment particularly important.

68–D. Ibuprofen and other nonsteroidal anti-inflammatory agents (NSAIDs) are associated with significant increases in plasma lithium levels, and patients who need both medications should be monitored closely. Diuretic medication also increases lithium levels.

69–B. Photosensitivity resembling sunburn is often associated with antipsychotic medication, especially phenothiazines. Patients using these medications must be warned to use sunblock and wear suitable protective clothing if they plan to spend extended periods in direct sunlight. Other ocular and dermal adverse effects from phenothiazines include cataracts, skin discoloration, and—only with thioridazine—pigmentary retinopathy. Most antipsychotic medications are associated with some weight gain, and those with anticholinergic blockade are associated with constipation and urinary hesitancy.

70–D. Atropine is administered 30 minutes before each session of electroconvulsive therapy (ECT) to reduce oral secretions that may interfere with airway maintenance and to reduce the postconvulsive bradycardia caused by vagal stimulation. A few seconds before ECT, an ultrashort barbiturate (e.g., methohexital) is administered to induce general anesthesia and is followed by administration of a muscle relaxant (e.g., succinylcholine) to prevent fractures caused by muscle contractions during the convulsion.

71–B. The age-group with the highest prevalence of alcohol abuse is young adults 18 to 22 years of age; some studies suggest that rates of binge drinking in this group may be as high as 35%. The rate for males in this group is at least 5 times higher than for females. Young adult alcohol abusers are most likely to engage in high-risk activities that are more dangerous when combined with alcohol. Most young adult alcohol abusers decrease their alcohol use spontaneously within several years.

72–D. Benzodiazepines, including diazepam, are associated with a high incidence of generalized seizures during withdrawal. Although methamphetamine, cocaine, cannabis, and pentazocine produce a variety of unpleasant symptoms during withdrawal, not one is as commonly associated with seizures or other serious complications as benzodiazepine.

73–A. The incidence of seizures with a daily dosage of clozapine greater than 600 mg is more than 5%. Agranulocytosis is another serious adverse effect of clozapine treatment, but the incidence is about 1%. Renal failure, pigmentary retinopathy, and anticholinergic delirium have rarely or never been associated with use of clozapine.

74–C. Destruction of the dorsal raphe nucleus severely affects sleep regulation. The locus ceruleus is also closely involved in regulating sleep. The hypothalamus, the amygdala, the hippocampus, and the cingulate gyrus are not as closely associated with sleep regulation.

75–E. The most effective method of preventing substance abuse has been teaching relevant social skills to children and adolescents. The other activities listed may have benefits or justifications but have not been demonstrated to be as effective in substance abuse prevention.

76–D. Symptoms of schizophrenia must be present for at least 6 months before schizophrenia can be diagnosed. Active phase symptoms, such as disorganization, hallucinations, and delusions, must be present during at least 1 of the 6 months. Mood symptoms are common in schizophrenia. Disorganized behavior and speech as well as auditory hallucinations are all common in schizophrenia, but no one symptom must always be present to make the diagnosis.

77–A. Tacrine is an acetylcholinesterase inhibitor that is moderately effective in improving cognitive performance in patients with mild dementia of the Alzheimer type. Over several weeks of treatment, it may return the patient's cognitive performance to a level present 6 months earlier in the course of the illness. It does not appear to slow the further progression of dementia. Because of potential hepatotoxicity, it is contraindicated in patients with liver disease. It has no known effect on dopamine levels and is not contraindicated in patient's with renal disease.

78–C. In psychodynamic terminology, primary process thinking is defined as a primitive mode of thinking that is not governed by considerations of external reality, such as cause-and-effect and logic. By 3 years of age, secondary process thinking, which is strongly influenced by logic and consistency, becomes the predominant mode of waking thought. Primary process thinking remains active during dreams and fantasies. Automatisms, complaining without cause, deductive reasoning, and obsessions are not examples of primary process thinking.

79–B. About 20% of adult sons of alcoholic fathers have alcohol dependence. The prevalence of alcohol dependence for the United States general population is about 5%.

80–D. Most cases of mild mental retardation are idiopathic and familial; there are higher rates of mild mental retardation in depressed socioeconomic groups. Mild physical and neurologic abnormalities are more common in individuals with mild mental retardation. Specific genetic, chromosomal, and developmental lesions are the most common causes of more severe mental retardation.

81–B. The doctrine of a least restrictive alternative is a common component of civil law mandating that treatment for mental illness must be selected based on the least restrictive, acceptably effective treatment, as opposed to selecting treatment based solely on effectiveness. Relative degree of restrictiveness is more easily determined in regard to treatment setting (e.g., a locked unit is more restrictive than an unlocked unit). Degree of restrictiveness is more difficult to determine in regard to other aspects of treatment (e.g., the use of various medications, therapies, and adjunctive interventions).

82–E. In psychodynamic terminology, mature defenses refer to those that involve less distortion of external reality and have a greater potential for facilitating adaptive responses. Sublimation is the most mature defense of those listed. It occurs when unacceptable impulses are channeled into more acceptable activities. Mature defenses are generally learned later and give way to more immature or primitive defenses during overwhelming stress.

83–A. These symptoms suggest atypical depression, which is characterized by mood reactivity (i.e., mood can transiently improve in pleasant circumstances); increased appetite, particularly for high-calorie foods; leaden paralysis (i.e., extreme motor fatigue); and hypersensitivity to interpersonal rejection. Clinical studies indicate that monoamine oxidase inhibitors, such as phenelzine, may be especially effective for treating this condition.

84–C. The symptoms suggest that the man remains dangerously suicidal. Severe suicidality as well as treatment failure with antidepressants is an indication for electroconvulsive therapy.

85–B. The woman's symptoms suggest Wilson disease, a copper metabolism disorder that presents with personality and cognitive changes, motor abnormalities, and endocrine disturbances. Treatment consists of a copper-restricted diet and the use of copper-chelating agents, such as D-penicillamine and zinc.

86–A. These symptoms suggest cobalamin (vitamin B_{12}) deficiency, which is characterized by the gradual onset of personality and cognitive changes, disturbances of dorsal tract motor reflexes, gait disturbances, peripheral neuropathies, and megaloblastic anemia. It is treated with cobalamin injections, because the etiology is usually a failure to absorb the vitamin from the ilium, because gastric mucosa fails to produce intrinsic factor.

87–A. The boy's symptoms suggest Asperger disorder, which is characterized by deficits in interpersonal development, restricted patterns of interest and behavior, and normal cognitive and speech development.

88–D. The girl's symptoms suggest Rett disorder, which is characterized by a period of normal development followed by decelerated head growth, severe language and cognitive deficits, psychomotor retardation, social withdrawal, gait disturbance, and loss of manual skills often accompanied by peculiar wringing or gripping movements. It has been described only in females.

89–E. Trazodone is associated with priapism, which may be disturbing and painful. It may require surgical intervention.

90–D. Thioridazine is the antipsychotic agent most strongly associated with retrograde ejaculation, during which semen is discharged into the bladder instead of through the penile meatus.

91–A. Negative symptoms of schizophrenia include alogia (poverty of speech), amotivation, and affectual flattening.

92–E. Positive symptoms of schizophrenia include auditory hallucinations and delusions.

93–B. The woman's symptoms suggest a depressive episode. Decreased rapid eye movement (REM) latency, the onset of REM quickly after falling asleep, often occurs during depressive episodes.

94–C. The man's symptoms suggest that he is spending more of his total sleep period in the awake state, a condition referred to as decreased sleep efficiency.

95–A. The woman's symptoms suggest benzodiazepine withdrawal, which is characterized by anxiety, insomnia, tremulousness, gastrointestinal distress, hallucinosis, and generalized seizures.

96–D. The man's symptoms suggest cocaine withdrawal, which is characterized by fatigue, dysphoria, hyper- or hyposomnia, disturbed dreams, and psychomotor agitation or retardation.

97–F. The man's symptoms suggest opioid withdrawal, which is characterized by dysphoria, generalized pain, rhinorrhea, lacrimation, yawning, nausea, vomiting, diarrhea, and piloerection. Heroin is the opioid most commonly associated with withdrawal.

98–I. Behavioral psychotherapy, especially systematic desensitization, is the treatment of choice for specific phobia. In this disorder, the patient's problematic behavior is well defined and measurable and lends itself to behavioral techniques. Behavioral therapy is also the treatment of first choice in many mental disorders of childhood.

99–H. Cognitive psychotherapy, especially assertiveness training, is a treatment of choice for social phobia. It is also used as a primary treatment modality in a number of depressive disorders, but rarely in those characterized by psychosis or melancholia.

100–B. Psychodynamic psychotherapy is often the most effective treatment for borderline personality disorder, although this treatment is demanding and requires significant patient motivation for success. Although psychodynamic psychotherapy may be a useful adjunct for many of the other disorders listed, it is rarely used as the primary treatment modality. Antipsychotic medication and supportive and social psychotherapies are usually indicated in bipolar disorder, major depressive disorder with melancholic features, obsessive-compulsive disorder, and schizophrenia. Dementia and cognitive disorder not otherwise specified may require supportive psychotherapy, but careful environmental structuring, skills retraining, and judicious use of various medications are critical components of effective treatment.

Index

Note: Page numbers in italics denote illustrations, those followed by *t* denote tables, those followed by Q denote questions, and those followed by E denote explanations.